PRINCIPLES OF
ENDOCRINE
PHARMACOLOGY

PRINCIPLES OF
ENDOCRINE
PHARMACOLOGY

John A. Thomas
Vice President, Corporate Research
Travenol Laboratories, Inc., Round Lake, Illinois
Adjunct Professor, Department of Pharmacology and
Adjunct Professor, Department of Urology
Northwestern University School of Medicine, Chicago, Illinois
Adjunct Professor, Department of Pharmacology and Toxicology
West Virginia School of Medicine, Morgantown, West Virginia
Lecturer, Department of Pharmacology
University of Illinois School of Medicine, Chicago, Illinois
Instructor, Department of Pharmacology
Rush-Presbyterian School of Medicine, Chicago, Illinois

and

Edward J. Keenan
Director, Hormone Receptor Laboratory
Associate Professor, Department of Surgery
Assistant Professor, Department of Pharmacology and
Adjunct Associate Professor, Department of Medicine (Medical Oncology)
School of Medicine
The Oregon Health Sciences University, Portland, Oregon

PLENUM MEDICAL BOOK COMPANY
New York and London

Library of Congress Cataloging in Publication Data

Main entry under title:

Thomas, J. A. (John A.), 1933–
  Principles of endocrine pharmacology.

  Includes bibliographies and index.
  1. Hormone therapy. 2. Endocrine glands—Effect of drugs on. 3. Hormones. I. Keenan,
Edward J. II. Title. [DNLM: 1. Endocrine Glands—drug effects. 2. Hormones—pharmacodynamics. WK 102 T458p]
RM288.T47   1986   615'.36   85-28251

ISBN-13: 978-0-306-42143-3   e-ISBN-13: 978-1-4684-5036-1
DOI: 10.1007/978-1-4684-5036-1

© 1986 Plenum Publishing Corporation
233 Spring Street, New York, N.Y. 10013
Softcover reprint of the hardcover 1st edition 1986
Plenum Medical Book Company is an imprint of Plenum Publishing Corporation

"Even our destiny is determined by the endocrine glands"

Albert Einstein

FOREWORD

The authors have provided an overview of the relationships between hormones that are physiologic constituents of the body as well as their pharmacologic use in replacement therapies and related endocrine dysfunction. *Principles of Endocrine Pharmacology* concerns itself with the therapeutic use of hormones, and hormonelike substances, or drugs that can act either by suppressing or enhancing the metabolism of certain glands of internal secretion. Other drugs used for nonendocrine therapies can likewise affect the endocrine system.

Endocrine pharmacology emerged in the early 1900s with the use of crude pituitary extracts. By the mid-1900s several investigators had isolated and begun to synthesize hormones or hormonelike substances. Recognizing the limited supply of hormones that could be obtained both from animal sources and human autopsy material, the search for so-called hormone substitutes also began early in the 1900s. Recently, recombinant DNA technologies have been used to provide alternative therapeutic sources of human insulin and human growth hormone.

Aside from insulin, perhaps no other use of hormonally-active substance is better exemplified by those drugs which affect fertility. The synthesis of an orally-effective steroid represented one of the first major breakthroughs in the chemical suppression of ovulation. Since the orally-active 19-norsteroids were introduced in the 1950s, several oral contraceptive steroid preparations have been marketed. Indeed, the advent of oral contraceptives for birth control has led to a renewed interest in endocrine pharmacology.

Principles of Endocrine Pharmacology provides not only some of the basic tenets of hormone action at the molecular level, but also describes the therapeutic and diagnostic indications and contraindications of various steroidal and nonsteroidal agents. The authors have grouped and assimilated various endocrine disorders in relation to their most responsive drug or hormone therapy.

Finally, *Principles of Endocrine Pharmacology* contains information about drug–hormone interactions which is not only valuable in discerning side effects but also provides some insight into the basic mechanisms of such interactions. The fact that hormones or substances with inherent hormonal activity can affect blood chemistry methodologies or otherwise interfere with analytical procedures is a valuable inclusion in *Principles of Endocrine Pharmacology*.

Victor A. Drill, M.D., Ph.D.

PREFACE

Principles of Endocrine Pharmacology is an expanded update of the field. Several areas of recent development in certain hormonal therapies are covered. The volume also presents an overview of the relationships between hormones that are normal constituents of the body in some instances and those that are therapeutic replacements or diagnostic tools in other clinical conditions.

Not only are basic mechanisms of hormonal action discussed, but drug-induced alterations of secretion of the glands of internal secretion are considered as well. Drug–hormone interactions as well as the effects of drugs on clinical chemistry tests are discussed. Finally, progress in the area of recombinant DNA technology and its impact on the field of endocrine pharmacology, as witnessed by the introduction of recombinant human insulin and recombinant human growth hormone into clinical medicine, is discussed in this volume.

John A. Thomas
Edward J. Keenan

Roundlake, Illinois
Portland, Oregon

CONTENTS

3. POSTERIOR PITUITARY HORMONES, OXYTOCICS, AND PROSTAGLANDINS

4. THYROID AND ANTITHYROIDAL DRUGS

5. PARATHYROID HORMONE AND CALCITONIN

6. ANDROGENIC AND ANABOLIC STEROIDS

9. ADRENOCORTICOSTEROID DRUGS

10. INSULIN AND ORAL HYPOGLYCEMIC AGENTS

11. EFFECTS OF DRUGS ON THE ENDOCRINE SYSTEM

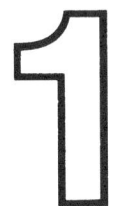

INTRODUCTION AND GENERAL MECHANISMS OF HORMONAL ACTIONS

1.1. HISTORY AND SCOPE OF ENDOCRINE PHARMACOLOGY

Claude Bernard's many brilliant contributions to medicine and science included the discovery of glycogen in 1857, but it was von Mering and Minkowski who performed the classic endocrine experiments involving the removal of the canine pancreas. During the intervening years, many unsuccessful attempts were made to isolate the active antidiabetic factor until Banting and Best infused an extract into a depancreatized dog on November 19, 1921 and brought about a reduction in blood sugar; it was this study that most likely gave way to the widespread acceptance of hormonal replacement therapy. About 4 years later, Abel successfully prepared crystalline insulin, which not only substantiated its importance in the etiology of diabetes mellitus, but for the first time introduced the concept that specific protein possessed inherent physiological activity. Of all the hormonal replacement therapies used in modern medicine, insulin treatment in the patient with diabetes mellitus remains of paramount importance. Recent successes in the synthesis of proteins with the same amino acid sequences as those found in human insulin have been achieved using bacterial systems. Such biochemical accomplishments could eventually lead to the obsolescence of using animal-derived insulins for the therapeutic management of diabetes mellitus in humans, thereby reducing the immunological differences between the pancreatic hormones obtained from different species.

Other classical endocrine experiments having less immediate clinical implication involved the concept of hormonal replacement. In 1929, Koch and associates used extracts of bull testes to demonstrate its stimulatory effects on comb growth in capons. The discovery of cortisone by Kendall in 1935 provided further impetus for the development of extraction and synthesis methodologies, culminating in the concept of hormonal therapies involving pathological states not characterized by hormone deficiencies. Nevertheless, it took more than a decade for sufficient amounts of cortisone to become available for the management of such diseases as rheumatoid arthritis. Hench, in 1948, is generally credited with the initial therapeutic use of cortisone in inflammatory states such as rheumatoid arthritis.

Although modern biochemistry continued to provide more highly purified hormone preparations, as well as the methodologies required for their chemical synthesis in some instances, the widespread use of hormones was not initiated until the 1950s or 1960s. This era witnessed the advent of synthetic hormones and the eventual development of the so-called "pill" or oral contraceptive. While interest in the control of fertility was referenced in the Ebers Papyrus in about 1550 BC, it was not until 1960 that the availability of an effective chemical suppressor of ovulation became a reality. On the basis of earlier observations, Pincus and co-workers established that steroids could effectively inhibit ovulation in rabbits. This inhibitory action was demonstrated using either natural progestogens or synthetic steriods such as norethynodrel (Enovid). By 1954, sufficient animal testing had been completed, and clinical trials were undertaken by Rock, Garcia, and Pincus in Puerto Rico. The U. S. Food and Drug Administration (FDA) approved the use of the first combination-type oral contraceptive, Enovid, a 10-mg preparation containing norethynodrel and mestranol, in November 1959. Many other oral contraceptive preparations have since been approved, and continuing modifications have been made in the doses and dosage formulations of these synthetic steroids. The history or the development of the pharmacology of oral contraceptives represents an excellent example of the ingenuity of the U.S. pharmaceuticals industry coupled with the scientific talents of its basic researcher and clinical investigator.

Many significant contributions in the field of endocrinology have not only resulted in a better understanding of hormonal disorders but have led to clinically useful therapies (Table 1-1).

Table 1-1. Chronology of Highlights in Endocrine Pharmacology

1897	Von Mering and Minkowski pancreatectomize dogs and produce characteristic symptoms of diabetes mellitus
1906	Dale discovers the uterine stimulatory actions of posterior pituitary extracts
1910	Bell and Hofbauer employ posterior pituitary extracts in humans
1914	Kendall isolates crystalline thyroxine from thyroid glands and shows that the molecule contains iodine
1921	Banting and Best discover insulin
1925	Collip succeeds in using parathyroid extracts to elevate serum calcium
1928	Aschheim and Zondek and Cole and Hart use gonadotropin substitutes
1929	Koch and associates use bull testes to produce comb growth in capons
1930	Huggins and co-workers demonstrate hormonal antagonism between androgens and estrogens
1931	Butenandt and co-workers isolate the first male sex hormone, androsterone
1931	Houssay and co-workers demonstrate the role of the anterior lobe of the pituitary gland in diabetes mellitus
1931	Doisy and co-workers isolate urinary estrogens
1934	Moore demonstrates that estrogens and progesterone inhibit the secretion of anterior pituitary gonadotropins
1935	Kendall isolates granules of cortisone from adrenal gland
1942	Jambon and co-workers discover oral hypoglycemic drugs
1943	Dunn and co-workers produce experimental diabetes with alloxan
1945	Astwood and co-workers discover antithyroidal agents
1945	Reinke and Turner discover that L-thyroxine is about twice as active as the racemic form
1947	Green and Harris discover hypothalamic releasing polypeptides
1948	Hench injects newly available cortisone into patients with rheumatoid arthritis
1949	Thorn and co-workers observe that ACTH causes remission of symptoms of rheumatoid arthritis
1953	Pincus and co-workers describe the pituitary inhibitory effects of synthetic steroids
1953	Dù Vigead and co-workers synthesize oxytocin
1956	Rock, Garcia, and Pincus demonstrate the ovulation inhibiting actions of "the pill"—norethynodrel—in women
1960	Sutherland and co-workers postulate the second messenger concept of hormonal action
1962	Jensen and Jacobsen describe the interaction of steroid hormones with their target organ receptors
1966	Li and co-workers disclose the amino acid sequence of growth hormone
1970s	Goeddel and co-workers produce human insulin by cloning of chemically synthesized DNA in *Escherichia coli*

(Continued)

Table 1-1.   Chronology of Highlights in Endocrine Pharmacology (*Continued*)

1970s	Guillemin, Schally, and Yalow independently characterize hypothalamic releasing hormones and develop sensitive radioimmunoassays for measuring hormones
1980	First dose of human rDNA insulin is administered to normal subjects, at Guy's Hospital, London
1981	Allison and co-workers describe the construction and identification of rDNA plasmids containing human calcitonin precursors of cDNA sequences
1980–1981	Clinical trials for human rDNA growth hormone are initiated in Europe and the United States
1982	U.S. FDA approves the use of human rDNA insulin for the treatment of diabetes mellitus
1984	Industrial scientists at biotechnology company express somatomedin C from *E. coli* and from yeast
1984	Scientific groups clone human FSH and LH
1985	U.S. FDA approves use of rDNA growth hormone

1.2.   GENERAL CONCEPTS OF HORMONE ACTIONS

1.2.1.   Hormone Receptor/Acceptors

While subsequent chapters will discuss more specific characteristics of a particular hormone's receptor or receptor sites, several general features commonly found among specific classes of hormones can be highlighted. For example, large protein hormones usually have receptor sites or at least interact with plasma membrance molecules. Smaller molecular-weight hormones such as the androgens (male sex steroids) or the estrogens (female sex steroids) possess steroidophilic molecules in the cytoplasm and in the nucleus of their target organ cells. Still other hormones such as thyroxine (T_3) have an affinity for molecular sites within the mitochrondria of the cell. There are several subcellular sites or loci on the plasma membrane of respective target organs where hormones can interact (Figure 1-1). Such an interaction between the particular hormone and its receptor site(s) ordinarily triggers a series of subsequent biochemical and metabolic events. In instances wherein the molecular size of the hormone is too large to permit free passage through the plasma membrane, the hormone may trigger a biochemical intermediate or a second messenger such as cAMP; the second messenger may in turn trigger several complex intracellular biochemical processes leading to an overall stimulatory action on the specific target organ cell. Membrane phospholipids such as the polyphosphoinosotides appear to play a central role in signal transmission for a wide variety of neurotransmitters and growth factors.

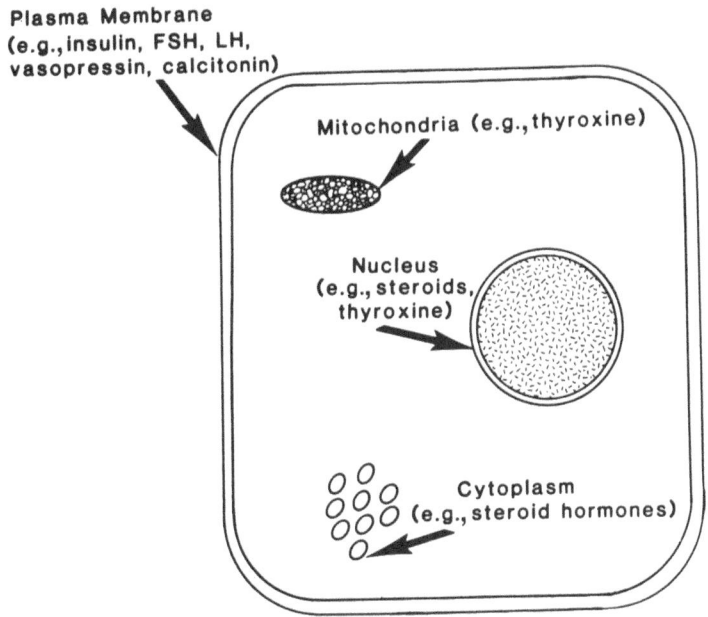

Figure 1-1. Cellular sites of action of different hormones. FSH, follicle-stimulating hormone; LH, luteinizing hormone.

The classic receptor concept suggests that the hormone interacts with some molecular structure often referred to as a receptor. Following the hormone–receptor interaction, a series of biochemical changes occurs producing either an increase or a decrease in metabolic activities. Several general criteria for receptors must be fulfilled in order to demonstrate hormone-mediated metabolic events. A receptor must possess structural and steric specificity not only for the particular hormone but for its close analogues as well. Receptors are saturable and limited, i.e., there is a finite number of sites. Hormone–receptor binding is cell specific in accordance with target organ specificity. The receptor must possess a high affinity for the hormone at physiological hormone concentrations. Once a hormone binds to its receptor, some recognizable early chemical event should be associated with the hormone's actions.

Progress in the isolation of soluble receptors for steroid hormones occurred during the early 1960s due to the availability of tritiated steroids containing a high specific activity of radioactivity. For the first time, it became possible to use almost physiological levels of the tritiated steroids in order to isolate and identify steroidophilic molecules or receptors. As a result of such experiments on radiolabeled steroids, receptor-site characteristics were disclosed for several of the steroid hormones (Table 1-2). Perhaps the most rapid progress was made in disclosing the receptor characteristics for the estrogens, since further biotransformation was minimal and target organ responsiveness was highly specific. Novel experimental models such as the toad bladder were exploited and ultimately led to a better understanding of the mineralocorticoid receptor(s) found in mammalian renal epithelial cells. Recently, steroid hormone systems have been discovered in yeast, but their biological and evolutionary significance awaits further investigation.

Several models have been postulated to explain the action of steroid hormones (Figure 1-2). A steroid receptor is defined as an intracellular component, usually proteinaceous, responsible for the specific and high-affinity binding of the particular hormone and playing an integral role in its metabolic actions. A steroid acceptor has been described as a nuclear component characteristically possessing a high affinity but a finite retention of the steroid–hormone complex in the chromatin.

Table 1-2. Selected Hormone Receptor/Acceptor Sites[a]

Hormone	Receptor sites
Androgens (testosterone, DHT)	Cytoplasm and nucleus of target organs (e.g., prostate)
Estrogen (estradiol)	Cytoplasm and nucleus of target organs (e.g., uterus)
Progesterone	Cytoplasm and nucleus of target organs (e.g., uterus)
Mineralocorticoids (aldosterone)	Cytoplasm and nucleus of renal epithelial cells
Glucocorticoids (cortisone, cortisol)	Cytoplasm and nucleus of several tissues (e.g, fibroblasts, lymphocytes, kidney, liver)
Insulin	Plasma membrane (e.g., adipocytes, monocytes)
Vasopressin	Plasma membrane (e.g., kidney)
HCG	Plasma membrane (e.g., lymphocytes)
Prolactin	Plasma membrane, ER, Golgi, nuclear membrane (e.g., breast, prostate)
Thyrotropin	At least two distinct sites bind TSH (e.g., thyroid)
TRH	Brain and spinal cord
Parathyroid hormone	Plasma membrane (e.g., kidney)
Glucagon	Plasma membrane (at least two sites) (e.g., hepatocyte)

[a] ER, endoplasmic reticulum; HCG, human chorionic gonadotropin; TRH, thyroid-releasing hormone; TSH, thyroid-stimulating hormone.

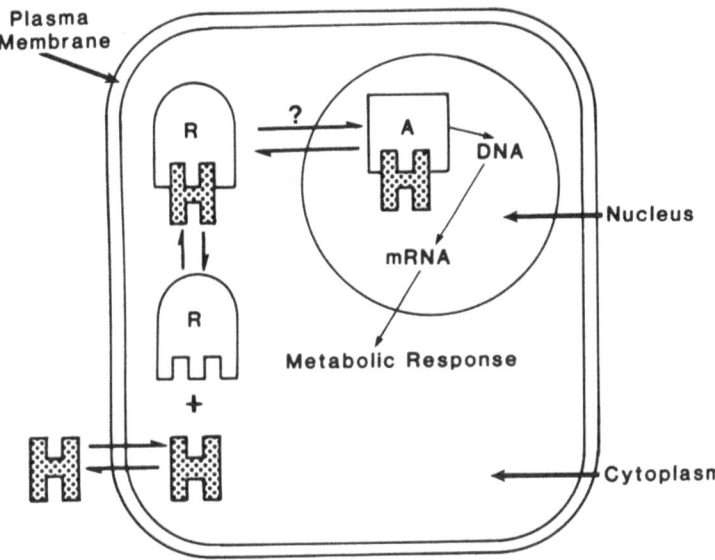

Figure 1-2. Hypothetical steroid receptor–acceptor interaction in target cell. The hormone (H) crosses plasma membrane where some of it can bind to steroidophilic molecules (R-receptor). The H-R complex appears to cross the nuclear membrane to an acceptor (A) site where it stimulates DNA and RNA synthesis culminating in specific metabolic responses.

Progress has also been made recently in disclosing some of the physicochemical characteristics of membrane-bound receptors of peptide hormones. Peptide hormones have specific receptors that are intrinsic proteins of the plasma membrane. Ordinarily, these peptide receptors have molecular weights greater than 10^5. Frequently they consist of several subunits. The binding of a peptide hormone to receptors located on the surface of the particular target cell causes the receptor to express its own intrinsic response. Oftentimes this initiation of response leads to a cascade of biochemical events mediated through a second messenger. The receptors therefore fulfill two principal functions: (1) recognition of the particular hormone, and (2) transfer of information. The magnitude of the signal transmitted to the target cell by its receptor is related to the concentration of the hormone–receptor complexes. Actually, the hormone concentration, the receptor concentration, and the receptor affinity are all physiologically important for the hormone's biological actions. Gonadal receptors that are highly specific for either luteinizing hormone (LH) or human chorionic gonadotropin (HCG) have been isolated from the plasma membranes of ovarian and testicular tissues. Spe-

cific receptors for the lactogenic hormones, prolactin, placental lacto-
gens, and primate growth hormones have been discovered in several
tissues and different species. Growth hormone binding sites have been
found in cultured human lymphocytes. Circulating lymphocytes have
been used as a model to study the interaction between insulin and its
receptor in man. Several other examples of receptor–hormone are dealt
with in more detail in subsequent chapters.

1.2.2. Hormone Substitutes

Until biochemical procedures became available whereby mixtures
of proteins could be separated and procedures were accomplished for
the synthesis of complex molecules, hormone substitutes generally con-
sisted of rather crude or semipurified forms of hormones extracted from
the endocrine glands of domestic animals. In addition, the urine of
domestic animals provided still another source of hormone substitutes.
Hormone substitutes such as pregnant mare serum (PMS) provided a
rich source of conjugated estrogens.

Hormone substitutes of human origin are, for all practical purposes,
limited to those hormonelike proteins isolated from the urine. Human
chorionic gonadotropin is readily extracted from the urine of pregnant
women during the first trimester of gestation. Human menopausal gonadotropin (HMG) is found in high titers in the urine of postmenopausal
women. While human pituitary glands obtained at necropsy were a
source of the various trophic hormones, extracts have never been sufficient to meet the amounts necessary to satisfy therapeutic needs. Since
ACTH can now be synthesized, it is no longer necessary to rely on either
naturally occurring animal or human ACTH.

Table 1-3 presents representative examples of both protein and ste-

Table 1-3. Examples of Different Hormones and Substances That Possess
Analogous Physiological and Pharmacological Properties

Hormone	Hormone substitute
Luteinizing hormone (LH)	Human chorionic gonadotropin (hCG)
Follicle-stimulating hormone (FSH)	Human menopausal gonadotropin (HMG)
Estradiol	Diethylstilbestrol (DES)
Adrenocorticotropic hormone (ACTH)	Synthetic ACTH
Thyroid-releasing hormone (TRH)	Synthetic TRF (a tetrapeptide)
Cortisol	Triamcinolone (a synthetic corticoid)
Progesterone	Norethynodrel (a synthetic progestagen)
Insulin	Tolbutamide (an oral hypoglycemic agent)

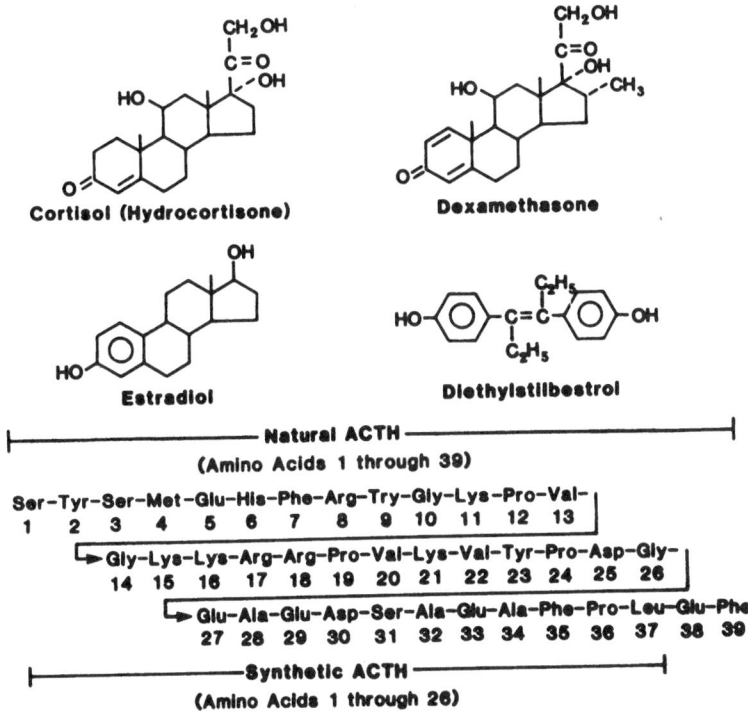

Figure 1-3. Hormone substitutes and agents mimicking hormonelike actions.

roid hormones along with their substitutes. In some instances the hormone substitutes are naturally occurring (e.g., HCG) while in other instances the hormone substitutes are commercially synthesized (e.g., 19-norsteroids). Not all hormone substitutes are chemically similar to their hormone counterpart. For example, diethylstilbestrol (DES) is a potent synthetic estrogen that does not possess the steroid molecule characteristic of natural estrogens (Figure 1-3). By contrast, there is no structural similarity between insulin and the oral antidiabetic agents, yet both can produce hypoglycemia. It is not uncommon for large protein hormones to possess a specific amino acid sequence from which its physiological actions are derived. Such an amino acid sequence need not necessarily encompass the entire molecule; e.g., naturally occurring ACTH contains 39 amino acids only 26 of which are required for biological activity (see Figure 1-3). Similarly, some of the hypothalamic-releasing hormone substitutes retain significant biological activity even though they contain fewer amino acids than do the naturally occurring polypeptides.

It is believed that in most instances, the hormone substitutes merely occupy the receptor site(s) ordinarily occupied by the naturally occurring hormone. This receptor occupancy concept, however, does not apply to the action of the oral antidiabetic agents, even though their hypoglycemic action partially resides in their ability to stimulate the release of endogenous insulin.

1.2.3. Hormone Antagonists

There are perhaps as many examples of competitive hormone antagonists as there are agents whose biological actions lead to the attenuation of a particular hormonal effect (Figure 1-4). Spironolactone can effectively antagonize the actions of aldosterone by competing with the mineralocorticoid's receptors in the kidney. Other agents can effectively antagonize the actions of an endogenous hormone's by simply interfer-

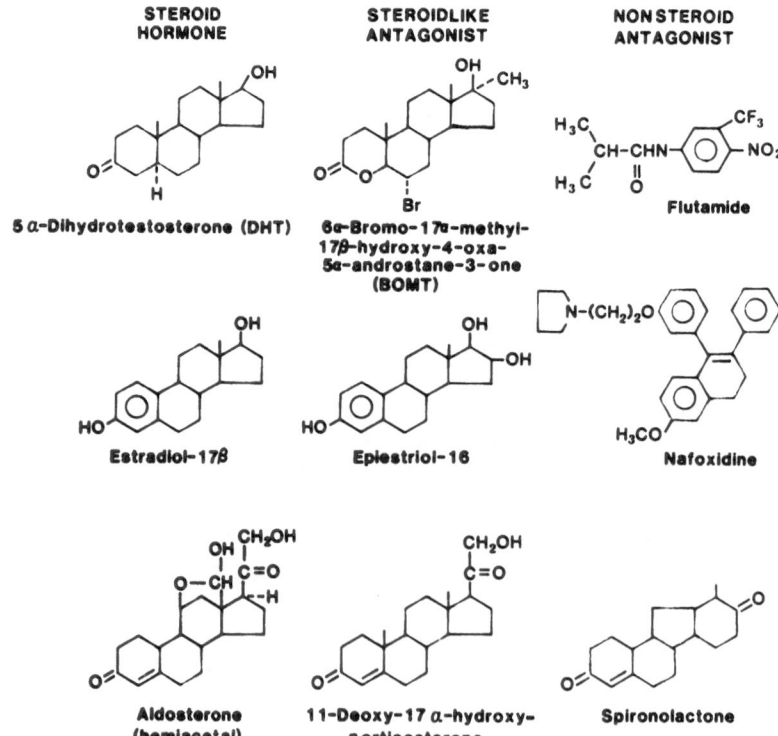

Figure 1-4. Examples of steroid hormones and their antagonists.

ing with the synthesis or secretion of the body's own hormone. Thus some of the so-called antithyroid agents (e.g., thionamides) antagonize or otherwise counteract the physiological actions of T_3 by inhibiting its synthesis. Estrogens can antagonize the actions of androgens and can do so not only by competition at the receptor site level within male sex hormone-dependent target organs but by exerting a physiological antagonism by suppressing pituitary gland gonadotropins as well.

Some hormone antagonists are naturally occurring substances (e.g., estradiol can antagonize testosterone), while others represent synthetic hormonal analogues or chemical entities that resemble the naturally occurring hormone. Hormone antagonists, more specificially those that act competitively at the hormone's receptor site, have not really gained widespread therapeutic usefulness (Figure 1-4). By contrast, those agents that produce a so-called physiological antagonist (e.g., antithyroidal drugs) occupy a more established role in the therapeutic management of thyrotoxicosis. Some agents that effectively suppress hormone secretion are too toxic for therapeutic use and are used principally for diagnostic tests (e.g., metyrapone). With the increased developments in protein chemistry, it is now possible to synthesize not only polypeptides that mimick hypothalamic releasing hormones, but tripeptides capable of releasing hormone antagonists (e.g., Wy-18,185).

1.2.4. Hormone Synthesis Inhibitors

A number of agents have the ability to reduce hormonally induced effects on different target organs. While some such drugs clearly act by inhibiting enzymes involved in synthesis of the hormone itself, other inhibitory effects or even toxic reactions produced by certain chemicals can also effectively interfere with a hormone's action by noncompetitive mechanisms. With the exception of the chemical class of antithyroidal agents called the thionamides, few of the inhibitory agents are of significant therapeutic usefulness. Antithyroid drugs such as methimazole (Tapazole) (Figure 1-5) carbimazole (Neomercazole), and propylthiouracil (see Chapter 4) possess more than a single mechanism of inhibitory action, but they are capable of interfering with thyroxine synthesis. Hence these agents can be used in the management of thyrotoxicosis.

Many drugs have been demonstrated to exert inhibitory action on certain enzymes involved in the metabolic conversion of cholesterol to hormonal steroids (see Figure 1-5). Metyrapone is capable of inhibiting 11β-hydroxylase and thus curtails the bioconversion of 11-deoxycortisol to cortisol and desoxycorticosterone to corticosterone. Metyrapone has been used disgnostically to assess pituitary–adrenal function. Cyano-

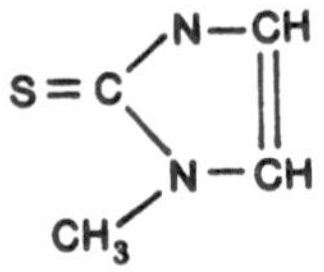

Methimazole

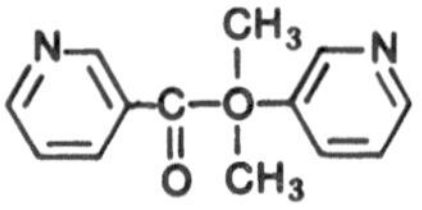

Metyrapone

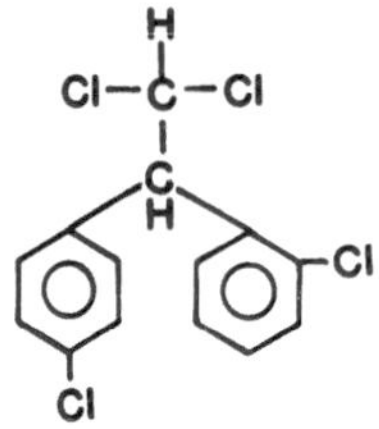

o,p-DDD

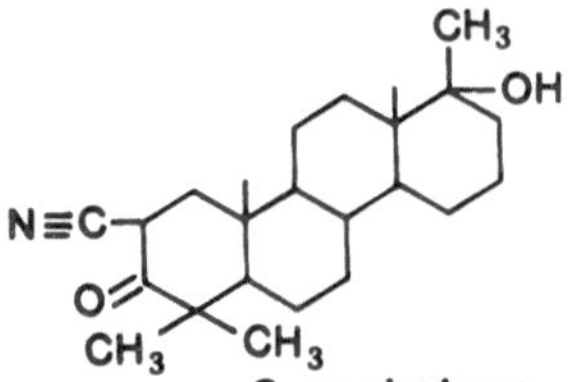

Cyanoketone

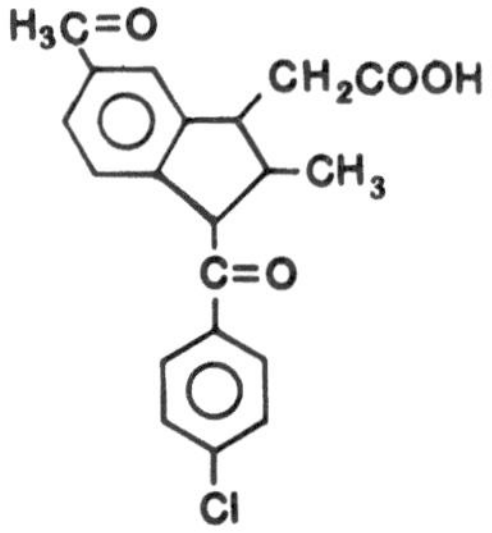

Indomethacin

Figure 1-5. Agents or drugs capable of inhibiting hormone synthesis.

ketone is too toxic to be of any therapeutic use, but it has been used as an experimental inhibitory agent in the study of steroidogenesis. Cyanoketone inhibits the conversion of Δ^5-3-ol steroids to Δ^4-3-oxo steroids by inhibiting the enzyme, 3β-hydroxysteroid dehydrogenase. Still another agent, aminoglutethimide, inhibits the bioconversion of cholesterol to pregnenolone by inhibiting 20α-hydroxylase. Unlike metyrapone, cyanoketone, or aminoglutethimide, o,p-DDD is not as enzyme specific in suppressing steroidogenesis. Nevertheless, o,p-DDD can inhibit steroid hydroxylase enzymes. Indomethacin, a nonsteroidal anti-inflammatory drug, is capable of inhibiting the synthesis of prostaglandins.

Protein inhibitory antibiotics such as puromycin, actinomycin D, or cyclohexamide can interfere with early biochemical events initiated by certain hormones. These agents can suppress protein synthesis and can interfere with hormone-induced stimulation of RNA and/or DNA within appropriate target organs.

The therapeutic usefulness of drugs that inhibit hormone synthesis is in those pathological states that involve hypersecretion of a particular hormone. The pharmacological inhibition of hormone synthesis, however, has not really been of any significance in the therapeutic management of endocrine disorders. Generally, these agents have been too toxic, and hypersecretory states are often amenable to surgery.

1.3. HORMONAL FEEDBACK SYSTEMS

A general understanding of how hormonal feedback systems can be manipulated or altered by pharmacological agents is crucial to the practice of good therapeutics (subsequent chapters develop specific hormonal feedback systems and to what extent various drugs can affect these particular relationships). Classically, most of the adenohypophyseal hormones stimulate their respective target organs, causing increased secretion of target organ hormone (Figure 1-6). The target organ hormone is released into the bloodstream, whence it can return to the hypothalamic–adenohypophyseal area and occupy receptors capable of modulating or suppressing the release and/or secretion of a particular trophic hormone. For example, LH, or interstitial cell-stimulating hormone (ICSH), can stimulate the testicular secretion of androgens. An-

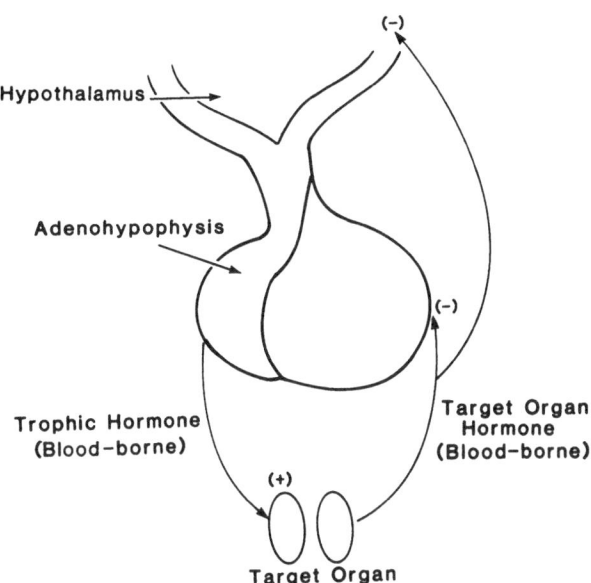

Figure 1-6. Hormonal feedback systems.

drogens, such as testosterone, are released into the bloodstream and act back upon receptors located in the hypothalamic–adenohypophyseal regions, resulting in a suppression or modulation of ICSH. This type of feedback system is also present between the thyroid gland and anterior pituitary. The feedback system becomes somewhat more complex in the case of estrogens and progesterone. Neither growth hormone nor prolactin exhibits clear-cut feedback systems, although both trophic hormones possess specific receptors within selected tissues.

Several drugs can alter some of these hormonal feedback systems. These alterations can frequently suppress the secretion of a particular trophic hormone. For example, the mechanism of action of oral contraceptive drugs is attributable to the inhibition of gonadotropic hormones. On the other hand, antithyroid drugs suppress thyroxine synthesis and lead to an increased secretion of thyroid-stimulating hormone (TSH), since circulating levels of thyroxine are no longer sufficient to exert their negative feedback actions.

RECOMMENDED READINGS

Aurbach, G. D., Polypeptide and amine hormone regulation of adenylate cyclase, *Annu. Rev. Physiol.* **44**:653–666, 1982.

Baxter, J. D., and Funder, J. W., Hormone receptors, *N. Engl. J. Med.* **301**:1149–1158, 1979.

Catalano, R. D., Stuve, L., and Ramachandran, J., Characterization of corticotropin receptors in human adrenocortical cells, *J. Clin. Endocrinol. Metab.* **62**:300, 1986.

Dufau, M. L., and Catt, K. J., Gonadotropin receptors and regulation of steroidogenesis in testes and ovary, *Vitamin Hormone* **36**:461–592, 1978.

Gorden, P., Carpentier, J. L., Freychet, P., and Orci, L., Internalization of polypeptide hormones: Mechanism, intracellular localization and significance, *Diabetologia* **18**:263–274, 1980.

Grody, W. W., Schrader, W. T., and O'Malley, B. W., Activation, transformation, and subunit structure of steroid hormone receptors, *Endocrine Rev.* **3**:141–163, 1982.

Katzenellenbogen, B. S., Dynamics of steroid hormone action, *Annu. Rev. Physiol.* **42**:17–35, 1980.

Lefkowitz, R. J., Wessels, M. R., and Stadd, J. M., Hormones, receptors and cyclic AMP: Their role in target cell refractoriness, *Curr. Topics Cell Regula.* **17**:205–230, 1980.

Marx, J. L., A new view of receptor action, *Science* **224**:271–274, 1984.

Means, A. R., and Chafouleas, J. G., Calmodulin in endocrine cells, *Annu. Rev. Physiol.* **44**:667–682, 1982.

O'Malley, B. W., Schwartz, R. J., and Schrader, W. T., A review of regulation of gene expression by steroid hormone receptors, *J. Steroid Biochem.* **7**:1151–1159, 1976.

Oppenheimer, J. H., Thyroid hormone action at the cellular level, *Science* **203**:971–979, 1979.

Roth, J., and Taylor, S. I., Receptors for peptide hormones: Alterations in diseases of humans, *Annu. Rev. Physiol.* **44**:639–651, 1982.

Sherman, M. R., and Stevens, J., Structure of mammalian steroid receptors: Evolving concepts and methodological developments, *Annu. Rev. Physiol.* **46**:83–105, 1984.

Tuomisto, J., and Mannisto, P., Neurotransmitter regulation of anterior pituitary hormones, *Pharmacol. Rev.* **37**:249, 1985.

2

PHARMACOLOGY OF ADENOHYPOPHYSEAL HORMONES

2.1. FACTORS MODIFYING ADENOHYPOPHYSEAL SECRETION: HYPOPHYSIOTROPHIC HORMONES

The modulation of anterior pituitary hormone secretion relies on the release of hypothalamic substances into the capillaries of the median eminence. The anatomical relationship between the hypothalamus and the anterior pituitary gland consists of a rather complex vascular network (Figure 2-1). The hypothalamus is adjacent to the pituitary stalk, and the general anatomical region is referred to as the median eminence. The pituitary stalk connects the hypothalamus to the adenohypophysis. A system of portal veins extending along the pituitary stalk serves as a connecting link of capillary plexuses in the median eminence and in the adenohypophysis. Most of the blood flowing into the adenohypophysis has initially traversed the capillary system situated in the median eminence region of the hypothalamus. A major portion of the blood supply to the anterior pituitary gland is derived from the superior hypophyseal arteries *via* the hypothalamus. Terminal arterioles from the superior hypophyseal arteries form a capillary network in the area of the median eminence of the hypothalamus. This portal system connecting the hypothalamus and adenohypophysis transports the hypophysiotrophic hormones from the median eminence to the anterior pituitary gland.

Several neurosecretory neurons terminate on or near the capillary loops of the median eminence. These neurosecretory neurons are capable of synthesizing hypophysiotrophic hormones. The secretion of

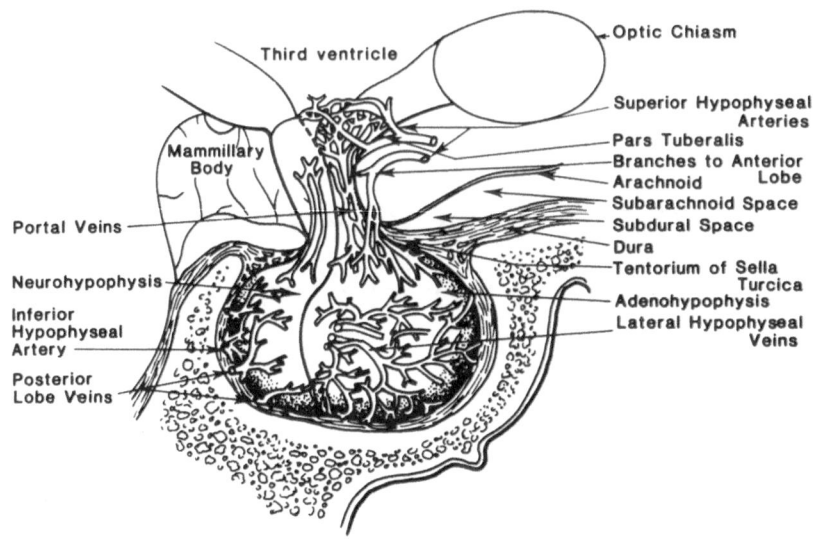

Figure 2-1. The hypothalamic–hypophyseal portal system.

hypophysiotrophic hormones is modulated, in part, by neurons releasing dopamine, norepinephrine, or serotonin. Once these hypophysiotrophic peptide hormones are synthesized, they are transported by the hypothalamic–hypophyseal portal system to the adenohypophysis, where they can either stimulate or inhibit anterior pituitary hormone secretion. Thus the hypophysiotrophic hormones modulate the secretion of trophic hormones emanating from the anterior pituitary gland.

Specific chromophilic cells (e.g., acidophils and basophils) located within the adenohypophysis are responsive to particular hypophysiotrophic hormones. These cells are capable of synthesizing, storing, and releasing trophic hormones upon command from various hormonal and nonhormonal stimuli. Once trophic hormones are released from the adenohypophysis, they are transported *via* the bloodstream to specific target organs, such as thyroid-stimulating hormone (TSH) to the thyroid gland, where they can accelerate metabolic events. In turn, target organ hormone secretions can act back upon the adenohypophysis, thereby exerting a positive or negative feedback action. This hormonal feedback loop (see Figure 2-2) acts to modulate the secretion of the adenohypophyseal hormone and the target organ hormone. There are two types of hormonal feedback system, named on the basis of the length of the loop. A long-loop feedback exists between the anterior pituitary gland and a specific target organ. For example, adrenocorticotrophic hormone

(ACTH) stimulates the biosynthesis of adrenocortical steroid hormones by the adrenal cortex. These steroids can act back upon the adenohypophysis (and hypothalamus) to suppress the secretion of ACTH and represent an example of the long-loop feedback system. A second type of hormonal feedback system, namely, a short-loop feedback, exists between the adenohypophysis and the hypothalamus.

Target organs or end organs such as the gonads (e.g., ovaries and testes), thyroid, and adrenal gland, rely to a large degree on circulating levels of adenohypophyseal hormones for their metabolic integrity. Through feedback systems, target organ hormones in the blood increase or decrease the secretion of anterior pituitary hormone(s). Not surprisingly, synthetic steroids, e.g., oral contraceptives, anti-inflammatory steroids, can mimic the actions of naturally occurring steroids, and thus affect the feedback system. In fact, oral contraceptives can exert a negative feedback on pituitary gonadotropin secretion, leading to an inhibition of ovulation (see Chapter 8). A negative feedback system is a situation in which the secretion of a target organ hormone (or pharmacologically administered amounts of hormone) decreases the secretion of the particular adenohypophyseal hormone. A positive feedback system, although less common, exists when a hormone, e.g., estrogen

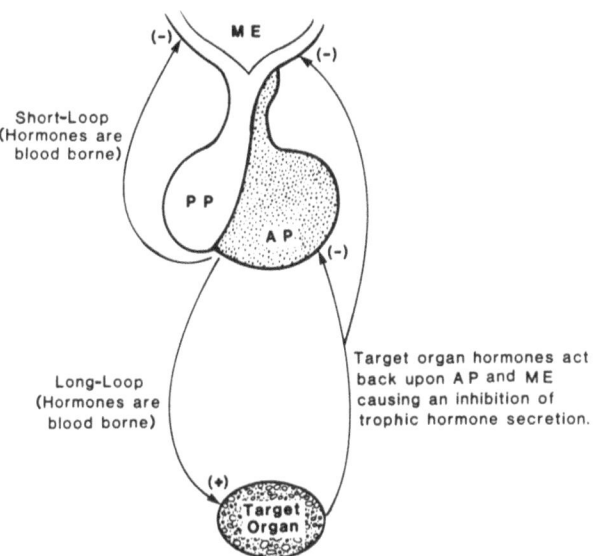

Figure 2-2. Hormonal feedback systems among median eminence (ME), the anterior pituitary (AP), and a target organ. PP, posterior pituitary.

accelerates the secretion of a particular adenohypophyseal hormone. Feedback systems are not restricted to the hypothalamic–hypophyseal–target organs but may be present elsewhere in the endocrine system (e.g., modulation of insulin secretion by blood glucose levels).

Hypothalamic peptide hormones are substances found in the hypothalamus, a neural structure situated at the base of the brain, which modulates the secretion of trophic hormones from the adenohypophysis. There are at least nine hypothalamic regulators of the anterior pituitary gland (see Table 2-1). The hypothalamic hypophysiotrophic substances were once referred to as releasing factors, but at least some of these peptides have fulfilled the criteria for a hormone. Consequently, those hypothalamic substances that fulfill these criteria are called hypothalamic releasing hormones, whereas those that do not completely fulfill these criteria may still be referred to as hypothalamic releasing (or inhibitory) factors. Releasing hormones affect specific trophic hormone-containing cells in the pituitary gland (see Figure 2-3).

The secretion of the hypothalamic peptides is modified by the actions of CNS neurotransmitters. Dopamine, norepinephrine, epinephrine, serotonin, and histamine can affect anterior pituitary hormone secretion by influencing hypothalamic peptides. Other CNS transmitters, such as acetylcholine (ACh) and γ-aminobutyric acid (GABA) can also influence the hypothalamic modulation of anterior pituitary hormone secretion. Those factors that can affect CNS transmitter levels, such as the environment (e.g., stress, cold), drugs, and certain disease states can alter the secretion and/or release of hypophysiotrophic hormones.

Table 2-1. Hypothalamic Hormones or Factors Controlling the Release of Anterior Pituitary Hormones

Nomenclature	Abbreviation
Corticotropin (ACTH)-releasing hormone	CRH
Thyrotropin-releasing hormone	TRH
Luteinizing hormone (LH)-releasing hormone/follicle stimulating hormone (FSH)-releasing hormone	LH-RH/FSH-RH (GnRH)
Growth hormone (GH)-inhibitory factor, somatostatin	GH-IF, SRIF
Growth hormone (GH)-releasing factor	GH-RF
Prolactin-inhibitory factor	PIF
Prolactin releasing factor	PRF
Melanocyte-stimulating hormone (MSH)-inhibitory factor	MIF
Melanocyte-stimulating hormone (MSH)-releasing factor	MRF

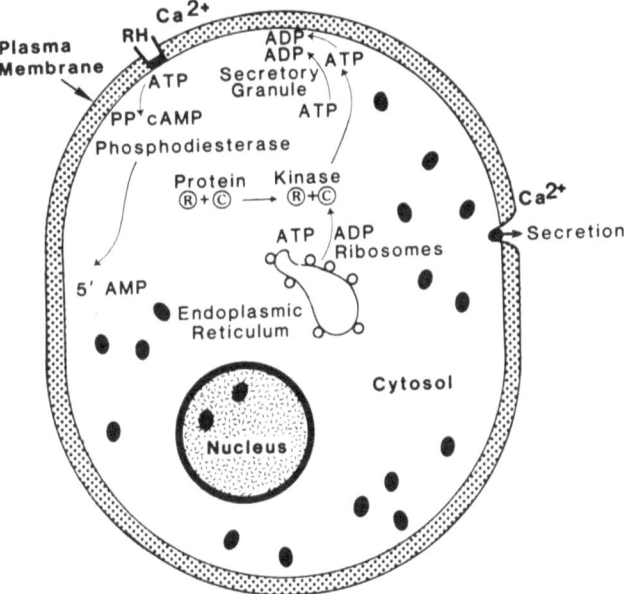

Figure 2-3. Mechanism of action of releasing hormones (RH). The particular RH interacts with a membrane receptor located on the cell's plasma membrane. Calcium is apparently required for its initial metabolic reactions.

2.1.1. CRH

Corticotropin-releasing hormone (CRH) is a 41-amino acid peptide; there may be subtle differences among various mammalian species. The sequence of human CRH precursor gene demonstrates that human and rat are identical, but different from ovine. Synthetic ovine CRH releases immunoactive ACTH and β-endorphin. The amino acid composition of CRH has been reported (see Figure 2-4).

Several substances within the CNS have been proposed as physiological stimulators of ACTH, including catecholamines, histamine, acetylcholine (ACh), and vasopressin. Although pharmacological amounts of vasopressin can effectively increase ACTH, it is most certainly not the physiological modulator of ACTH. Under certain experimental conditions, serotonin and ACh can stimulate the release of CRH and not of ACTH. This response to serotonin-induced release of CRH can be blocked by hexamethanium and atropine, suggesting that it is mediated by a cholinergic interneuron. Norepinephrine, melatonin, and GABA reportedly can block CRH release in some species. It is possible that

```
 1                                      10
H–Ser–Gln–Glu–Pro–Pro–Ile–Ser–Leu–Asp–Leu–Thr–Phe–His–Leu–Leu–
      20                                              30
Arg–Glu–Val–Leu–Glu–Met–Thr–Lys–Ala–Asp–Gln–Leu–Ala–Gln– Gln–
                                          40 41
     Ala–His–Ser–Asn–Arg–Lys–Leu–Leu–Asp–Ile–Ala–NH₂
```

Figure 2-4. Amino acid sequence of corticotropin-releasing hormone (CRH).

CRH not only releases ACTH but might cause the release of β-lipoprotein and β-endorphin as well. CRH can stimulate the secretion of β-endorphinlike immunoactivity (β-End-LI).

CRH is not yet available for clinical use. The eventual clinical usefulness may be restricted to diagnostic tests of pituitary function and possibly to counteracting pituitary suppression in patients who have received intensive adrenal cortical steroid therapy.

2.1.2.   TRH

Thyrotropin-releasing hormone (TRH) was the first of the hypophysiotrophic hormones to be characterized structurally:

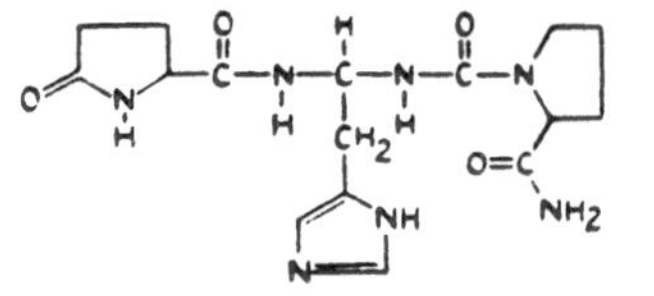

pyroGlu-His-Pro-NH₂
TRH

It is commercially available as Protirelin, Relefact TRH, Thymone and Thypinone. Synthetic pyroGlu-His-Pro-NH₂, a tripeptide, has been demonstrated to stimulate the release of thyrotropin in all mammals investigated including rodents, cows, sheep, goats, and humans. Still other synthetic derivates display TRH activity as well (see Figure 2-5). Other small peptides actually possess anti-TRH activity (see Figure 2-5).

The highest concentration of TRH is found in the median eminence. Neuronal cell bodies exhibiting TRH immunoreactivity have been detected in the hypothalamic dorsomedial nucleus and perifornical area. Immunoreactive TRH has been found in blood, cerebrospinal fluid (CSF), and urine.

TRH is orally active, but doses many times greater than parenteral routes of administration are required to increase TSH. TRH can also enhance the secretion of prolactin in animals and humans. It can also stimulate the secretion of the growth hormone.

Synthetic Analogues of TRH

a. pyr-Glu-His-Pro-NH$_2$

b. $[(N^{3im}-Me-His)^2]-TRH$

c. $[\beta-(pyrazolyl-l)-Ala^2]-TRH$

Figure 2-5. Chemical structure of synthetic thryotropin-releasing hormone (TRH) and some TRH antagonists.

Antagonists of TRH

d. (cpc-His-pyr)

e. cpc-Thi-pyr$[Thi=\beta-(2-thienyl)-L-alanine]$

The mechanism of action of TRH seems to involve specific binding to receptors located on the external surface of the plasma membrane of pituitary TSH-secreting cells. Analogues of TRH that have a high affinity for these receptors also possess the ability to stimulate TSH and prolactin. Apparently intracellular mechanisms initiated by the interaction between TRH and its receptor are comparable to those that mediate secretory events of other endocrine cells and involve cAMP. It is probable that cAMP acts as a mediator of the action of TRH on the TSH-containing pituitary cell.

TRH is used clinically for the differentiation between hypothalamus and pituitary hypothyroidism and for the diagnosis of mild hyper- and hypothyroidism. The evaluation of the pituitary TSH response to TRH is significant, since basal serum TSH values fail to provide proper differentiation between normal and hyperthyroid patients or between euthyroid subjects and those with diminished TSH secretory capacity. The TSH response to TRH (200 μg IV) results in a rapid increase in serum TSH (see Figure 2-6). The normal TRH response is usually witnessed by a peak of TSH at about 20 min, followed by a significantly lower 60-min postinjection level. At 2 hr, serum (triiodothyronine (T$_3$) in euthyroid

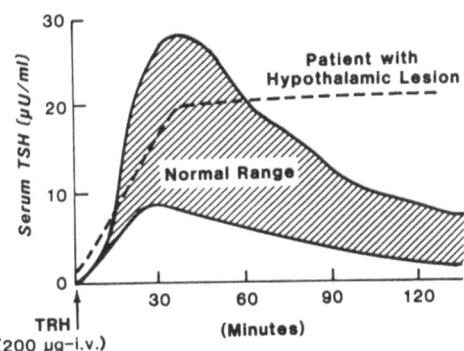

Figure 2-6. Representative responses of normal human subjects to thyrotropin-releasing hormone (TRH).

subjects increases by about 50%, with serum thyroxine (T_4) only increasing about 20%. There are several modifications of the TRH test employing different doses of TRH and other routes of administration, e.g., intramuscularly. Bolus administration of TRH is free of serious side effects, although some subjects experience nausea, malaise, flushing, and the urge to micturate. TRH administration can lead to increased secretion of prolactin. TRH can also increase the secretion of growth hormone levels in patients with acromegaly, renal failure, and mental depression. TRH may alleviate symptoms associated with amyotrophic lateral sclerosis; it is not a cure.

2.1.3. LH/FSH-RH (GnRH)

In all probability, luteinizing hormone-releasing hormone (LH-RH) is also follicle-stimulating hormone releasing hormone (FSH-RH). In other words, LH-RH is most likely the physiological modulator of FSH-RH. LH-RH can cause the release of enough FSH to induce follicular maturation. It is commercially available as Gonadorelin.

Biochemical and immunocytochemical findings demonstrate that LH-RH is present in high concentrations in the median eminence, where it is localized in nerve terminals that end on capillary loops of pituitary portal vessels. LH-RH might also be present at other anatomical sites. LH-RH activity can be detected in a number of subcellular sites, including the mitochondria.

Most likely, the chemical structure of porcine, bovine, ovine, rat, and human LH-RH is the same. The complete decapeptide structure is necessary for biological activity, and the removal of a single amino acid from the C-terminal end results in a 90% loss of activity.

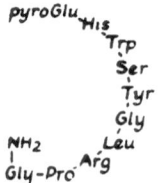

The fact that ovulation can be induced with LH-RH indicates that decapeptide can release sufficient amounts of FSH to produce follicular maturation.

LH-RH is evidently released in a pulsatile manner. Once released, it is readily inactivated in the bloodstream and excreted by the kidney. The mechanism of action of LH-RH remains to be resolved, but cAMP may mediate some of its action (see Figure 2-3). Its mechanism of action involves an interaction with pituitary plasma membrane receptors. Synthetic analogues of LH-RH, as well as LH-RH antagonists, appear to use the same pituitary plasma membrane receptor as those normally occupied by LH-RH itself.

Gonadotropin-releasing hormone (GnRH) most likely acts on a specific gonadal binding site(s) to directly modulate gonadal function. Various steroidogenic enzymes are affected by GnRH. GnRH-induced decreases in progesterone production may result from the inhibition of progesterone biosynthesis and/or increases in the conversion of progesterone to inactive metabolites. The mechanism wherein GnRH inhibits FSH-stimulated progesterone production is undoubtedly similar to the mechanism(s) induced either by prolactin or by β-adrenergic agonists.

The clinical use of LH-RH has been in determining pituitary LH and FSH reserve. It has also been used to induce ovulation in amenorrhea as well as in the therapeutic management of oligospermia. Sometimes LH-RH can be used in conjunction with human menopausal gonadotropins (HMG) in the management of infertility, with LH-RH avoiding superovulation (hence the incidence of multiple births) in those patients.

Several analogues of LH-RH (e.g. Histrelin) have been synthesized, some of which inhibit its actions and others that markedly enhance its potency beyond that of the natural peptide. Regimens of intermittent LH-RH therapy given either subcutaneously, intranasally, or preferably by pulsatile minipumps mimic the physiological pulsatile surges of LH-RH. Several clinical indications for LH-RH have been suggested (see Table 2-2). The LH-RH agonist, naforelin acetate, has been used as a contraceptive agents. Leuprolide acetate (Lupron), another LH-RH an-

Table 2-2.   Clinical Indications for LH-RH

Precocious puberty
Central precocious puberty (secondary to neurofibromatosis and/or optic gliomas)
Cryptorchidism
Delayed puberty
Hypogonadism
Anovulation
Secondary amenorrhea
Premenstrual syndrome
Insufficient luteal function
Endometriosis
Acute intermittent porphyria
Certain hormone-dependent tumors
Prostatic cancer

alogue, is used in the treatment of prostatic cancer. Leuprolide was developed by substituting the D-isomer of leucine for glycine at position 6 of the natural occurring LH-RH, by deleting the 10th amino acid and by adding an ethylamide moiety to the proline at position 9. Leuprolide is designated by the notation D-Leu6,DES-Gly-NH2-10,proethylamide.

The administration of GnRH intravenously or intramuscularly does not generally produce any serious side effects. Occasionally, subcutaneous injections can produce a transient discomfort and a localized area of erythemia at the site of administration. Continuous injections of GnRH of about 1 mg for periods up to about 2 years have not generally resulted in any significant production of antibodies.

Comparison of different routes of LH-RH administration have been evaluated primarily in normal male subjects. Regardless of the route of administration (*viz.* intravenously, intramuscularly, or subcutaneously), a 100-g dose of synthetic LH-RH produces a quantitively similiar pattern of blood LH and FSH time course. The evaluation and decline in LH and FSH in the blood lasts approximately 4–6 hr, with a somewhat more sustained release occurring after an intravenous infusion. The intranasal application of LH-RH results in a release of LH and FSH, although the relative effect is much less than if LH-RH is injected. While LH-RH can be administered by several routes of administration (e.g., intravenously, subcutaneously, and orally), considerably higher doses are required if it is not administered parenterally. Analogues of LH-RH (Figure 2-7) generally have a more extended duration of action and result in a more

LH–RH Analogues

$[\text{D-Ala}^6, \text{ des-Gly-NH}_2^{10}]$-LH–RH ethylamide

$[\text{D-Leu}^6\text{-des-Gly-NH}_2^{10}]$-LH–RH ethylamide

$[\text{D-Ser (Bu}^t)^6, \text{ des-Gly-NH}_2]$-LH–RH ethylamide

$[\text{D-Trp}^6]$-LH–RH

LH–RH Antagonists

$[\text{des-His}_2]$-LH–RH

$[\text{Leu}^3]$-LH–RH

$[\text{des-His}^2, \text{des-Gly-NH}_2^{10}]$-LH–RH ethylamide

$[\text{des-His}^2, \text{ D-Ala}^6]$-LH–RH

$[\text{D-Phe}^2]$-LH–RH

$[\text{D-Phe}^2, \text{D-Trp}^3, \text{ D-Phe}^6]$-LH–RH

Figure 2-7. Chemical structures of some analogues of luteinizing hormone-releasing hormone (LH-RH) and LH-RH antagonists.

protracted stimulation of release of LH and FSH. The synthetic analogues of LH-RH are also pharmacologically active by several modes of administration, including the oral route.

Potentially, some of the highly pharmacologically active analogues could be used as either a pre- or a postcoital contraceptive, since their extended duration of action could interfere with the physiological timing of ovulation. Furthermore, certain LH-RH antagonists (Figure 2-7) or inhibitory peptides are capable of blocking ovulation. Only selected modifications of the chemical structure of the decapeptide of LH-RH (*viz.* modifications in amino acids in positions 1, 2, and 3) lead to molecules that are LH-RH antagonists. Increased research efforts may lead to the development of clinically useful LH-RH as another approach to contraception.

Finally, it has been suggested that Kalman's syndome may represent a congenital absence of LH-RH and, as such, might also represent another clinical indication for this decapeptide.

2.1.4. GH-RF and GH-IF (SRIF)

The secretion of growth hormone (GH) is regulated by a dualistic system of hypophysiotrophic factors—one inhibitory and one stimulatory. This inhibitory factor (GH-IF or SRIF), also known as somatostatin, is a tetradecapeptide that can be isolated from the median eminence (see Chapter 10). Thus, the inhibition of GH secretion is mediated by somatostatin.

Hypothalamic extracts contain a substance that releases GH both *in vivo* and *in vitro*. Unlike certain other hormones, growth hormone secretion is intermittent and episodic rather than continuous. Unlike many of the other hypophysiotrophic hormones, the precise physiological and biochemical characteristics of GH-RF remain to be elucidated. Efforts to purify GH-RF have not been entirely successful because of the concomitant presence of SRIF and SRIF-like substances. GH-RF appears to be localized in the lateral region of the ventromedial nucleus.

Many substances found in the hypothalamus and adjacent regions, such as serotonin, vasopressin, substance P, norepinephrine and TRH, can stimulate the release of growth hormone, but it is not entirely clear whether such responses are mediated *via* GH-RF. Growth hormone itself can be increased by a number of factors, including hypoglycemia, nonspecific stress, and drugs (see Section 2.2.2).

Should GH-RH become available for clinical use, it would presumably be effective in the therapeutic management of pituitary dwarfism by providing a stimulus for growth hormone secretion. GH-RH also has the pharmacological potential for promoting protein anabolism.

2.1.5. PRF and PIF

Both prolactin-releasing factor (PRF) and Prolactin inhibitory factor (PIF) are involved in modulating the physiological secretion of prolactin, although PIF seems to exert a more influential role in mammals. There is also some evidence that TRH may have a physiological role in the secretion of prolactin. Pharmacologically, TRH and analogues of TRH can cause an increase in the secretion of prolactin.

Several drugs can cause an increase in prolactin (see Section on 2.2.5), but it is unclear whether PRF is directly or indirectly involved in the mediation of this increased release. Evidence points to serotonin as a neurotransmitter involved in the modulation of PRF. cAMP and prostaglandins can also affect the cellular release of prolactin. Until the physiological significance and the chemical properties of PRF can be established, its pharmacological value remains in doubt.

There is evidence that dopamine inhibits prolactin by exerting a direct effect on the pituitary. Several substances are present in the brain and/or hypothalamus that can exert prolactin inhibitory activity. Acetylcholine may inhibit prolactin, while serotonin may act in a stimulatory fashion. Under certain experimental conditions and in supraphysiological doses, GABA can inhibit prolactin release by a direct action on the pituitary gland. Drugs such as apomorphine, perphenazine, MAO inhibitors, L-DOPA, and α-bromoergocriptine can inhibit the release of prolactin.

2.1.6. MRF and MIF

The release of melanocyte stimulatory hormone (MSH) from the pars intermedia of the pituitary gland is regulated by the hypophysiotrophic factors melanocyte releasing factor (MRF) and melanocyte inhibitory factor (MIF). MIF appears, however, to exert a more dominant role in the regulation of MSH. Two polypeptides have been isolated from the cells of the pars intermedia: α-MSH and β-MSH. Both cause a dispersion of melanin granules in pigment cells.

MIF has been isolated from the hypothalamus of domestic animals. This polypeptide has been identified in some species as having the following amino acid sequence: $H-Pro-Leu-Gly-NH_2$. Interestingly, incubation of oxytocin with endopeptidase extracted from the hypothalamus leads to the formation of this tripeptide with MIF activity. It is also possible that this tripeptide with MIF activity exerts an action on the pineal gland. MIF may enhance dopamine synthesis in the brain. A number of synthetic polypeptides have now been examined for their

MIF activity. Because these polypeptides can induce dopamine synthesis in the brain, they have the therapeutic potential to be used clinically in the management of Parkinson's disease or in certain forms of depression.

It is quite probable that MRF has the following amino acid sequence: H-Cys-Tyr-Ile-Gln-Asn-Cys-OH. This sequence of amino acids also constitutes the opened N-terminal ring of oxytocin. There is evidence to indicate that the release of MIF is under adrenergic regulation. Despite some progress indentifying polypeptides with either MIF or MRF activity, many uncertainties remain with regard to their physiological role and pharmacological potential.

2.2. PHARMACOLOGY OF ANTERIOR PITUITARY HORMONES

2.2.1. TSH

Although throid-stimulating hormone (TSH) has not been completely purified and chemically characterized, it is known to consist of two peptide chains. One peptide chain, the α-chain, has an amino acid sequence similar to that of LH and α-FSH. The β-subunit confers on the hormone its biological specificity; it is the major determinant of immunological specificity. TSH is a glycoprotein containing glucosamine and galactosamine. It has a molecular weight of approximately 28,000.

TSH is synthesized and stored in the thyrotrophs, a cell line that constitutes approximately one-tenth of the cells of the adenohypophysis. The production of TSH is modulated by TRH and by the concentration of circulating hormones. The hormonal relationship among TRH, TSH, and the thyroid gland reveals a rather complex feedback system (Figure 2-8). TRH stimulates the thyrotroph, which in turn enhances the synthesis/secretion of TSH; this leads to a stimulation of the thyroid gland and results in the release of thyroid hormone (T_4 and T_3) into the bloodstream. Blood concentrations of thyroid hormone act back upon the adenohypophysis (and perhaps the hypothalamus) to inhibit the secretion and/or release of TSH (Figure 2-8). SRIF, or somatostatin, may act to suppress the activity of the thyrotroph. A number of other factors, such as environmental influences (e.g., heat or cold, stress) and the peripheral metabolism of thyroid hormone, can affect the feedback system involving TSH secretion.

TSH exerts its major physiological effects by regulating the synthesis and release of T_4 and T_3 (see also Chapter 4). TSH stimulates the uptake of iodine by the thyroid gland. TSH can also accelerate the uptake of glucose and amino acids by the thyroid.

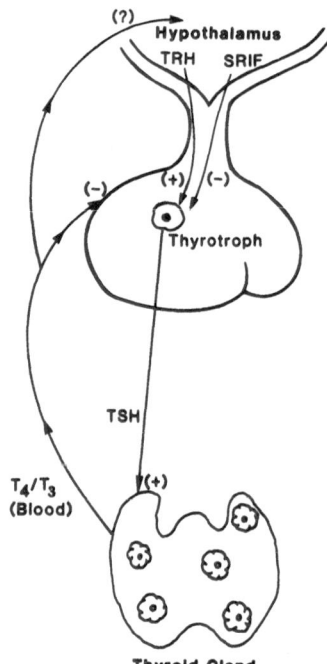

Figure 2-8. Hormonal relationship among the hypothalamus, adenohypophysis, and the thyroid gland. SRIF, somatostatin; T_3, triiodothyronine; T_4, thyroxine; TRH, throtropin-releasing hormone; TSH, thyroid-stimulating hormone.

The mechanism of action of TSH on the thyroid gland is not entirely understood. Nevertheless, its actions on the thyroid gland, are known to be mediated *via* specific TSH receptors located on the cell membrane. This TSH receptor, at least in some species, is a glycoprotein containing sialic acid. Sialic acid is necessary for receptor responsiveness. Once TSH binds to its glycoprotein receptor, it interacts with a specific ganglioside in the membrane, resulting in a conformational change. This conformational change seems to induce the stimulation of membrane-bound adenylate cyclase and cAMP. Subsequent metabolic events include an increase in the transport of iodide into the thyroid gland and in the synthesis of rRNA and mRNA. Calcium ion is somehow involved in the binding of TSH to its receptor and to some of the subsequent metabolic actions of the hormone. Many substances, including epinephrine and prostaglandins, can mimic the action of TSH on the thyroid gland, but not *via* TSH receptors. Long-acting thyroid stimulate (LATS) an IgG, also known as thyroid-stimulating immunoglobulin (TSI), can stimulate adenylate cyclase activity of the thyroid gland, mimicking the action of TSH. Other thyroid-stimulator proteins, such as chorionic thyrotropin and human placental thyrotropin (HCT), which emanate from the placenta, can also act in a manner that can mimick some of the actions of TSH.

The clinical significance of the TSH determination is to differentiate between primary (thyroid) and secondary (pituitary) hypothyroidism. Primary hypothyroidism due to a decrease in thyroid hormone feedback is characterized by an increased secretion of TSH and elevated serum TSH. Testing the TSH response to exogenous TRH will differentiate pituitary- from hypothalamic-induced hypothyroidism. An intravenous injection of TRH (500 µg) into normal subjects produces a rapid rise in serum TSH in about 30 min.

The pharmacological use of TSH (thyrotropin) is relegated primarily to the diagnosis of thyroid disorders, although it has been employed therapeutically as an adjunct (Table 2-3) Thyrotropin is available for injection (subcutaneous or intramuscular) in strengths of 10 IU/vial (e.g., Thytropar). In assessing thyroid functional capacity, 10 IU can be administered intramuscularly on three successive days; a ^{131}I uptake test is performed on the last day of treatment. A 24-hr ^{131}I uptake of more than 10% is an indication of functional thyroidal cells. TSH therapy is of no value in the therapeutic management of either secondary or tertiary hypothyroidism.

Some side effects have been reported following TSH therapy. Faintness, itching, skin rash, local hyperemia at the site of injection, and symptoms associated with hyperthyroidism (i.e., overdose), such as chest pain, irritability, nervousness, tachycardia, and sweating, can occur in response to the injection of TSH. TSH must be used with discretion in patients with cardiovascular disease and in cases of adrenocortical insufficiency. If adrenocortical insufficiency is left untreated before instituting TSH therapy, thyrotropin can actually aggravate acute adrenocortical insufficiency.

2.2.2. STH or GH

Somatotropin (STH), or growth hormone (GH) (Somatrem), is essential to the metabolic processes and plays an important role in the

Table 2-3. Indications for Thyrotropin

Aid in diagnosis of subclinical hypothyroidism or low thyroid reserve
Differentiation between primary and secondary hypothyroidism
Differentiation between primary hypothyroidism and euthyroidism in patients whose thyroid has been suppressed by T_4/T_3 replacement therapy
Aid in diagnosis of thyroid carcinoma
Adjunct therapy in metastatic thyroid carcinoma

---

growth and proliferation of cells. Growth hormone affects the rate of skeletal growth and gain in body weight. It is synthesized in the adenohypophysis. The chemical structure of growth hormone varies with the particular animal species. Human growth hormone (HGH) contains 191 amino acids and has a molecular weight of 21,500 (see Figure 2-9). Growth hormone from the rhesus monkey has a molecular weight of about 25,000, whereas it is nearly two times heavier in the cow (46,000 M_r). Human growth hormone (Somatrem, Protopin) has recently been cloned in bacteria, using rDNA technology and has recently been approved for clinical use.

A number of endogenous hormones influence the rate of GH secretion. These hormones include TRH, GH-RF, and a β-endorphin. GH-IF (SRIF or somatostatin) inhibits the release of somatotropin.

The principal physiological action of STH is to promote protein synthesis and cellular growth. Not all the actions of growth hormone are mediated directly on the cell, as somatomedin, or sulfation factor, which probably emanates from the liver, enhances cartilage growth. Somatomedins are small peptides circulating in the blood that bear some chemical resemblance to proinsulin. Growth hormone stimulates the synthesis of RNA and acts to mobilize fatty acids from stored lipids.

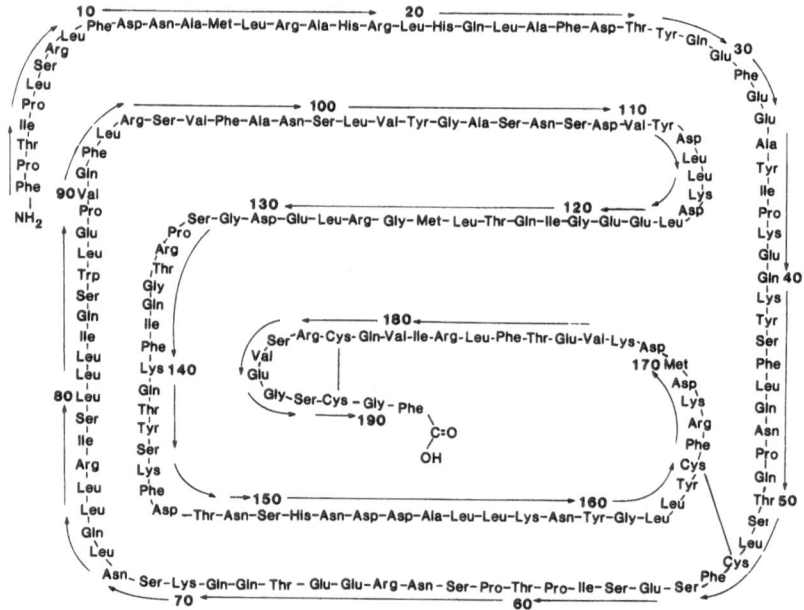

Figure 2-9. Amino acid sequence of growth hormone.

Growth hormone exerts both anti-insulin (e.g., hyperglycemia) and insulinlike action (e.g., stimulation of amino acid uptake).

The mechanism of action of STH appears to be mediated *via* cAMP. Growth hormone receptors have been isolated from a number of tissues. The receptor(s) for GH are located on the plasma membrane. Growth hormone seems to bind to its cell surface receptor with some degree of biological discrimination. While the binding of STH to its receptor on the plasma membrane can initiate certain intermediate biochemical events such as activating the cAMP-adenyl cyclase system, little is known about subsequent metabolic events that culminate in increased growth and proliferation by the cell.

The hypersecretion of GH in children can lead to gigantism, while this condition in adults can lead to acromegaly. Excessive production of GH can also occur in certain pituitary adenomas.

A congenital absence or defective synthesis/secretion of GH can result in dwarfism. About 10% of all cases of dwarfism in children may be caused by hyposecretion of GH. The early diagnosis and establishing the etiology of dwarfism as being due to GH deficiency is important, since these children can benefit from pharmacological replacement therapy with GH. The radioimmunoassay of GH as well as provocative tests revealing the pituitary reserve (or lack of) of STH can aid in establishing the diagnosis of GH disorders. Although serum levels of GH are subject to wide and sometimes rapid fluctuations, normal fasting and ambulatory human subjects may have the following baseline zinc levels: adult male < 10 ng/ml, adult female <15 mg/ml and children <10 ng/ml.

Several agents or factors can stimulate the secretion of GH and are therefore of diagnostic value in assessing pituitary research. Among the agents that stimulate or provoke the release of GH are insulin, arginine, clonidine, glucagon, β-adrenergic blocking drugs, and L-DOPA. Dopamine stimulates the secretion of GH acutely by a CNS-mediated mechanism. The dopaminergic agent, bromocriptine mesylate (Parlodel), is sometimes useful in the therapeutic management of acromegaly. Bromocriptine possesses other pharmacological properties and has been indicated in the prevention of postpartum lactation (see Section 2.2.5).

Somatotropin (Asellacrin, Crescormon) is a preparation of GH, extracted from the human pituitary glands of cadavers, sterilized, and lyophilized. Somatropin may be indicated in growth failure due to a hypersecretion of GH (Table 2-4). Somatotropin is of no value in patients with closed epiphyses or in those patients who are unable to secrete somatomedin after stimulation with GH.

Somatotropin is injected intramuscularly initially in doses of 2 IU, three times per week allowing for a minimum of 48 hr between admin-

Table 2-4. Clinical Indications
for Growth Hormone

Normal variant short stature
Infantile hypoglycemia
Turner's syndrome
Would healing
Burn trauma
Stress ulcers
Cartilage healing
Fracture healing
Osteoporosis
Juvenile rheumatoid arthritis
Hypercholesterolemia

---

istrations. If there has not been any evidence of significant growth over a 6-month treatment period, the dose may be doubled to 4 IU. If there is no evidence of significant body weight and height growth after this treatment interval at the higher dose regimens, the patient should be diagnostically reevaluated. Successful therapy usually culminates in closure of the epiphyseal plates at a height of about 5 ft (150 cm) or a reasonable adult height.

Somatotropin possesses some side effects. It may cause hyperglycemia and ketosis. It must be administered with care to diabetic dwarfs or to those children with a familial history of diabetes mellitus. Because supplies of somatotropin are limited, the cost of long-term therapy can be very expensive. Accordingly, it is of utmost importance to reaffirm the etiology of the dwarfism before embarking on an extended therapeutic regimen. Recently, HGH has been genetically engineered using recombinant DNA. This rDNA hormone (Somatonorm, Protropin) is currently being used clinically since cadaveric HGH use has been suspended.

2.2.3. ACTH

The secretion of adrenocortical steroids particularly the glucocorticoids, relies on stimulation by corticotropin, or ACTH (see Chapter 9). ACTH is secreted by the adenohypophysis and modulates the secretory activity of the adrenal cortex. This hormonal relationship is accomplished by a feedback system (see Figure 2-2). The secretion of ACTH is regulated by CRH and by the negative feedback control exerted by glucocorticoids secreted from the adrenal cortex. The integration of all these hormonal influences results in a diurnal rhythm of ACTH secretion, with elevated levels in the morning and lower levels in the evening. A host of factors, such as stress, surgery, hypoglycemia, and pyrogens can produce an elevation in ACTH, as can various pharmaceutical agents (see Chapter 11).

Corticotropin (Acthar, Cortrophin gel) is a straight-chain polypeptide consisting of 39 amino acids (see Figure 2-10). It has a molecular weight of 4566. Species variation in amino acid sequencing are limited to the region of amino acid residues 25–32. The first 24 amino acid residues are common to many species, including man, and this portion contains as much biological activity displayed by the parent hormone (i.e., the 39-amino acid residue polypeptide). Commercially available synthetic ACTH-like molecules contain between 18 and 24 amino acid residues. Cosyntropin (Cortrosyn), a synthetic analogue of ACTH, contains that first 24 amino acid residues of the parent hormone. Interestingly, loss of a single amino acid from the N-terminal end of the parent hormone by hydrolytic cleavage was found to abolish biological activity, while loss of C-terminal amino acids has little effect on biological activity.

The amino acid sequence of certain portions of the ACTH molecule can also be found in several other hormones. For example, the first 13 amino acids of ACTH are also contained in the sequence of α-melanocyte-stimulating hormone (α-MSH). The polypeptide precursor of ACTH contains the amino acid sequences of a number of other peptides, including β-lipoprotein (β-LPH), β-LPH, β- and γ-endorphin, and met-enkephalin. Corticotropin-like intermediate lobe peptide (CLIP) contains a 22-amino acid peptide that is the same as residues 18–39 of ACTH itself.

The mechanism of action of ACTH resides in the fact that it can stimulate the secretion of cortisol and its precursors. The rate-limiting step involved in adrenal steroidogenesis that is affected by ACTH appears to be the conversion of cholesterol to pregnenolone.

Although the precise mechanism of action of ACTH on the adrenal cortex is unknown, a number of early molecular events, including increases in permeability to glucose and certain ions and activation of adenyl cyclase, can occur after the administration of this hormone. cAMP,

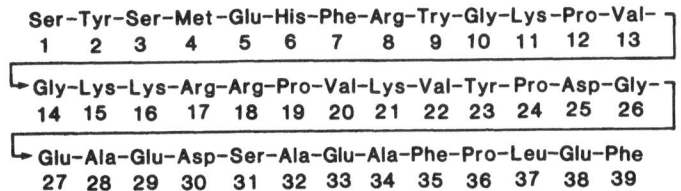

Figure 2-10. Chemical structure of ACTH.

in turn, activates dephosphorylase kinase, leading to an increase in active phosphorylase in the zona fasciculata of the adrenal cortex (see also Chapter 9). cAMP is capable of stimulating steroidogenesis, probably by enhancing the production of energy substrate and NADPH. Drugs acting on phosphodiesterase to cause its inhibition can enhance the action of ACTH upon steroidogenesis. ACTH can also induce morphological changes in adrenal mitochondria. A biochemical event previously used as a bioassay for this trophic hormone involved the ability of ACTH to cause the depletion of adrenal ascorbic acid.

ACTH is used in clinical medicine both for its therapeutic value and for diagnostic purposes (Table 2-5). ACTH or its synthetic analogues can be used diagnostically to determine the competency of the hypophyseal–adrenal axis. Several agents can provoke ACTH secretion, and oftentimes vasopressin is employed to examine the pituitary reserve of ACTH. Corticotropin has been used to treat glucocorticoid-responsive diseases in patients with functional adrenal glands, but it is generally not as effective as simple steroid replacement with cortisone or cortisonelike drugs. Furthermore, adrenocortical steroids are pharmacologically active by the oral route, whereas corticotropin must be administered parenterally.

In addition to the occasional use of ACTH for selected anti-inflammatory states, it is also used for certain types of epilepsy. More specifically, ACTH has been indicated in selected forms of infantile seizures.

ACTH and its synthetic analogues possess some side effects, including sodium retention and potassium loss. Such electrolyte changes are due to ACTH-induced increases in adrenocortical steroid secretion. Hypersensitivities, mild fever, and occasionally anaphylaxis can occur with ACTH preparations of animal origin, but generally not with synthetic preparations.

2.2.4. FSH/LH

The adenohypophyseal hormones that modulate ovarian and testicular function are referred to as gonadotropins. Actually, there are five gonadotropins, two of pituitary origin, *viz.* follicle-stimulating hormone

Table 2-5.   Indications for ACTH and Its Analogues

Differential diagnosis of adrenocortical insufficiency (ACTH provocative test)
Management of certain anti-inflammatory states
Selected infantile seizures

(FSH) and luteinizing hormone (LH) and three of placental origin, *viz.* chorionic gonadotropin (CG), chorionic follicle-stimulating gonadotropin (CFSH), and pregnant mare serum (PMS). In the female, FSH enhances the growth of the graafian follicles of the ovary. It primes the young ovarian follicles to develop multiple layers of granulosa and to form antra. In the male, FSH stimulates the seminiferous tubules of the testes, thereby stimulating the process of spermatogenesis. FSH appears to localize in the Sertoli cells, where it may affect steroidogenesis. While FSH is important in enhancing the process of spermatogenesis, it appears that LH regulates the overall process. FSH has no effect on the Leydig cells of the testes.

LH acts synergistically with FSH, stimulating the secretion of estrogens by follicles undergoing maturation. LH is believed to be the hormone responsible for ovulation. LH possesses a luteotrophic action in certain subhuman species.

In the male, LH stimulates the interstitial cells of the testes, also called the Leydig cells. LH is sometimes referred to as interstitial cell-stimulating hormone (ICSH) in the male. By virtue of its actions on the Leydig cells, LH causes secretion of testicular androgen (e.g., testosterone).

Most of the biological actions of LH depend to some extent on the primary actions of FSH. Indeed, and in order to achieve optimal biological responsiveness of the endocrine target organ, both gonadotropins must be operant. The regulation of FSH and LH by the pituitary is complex, but both hormones necessarily act in concert in order to modulate the secretion of male and/or female sex steroids.

FSH and LH, as well as TSH, are glycoproteins. FSH is composed of two polypeptide chains. The α-chain of FSH is similar to that of LH (see Figure 2-11). FSH and LH have comparable molecular weights of approximately 32,000, and each has a carbohydrate content of about 18%. FSH and LH are composed of two chemically dissimilar subunits possessing a molecular weight of about 16,000. The α- and β-subunits are noncovalently bound and can be readily dissociated by a number of physicochemical conditions. It is the β-subunit that conveys the hormone's inherent specificity. The α-subunits of FSH and LH (as well as TSH) are structurally similar.

HCG, often used as a hormone substitute for LH, appears also to be composed of two polypeptide chains. It, too, is a glycoprotein and possesses a molecular weight of approximately 27,000. Chorionic follicle-stimulating hormone (CFSH) has also been characterized as a glycoprotein; it is synthesized in the placenta and has a carbohydrate content of about 30%. PMS is likewise a glycoprotein and is composed of nearly

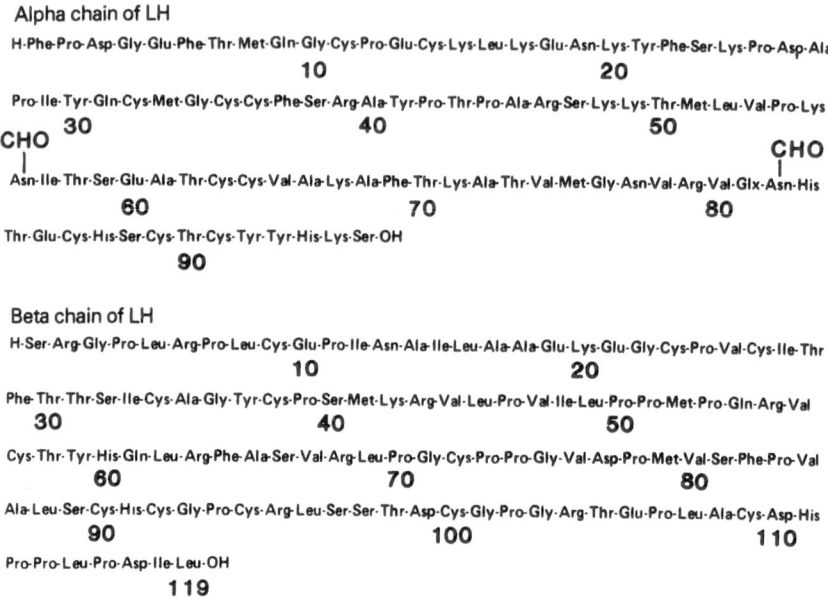

Alpha chain of LH

H-Phe-Pro-Asp-Gly-Glu-Phe-Thr-Met-Gln-Gly-Cys-Pro-Glu-Cys-Lys-Leu-Lys-Glu-Asn-Lys-Tyr-Phe-Ser-Lys-Pro-Asp-Ala
                              10   20

Pro-Ile-Tyr-Gln-Cys-Met-Gly-Cys-Cys-Phe-Ser-Arg-Ala-Tyr-Pro-Thr-Pro-Ala-Arg-Ser-Lys-Lys-Thr-Met-Leu-Val-Pro-Lys
CHO   30   40   50
 | CHO
 | |
Asn-Ile-Thr-Ser-Glu-Ala-Thr-Cys-Cys-Val-Ala-Lys-Ala-Phe-Thr-Lys-Ala-Thr-Val-Met-Gly-Asn-Val-Arg-Val-Glx-Asn-His
                              60   70   80

Thr-Glu-Cys-His-Ser-Cys-Thr-Cys-Tyr-Tyr-His-Lys-Ser-OH
                              90

Beta chain of LH

H-Ser-Arg-Gly-Pro-Leu-Arg-Pro-Leu-Cys-Glu-Pro-Ile-Asn-Ala-Ile-Leu-Ala-Ala-Glu-Lys-Glu-Gly-Cys-Pro-Val-Cys-Ile-Thr
                              10   20

Phe-Thr-Thr-Ser-Ile-Cys-Ala-Gly-Tyr-Cys-Pro-Ser-Met-Lys-Arg-Val-Leu-Pro-Val-Ile-Leu-Pro-Pro-Met-Pro-Gln-Arg-Val
       30   40   50

Cys-Thr-Tyr-His-Gln-Leu-Arg-Phe-Ala-Ser-Val-Arg-Leu-Pro-Gly-Cys-Pro-Pro-Gly-Val-Asp-Pro-Met-Val-Ser-Phe-Pro-Val
       60   70   80

Ala-Leu-Ser-Cys-His-Cys-Gly-Pro-Cys-Arg-Leu-Ser-Ser-Thr-Asp-Cys-Gly-Pro-Gly-Arg-Thr-Glu-Pro-Leu-Ala-Cys-Asp-His
       90   100   110

Pro-Pro-Leu-Pro-Asp-Ile-Leu-OH
       119

Figure 2-11   Chemical structure of luteinizing hormone.

50% carbohydrate. PMS, like the other gonadotropins, is composed of two subunits.

Little is known about the metabolism of either FSH or LH. Only about 15% of the amount of secreted FSH can actually be chemically or immunologically identified. The mechanism of action of LH and FSH appears to be initiated after these hormones have interacted with their respective receptors. These receptors are quite specific for their particular gonadotropin and reside in particular fractions obtained from either the testes or the ovary. Either FSH or LH stimulates its target organ(s), causing an increase in cAMP. In turn, cAMP can act to stimulate steroidogenesis. Whether prostaglandins are involved in the mechanism of action of the gonadotropins has not been definitely established (see Chapter 3).

Because sufficient amounts of human FSH and/or LH have not been available for the widespread clinical management of certain endocrine dysfunctions, HCG and HMG can effectively be used in place of FSH or LH. Soon LH and FSH may be made by rDNA technologies

There are several indications for the clinical use of gonadotropins (see Table 2-6). If available, human FSH and LH can be sequentially administered in order to create pharmacologically a hormonal milieu conducive to ovulation. Sometimes gonadotropin substitutes (*viz.* HMG and HCG) are used to achieve ovulation. Dosing and timing during the menstrual cycle are important to the success of gonadotropin therapy. Before initiating any hormonal therapy, the primary cause of female infertility should be established. Infertility due to organic disease or anatomical obstruction will not respond to hormonal therapies.

Three agents are currently available to treat ovulatory failures: clomiphene citrate (Clomid, Serophene), HMG, and HCG. Clomiphene may be used alone or in combination with these gonadotropins. HMG and HCG are commonly used in combination with one another. HCG and HMG, substitutes for LH and FSH, respectively, represent replacement hormonal therapy in those anovulatory women experiencing abnormal menstrual cycles or reduced gonadotropin secretion. On the other hand, clomiphene exerts its pharmacological action(s) by stimulating the release of endogenous FSH and/or LH, thereby producing ovulation. Dose regimens of these various agents vary, depending on the hormonal state of the patient. Urofollitropin (Metrodin) is also used in the treatment for the induction of ovulation. This agent contains amounts of FSH that are comparable to Pergonal, but contains less LH. In general, the more severe the ovulatory dysfunction, the more difficult and less successful the hormonal therapy.

Clomiphene citrate (Clomid) is a nonsteroidal agent possessing very weak estrogenic actions (Figure 2-12). Clomiphene competes with estrogens for their receptors located in the hypothalamus and the adenohypophysis. Clomiphene, like tamoxifen, has also been categorized as an antiestrogen because of its receptor competitive properties. This competitive effect blocks the actions of endogenous estrogens, causing the hypothalamus to interpret such a presumed reduction in female sex steroids, which leads to an outpouring of LH and FSH. This surge can often lead to ovulation. Patients best suited for clomiphene therapy are those who secrete gonadotropins and estrogens but who fail to ovulate due to abnormality in the cycling mechanism that modulates gonadotropin secretion. A representative dose regimen for clomiphene is depicted in Figure 2-13. Clomiphene therapy is ordinarily initiated at the lowest dosage (50 mg/day for 5 days) and is increased in gradual increments until an ovulatory response is attained. With individually pat-

Table 2-6.   Indications for FSH/LH

FSH (or HMG) used to induce ovulation (with LH or HCG)
LH (or HCG) used to induce ovulation (with FSH or HMG)
Male hypogonadism
Cryptorchidism
HCG stimulation test to diagnose anorchia (?)

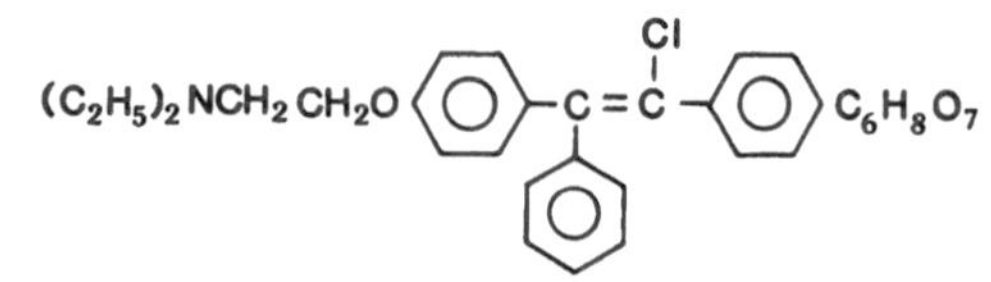

$$(C_2H_5)_2\,NCH_2\,CH_2O \bigcirc -C = \overset{\overset{\displaystyle Cl}{|}}{C} -\bigcirc\; C_6H_8O_7$$

Figure 2-12.   Chemical structure of clomiphene citrate (Clomid).

terned dose regimens of clomiphene therapy, the ovulatory rate can be as much as 70%. Despite this improved ovulatory rate in infertile women, the pregnancy rate is unfortunately only about 40%.

Clomiphene will produce several side effects depending on the duration of therapy and dosage. Side effects include hot flashes, nausea, vomiting, ocular disturbances, CNS symptoms, breast tenderness, weight gain, urinary frequency, and heavy menses. It may also cause ovarian enlargement and abdominal pain. The incidence of multiple pregnancy is about 10%. Clomiphene is only effective in those patients whose pituitary glands are capable of releasing gonadotropins.

Therapy with menotropins (*viz.* HMG) is most often difficult and complex due to the usual concomitant hormonal imbalances in many of these patients. Induction of ovulation with HMG is indicated in those

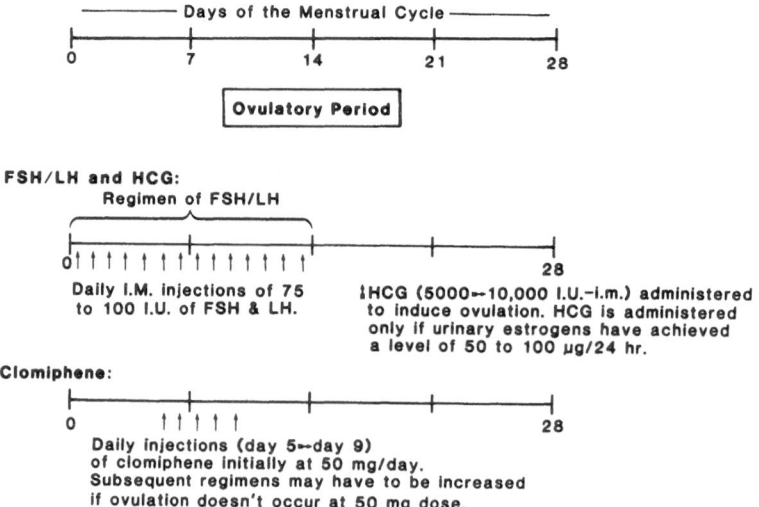

Figure 2-13.   Representative dosing regimens employed in the clinical management of anovulatory patients. FSH, follicle-stimulating hormone; HCG, human chorionic gonadotropin; LH, luteinizing hormone.

patients who require administration of exogenous gonadotropins in order to become pregnant. The dosage varies considerably and is based on the patient's endocrine status. HMG (Pergonal) is a lyophilized preparation containing 75 IU of FSH and 75 IU of LH. HMG can cause ovarian enlargement and is associated with an increased incidence of multiple births. HMG is only indicated (alone or in combination with HCG) in those cases of female infertility due to ovulatory failure. Various dose regimens of HMG have been used to prime the ovary during the early portion of the cycle (see Figure 2-14).

HCG (Antuitrin-S, APL, Profasi, Follutein, Pregny) possesses luteotropin properties and may also trigger ovulation. HCG is often used in combination with FSH for the induction of ovulation. It may also be used in combination with HMG and clomiphene. In addition, HCG can be used diagnostically to determine the ability of the ovaries to secrete estrogens and progestogens.

Many of the same hormones (or hormonal substitutes, such as HCG) and drugs used to treat female infertility are also used in the clinical management of male infertility. HCG, either alone or in combination with HMB and clomiphene, has been used with some success in stimulating spermatogenesis in men with reduced endogenous gonadotropins.

2.2.5. PRL

Prolactin (PRL) is necessary for the initiation of lactation in mammals at parturition. In some species, PRL also enhances the secretion of milk. Other hormones, such as estrogen, cortisol, and insulin, appear to act synergistically with PRL, leading to growth and proliferation of the mammary gland. Once the mammary gland has developed, PRL, insulin, and cortisol are required to maintain milk secretion. Estrogen can antagonize the stimulation of milk production by PRL (see also Chapter 7). In some instances, elevated levels of PRL leads to infertility. Several drugs can affect the secretion of PRL and thus affect lactation (see Chapter 11). Still other nondrug factors, such as stress, coitus, suckling, and pregnancy, can increase the secretion of PRL.

The physiological role of PRL in the male is poorly understood. In some instances, PRL may act synergistically with androgens, leading to increases in the growth and proliferation of the male sex accessory organ. Whether production plays a pathological role in the genesis of abnormal growth of the prostate gland remains to be established.

In nonprimates, PRL exerts a luteotropic action. For example, PRL can maintain the corpus luteum in rodents. Birds are particularly sen-

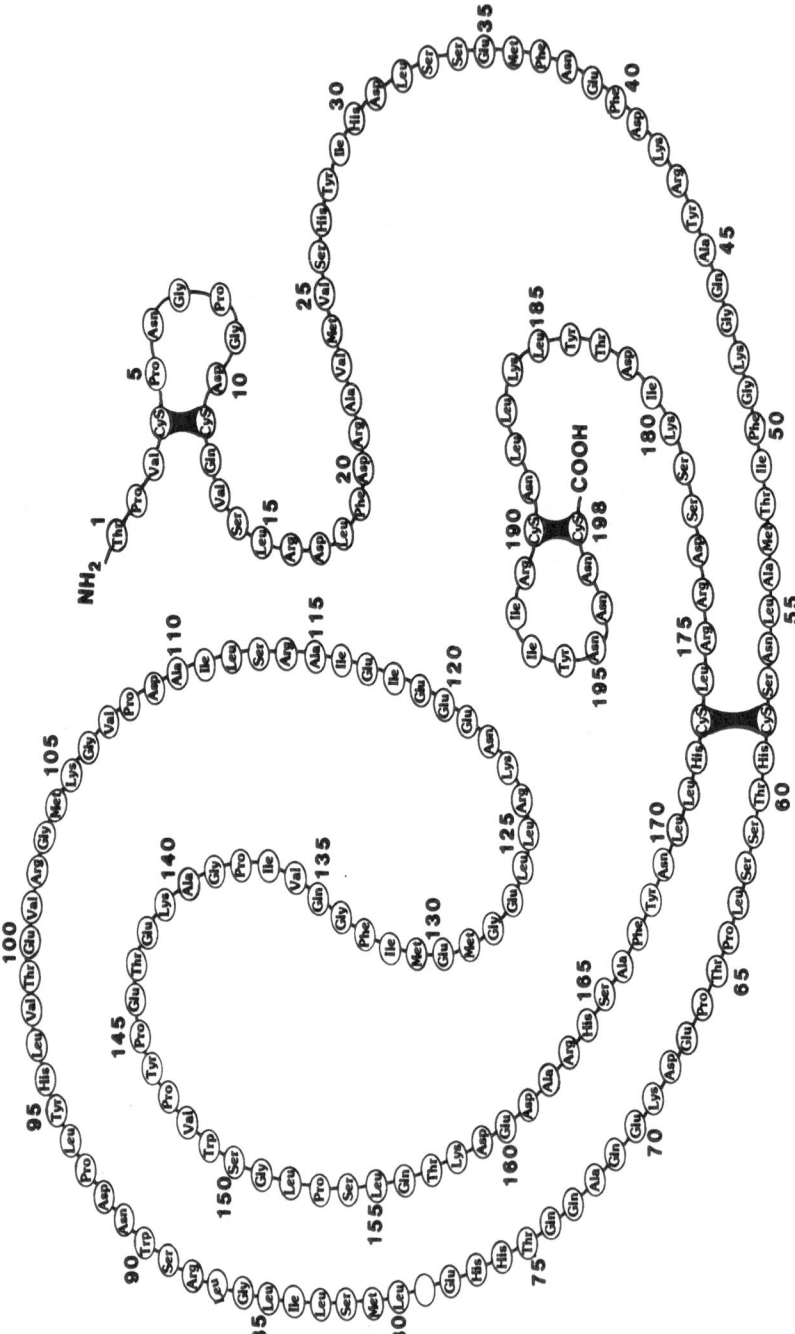

Figure 2-14. Amino acid sequence of ovine prolactin.

sitive to PRL. The term prolactin originated for the hormone responsible for the secretion of milk by the crop-sac gland of the pigeon. Before the radioimmunoassay of PRL, the pigeon crop-sac bioassay for PRL was used extensively in experimental endocrinology. Prolactin also can affect sexual behavior in lower animals. It also affects salt and water metabolism in invertebrates.

The human placenta contains substance(s) that possesses both growth-promoting properties and lactogenic activity. Human placental lactogen (HPL) seems to have chemical properties similar to human growth hormone, but its physiological function is poorly understood.

Elucidating the precise chemical identity of human PRL has been slow because it is difficult to isolate completely from GH. Ovine prolactin, however, has been characterized extensively. The amino acid sequence of ovine PRL has been established (see Figure 2-14). Ovine and bovine PRL appear to possess similar molecular weights of about 24,000. Neither contains any carbohydrate.

Receptors for PRL have been isolated from several different organs, including the mammary glands and reproductive tissues. The receptor(s) is located on the plasma membrane. Once PRL binds to its specific receptor, subsequent events lead to enhanced cellular proliferation and differentiation. It can cause a rapid increase in RNA synthesis and the induction of enzymes and proteins involved in the process of lactation.

Because human PRL is not available for therapeutic use and because PRL obtained from domestic animals (e.g., ovine, bovine) is immunologically dissimilar, this hormone is currently not employed pharmacologically. Interestingly, preparations of HGH with high PRL activity have been administered successfully in an effort to enhance milk production in lactating women.

RECOMMENDED READINGS

Abboud, C. F., Laboratory diagnosis of hypopituitarism, *Mayo Clin. Proc.* **61**:35, 1986.

Baird, D. J., Endocrinology of female infertility, *Br. Med. Bull.* **35**:193, 1979.

Burger, H. G., and Patch, Y. C., Thyrotropin releasing hormone—TSH, *Clin. Endo. & Metab.* **6**:83, 1977.

Chawla, R. K., Parks, J. S., and Rudman, D., Structural variants of human growth hormone: Biochemical, genetic and clinical aspects, *Annu. Rev. Med.* **35**:519–547, 1983.

Chrousos, G. P., Schuermeyer, T. H., Doppman, J., Oldfield, E. H., Schulte, H. M., Gold, P. W., and Loriaux, D. L., Clinical applications of corticotropin-releasing factor, *Ann. Intern. Med.* **102**:344–358, 1985.

Conn, P. M., Hsueh, A. J. W., and Crowley, W. F., Gonadotropin-releasing hormone; molecular and cell biology, physiology, and clinical applications, *Fed. Proc.* **43**:2351–1261, 1984.

Cutler, G. B., Hoffman, A. R., Swerdloff, R. S., Santen, R. J., Meldrum, D. R., and Comite, F., Therapeutic applications of luteinizing-hormone-releasing hormone and its analogues, *Ann. Intern. Med.* **102**:643–657, 1985.

de Kretser, D. N., Endocrinology of male infertility, *Br. Med. Bull.* **35**:187, 1979.

Garcia, J., Jones, G. E., and Wentz, A. C., The use of clomiphene citrate, *Fertil. Steril.* **28**:707, 1977.

Glode, L. M., The biology of gonadotropin-releasing hormones and its analogs, *Urology* **27**:16, 1986.

Hsueh, A. J. W., and Jones, P. B. C., Gonadotropin releasing hormone—Extrapituitary actions and paracrine control mechanisms, *Annu. Rev. Physiol.* **45**:83–94, 1983.

Kolesnick, R. N., Gershengorn, M. C., Thyrotropin-releasing hormone and the pituitary, *Am. J. Med.* **79**:729, 1985.

Krulich, L., Central neurotransmitters and the secretion of prolactin, GH, LH and TSH, *Annu. Rev. Physiol.* **41**:603, 1979.

Leong, D. A., Frawley, S., and Neill, J., Neuroendocrine control of prolactin secretion, *Annu. Rev. Physiol.* **45**:109–127, 1983.

McCann, S. M., Physiology and pharmacology of LHRH and somatostatin, *Annu. Rev. Pharmacol. Toxicol.* **22**:291, 1982.

Rosenberg, E., Clinical studies of gonadotropins in the male. *Pharmacol. Ther.* **2**:1, 1977.

Schulte, H. M., Chrousos, G. P., Booth, J. D., Oldfield, E. H., Gold, P. W., Cutler, G. B., and Loriaux, D. L., Corticotropin-releasing factor: Pharmacokinetics in man, *J. Clin. Endocrinol. Metab.* **58**:192, 1984.

Vale, W., and Greer, M., Corticotropin-releasing factor, *Fed. Proc.* **44**:145, 1985.

Wehrenberg, W. B., Baird, A., Zeytin, F., Esch, F., Bohlen, P., Ling, N., Ying, S. Y., and Gyillemin, R., Physiological studies with somatocrinin, a growth hormone-releasing factor, *Ann. Rev. Pharmacol. Toxicol.* **25**:463–483, 1985.

Yasuda, N., Greer, M. A., and Aizawa, T., Corticotropin-releasing factor, *Endocrine Rev.* **3**:123–140, 1982.

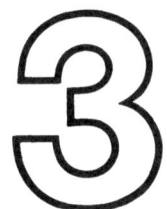

POSTERIOR PITUITARY HORMONES, OXYTOCICS, AND PROSTAGLANDINS

3.1. POSTERIOR PITUITARY HORMONES

3.1.1. History

The posterior pituitary hormones were the first biologically active peptides to be isolated, to be characterized for their amino acid sequence, and to be subsequently synthesized, by du Vigneaud. However, interest in the biological actions of secretions of the neurohypophysis date back nearly 200 years. Oliver and Schaffer described the pressor effects of pituitary extracts as early 1894. Three years later, Howell tracked these pressor substances of the pituitary gland to the neurohypophysis itself. Shortly after the discovery of the vasopressor actions of these neurohypophyseal extracts, the antidiuretic properties of posterior lobe extracts were described. In 1906, Sir Henry Dale reported that extracts of the posterior pituitary caused a stimulation of uterine smooth muscle. Although an awareness of the differences between diabetes insipidus and diabetes mellitus was recognized during the late 1700s, it was not until 1913 that injections of posterior pituitary extracts were observed to cause an improvement in the treatment of diabetes insipidus.

By 1928, Kamm had accomplished the separation of the octapeptides vasopressin and oxytocin. Shortly after World War II, oxytocin was purified and, by the 1950s, du Vigneaud and co-workers not only established the amino acid sequence of these octapeptides, but succeeded in synthesizing these polypeptides. The development of peptide chemistry made it possible to synthesize a large number of analogues of ADH and to assess them for their pharmacological activity. Some of these analogues (e.g., 1-deamino-8-D-arginine vasopressin-dDAVP, or desmopressin) are particularly useful in the therapeutic management of ADH-sensitive diabetes insipidus. More recently, other analogues, such as 1-deamino-4-valine-8-D-arginine vasopressin (dVDAVP) have been synthesized and have been found to be devoid of pressor activity, hence more desirable for the treatment of diabetes insipidus. There has also been considerable progress in actually synthesizing antagonists to oxytocin (e.g., 1-deaminopenicillamine oxytocin). It should be evident that the history of the development of the posterior pituitary hormones represents a successful progression of events, beginning with the use of crude extracts in replacement therapies to the use of synthetically derived peptide analogues specifically designed for the management of diabetes insipidus.

3.1.2. Synthesis, Transport, and Release

The hypophysis or pituitary gland is composed of anterior (adenohypophysis) (see Chapter 2) and posterior (neurohypophysis) lobes and the intermediate lobe (pars intermedia). The neurohypophysis is directly innervated by axons from the hypothalamus. There is little functional relationship between the adenohypophysis and the neurohypophysis. The posterior pituitary gland is the principal site of storage of ADH and oxytocin. ADH is synthesized primarily in regions of the paraventricular nucleus. The anatomical and functional relationship between the hypothalamus and the pituitary gland is depicted in Figure 3-1. Vasopressin and oxytocin are synthesized and released by these neurons of the hypothalamoneurohypophyseal system. The neurohypophysis is richly served with neuronal processes, and nearly one-half its total volume is composed of axons and axon terminals. Such neuronal processes originate from large neurons situated in the supraoptic and paraventricular nuclei of the hypothalamus.

The neuronal terminals in the neurohypophysis store peptide hormones (e.g., ADH and oxytocin) and release them into blood vessels. Separate populations of neurons, namely, the paraventricular and supraoptic regions, are involved in the synthesis of these octapeptides. ADH and oxytocin are stored in secretory granular (or vesicles) along with so-called carrier proteins referred to as neurophysins. They neurophysins have molecular weights of about 20,000; they contain cysteine residues linked by disulfide bridges.

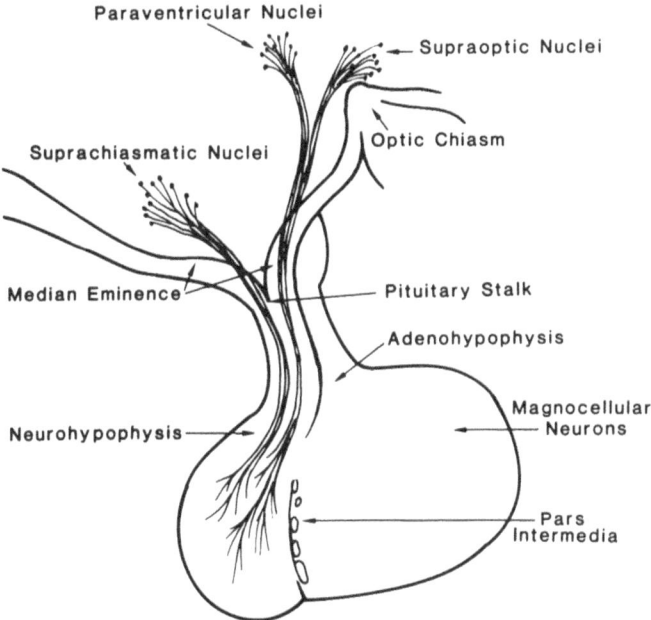

Figure 3-1. Anatomical and functional relationship of the hypothalamoneurohypophyseal system.

Vasopressin along with its carrier protein are believed to be synthesized in the cell body as a portion of a common precursor protein. The precursor protein is presumed to be synthesized by a ribosomal mechanism on the rough endoplasmic reticulum (RER), sacculated into vesicles *via* the Golgi apparatus, and subsequently processed into biologically active peptides. These biosynthetic and processing events are depicted schematically in Figure 3-2. The translation of mRNA takes place in the RER, resulting in the synthesis of a precursor protein or propeptide in the cisternal space of the endoplasmic reticulum. The sacculation (i.e., packaging) or precursor protein into vesicles occurs within the Golgi apparatus. The post-translational processing of precursor protein to smaller peptide(s) occurs within the storage vesicle. The peptides are subsequently stored in the granules in the nerve endings of the neurohypophysis. The secretory granules containing both propeptide and peptide travel down to the axon by axoplasmic flow, eventually released by a mechanism involving depolarization of the nerve membrane and calcium ion. Presumably the secretory granules contain the enzymes necessary to convert pro-oxyphysin and pro-pressophysin

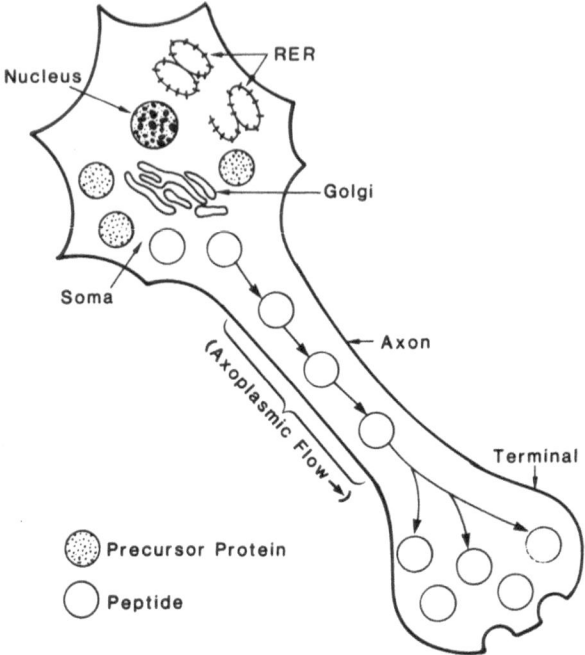

Figure 3-2. Proposed synthesis, transport, and release of neurohypophyseal hormones (e.g., vasopressin). RER, rough endoplasmic reticulum.

to oxytocin and vasopressin, respectively. Pro-pressophysin appears to contain a glycoprotein moiety. It should also be noted that a polypeptide complex isolated from the bovine neurohypophysis called coherin is capable of inhibiting gastrointestinal activity.

The precise mechanism whereby the octapeptide is released remains to be elucidated, but it seems apparent that the propeptide (or prohormone) lacks significant biological activity upon either the kidney or upon uterine smooth muscle.

3.1.3. Antidiuretic Hormone

3.1.3.1. Chemistry and Metabolic Fate

The chemical structure of antidiuretic hormone (ADH), or arginine vasopressin, and other neurohypophyseal octapeptides is shown in Figure 3-3. While vasopressin and oxytocin are found in mammals, vasotocin is produced by amphibians and certain fishes. The chemical structure of vasopressin and oxytocin differ only by a single amino acid and an amino acid ring structure is formed by the closure of a disulfide bond between number 1 and number 6 cysteine molecules to form cystine. Arginine vasopressin is present in humans, sheep, and horses, while lysine vasopressin can be found in the pig. The molecular weight of arginine vasopressin is 1100.

Several analogues of vasopressin, oxytocin, and melanocyte-stimulating hormone (α-MSH and β-MSH) have now been synthesized and evaluated for their biological activity. A number of critical features are necessary for retaining the biological activity of these peptides, including a chain length of nine amino acid residues, the cyclic moiety of the molecule, the position of the proline (position 7), and the presence of amide groups (positions 4 and 5). Other structural features are also necessary, such as the phenylalanine residue (position 3) for vasopressor activity and amino acids with aliphatic side chains (position 8) for oxytocic activity. Analogues containing additional residues at the amino terminus tend to prolong the duration of biological action.

The degradation of the naturally occurring peptides, i.e., oxytocin and arginine vasopressin, is rapid. The principal organ involved in the enzymatic breakdown of the neurohypophyseal hormone is the kidney, although the liver may also contribute to their loss of biological activity. Vasopressin disappears from the blood very quickly and possesses a half-life of about 10 min. The blood serum obtained from pregnant humans can readily inactivate both oxytocin and vasopressin. Aminopeptidase oxytocinase is capable of cleaving both octapeptides, although there is evidence for still another aminopeptidase that is quite selective for destroying vasopressin. Oxytocinase activity is higher in the first trimester of pregnancy and slowly declines through the mid- and last trimester. At least four sites of enzymatic degradation on the octapeptide

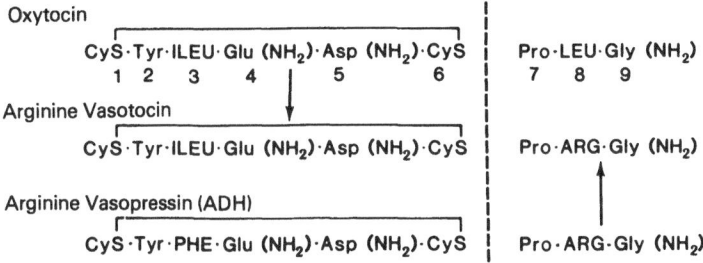

Figure 3-3. Chemical relationships between various neurohypophyseal hormones. The relationship of arginine vasotocin to oxytocin and to vasopressin is shown.

molecule(s) have been identified, with the linear portion of the hormone(s) being most vulnerable to cleavage.

3.1.3.2. Mechanism of Action and Biochemical Effects

Nerve terminals of hypothalamoneurohypophyseal neurons store and release vasopressin. The actual secretion of vasopressin is influenced by several different stimuli, including changes in osmotic pressure in the blood, adrenocortical hormones, alterations in the renin-angiotensin system and actions upon the CNS (e.g., emotional states, pain, trauma). In addition, several drugs can affect the secretion of vasopressin (Table 3-1).

Regardless of the physiological or pharmacological stimuli, cation potentials generated in the cell bodies of the hypothalamic neurons serve as the primary signal to the release of vasopressin and possibly modulate the rate of hormone release. Calcium ions are believed to provide the crucial link between excitation and secretion of vasopressin. The release of vasopressin from the neurosecretory nerve terminals is quite similar to neurotransmitter release, particularly with regard to the calcium dependence of the secretory process.

Vasopressin causes a marked increase in water uptake through the skin of amphibians (e.g., frogs and toads). The effect of vasopressin appears to be due to the acceleration of the passive osmotic movement of water across the skin. In other words, vasopressin facilitates the move-

Table 3-1. Drugs Affecting Vasopressin Release/Secretion

Drug	Effect
Estrogen	Increase[a]
Nicotine	Increase[a]
Angiotensin	Increase
Renin	Increase
ACTH	Increase
Atropine	Increase
Ether (stress)	Increase
Epinephrine	Increase
Morphine	Increase
Chlorpropamide	Increase
Acetaminophen	Increase
Ethanol	Decrease

[a] Demonstrated to stimulate the release of neurophysin.

ment of water in the direction of the osmotic gradient. The action of vasopressin is mostly independent of sodium movement, and its actions do not appear to require an expenditure of energy.

The mechanism of action of vasopressin involves its interaction with specific receptors. Such receptors have been found in the skin of amphibians and in the mammalian kidney. Vasopressin stimulates the production of 3'5'-cyclic adenylic acid (cAMP). There is evidence to indicate that vasopressin may exert its mechanism of action by enhancing protein kinase(s), leading to the phosphorylation of membrane constituents. Such events presumably result in conformational changes in the membrane, altering its permeability to water. Electron photomicrographs tend to support these vasopressin-induced conformational changes in the epithelial cell.

Not only is cAMP somehow involved in vasopressin-induced permeability changes in the distal convoluted tubules and collecting ducts of the kidney, but this cyclic nucleotide may also play a role in the neurohypophyseal release of vasopressin. Three basic mechanisms may be involved in the action of cAMP on the release of vasopressin, as well of oxytocin: (1) cAMP maintains intracellular calcium at a low level in the nondepolarized neural lobe, (2) residual cAMP acts to modulate stimulus–secretion coupling by regulating the sensitivity of the release process involving the intracellular levels of calcium ion; and (3) cAMP appears to promote calcium influx in the depolarized neural lobe by acting at an extracellular site. Thus, cAMP influences the state of activation of the neurohypophyseal secretory mechanism by modulating calcium fluxes and by regulating the magnitude of activation of this process, depending on the levels of intracellular calcium.

Vasopressin is capable of exerting a number of biological actions (Table 3-2). The vasoactive properties of vasopressin are attributable to its ability to constrict peripheral arterioles and capillaries. Some species

Table 3-2. Biological Actions of Posterior Pituitary Hormones

Parameter[a]	Antidiuretic hormone	Oxytocin
Blood pressure	Elevates	Slight decrease
Diuresis	Inhibits	—
Blood vessels	Constricts	Mild vasodilation
Gastrointestinal smooth muscle	Contracts	—
Uterine smooth muscle	Contracts	Contracts
Milk letdown	Stimulates (slightly)	Stimulates

[a] Biological response is dose dependent and varies to some extent among various species.

are particularly sensitive to the vasoconstrictor properties of vasopressin. In general, it requires supraphysiological amounts of the hormone in most mammals in order to produce hypertension. The hypertensive dose is several fold higher than that amount required to produce an antidiuretic effect. The vasoactive properties differ depending on the locale, as evidenced by vasoconstriction in the coronary and pulmonary vessels and an actual dilation in the cerebral and renal vascular systems.

The antidiuretic action of vasopressin is due to its ability to enhance water reabsorption by affecting the distal region of the nephron, the distal convoluted tubule, and the collecting duct. Such actions lead to excretion of highly concentrated urine containing sodium, chloride, and inorganic phosphate. While urine volume is diminished, there may be an increased loss of chloride ion. Dehydration (or increased salt intake) can elevate the osmotic pressure in the blood and evoke the secretion of vasopressin, leading to antidiuresis.

The oxytocinlike action of vasopressin is more evident in certain species such as the rabbit. Most commonly, the smooth muscle-contracting properties of vasopressin on the GI tract and on the uterus are evident at pharmacological levels of the hormone. Finally, supraphysiological amounts of vasopressin can stimulate the release of ACTH (see Chapter 2).

3.1.3.3. Therapeutic Uses and Preparations

The principal therapeutic use of vasopressin is in the management of diabetes insipidus (Table 3-3). Diabetes insipidus is a disorder or water

Table 3-3. Drugs Useful in the Management of Diabetes Insipidus

Drug	Trade name	Dose ranges[a]
Vasopressin injection	Pitressin	5–10 pressor units (IM or SC) 3–4 times/day
Vasopressin tannate injection	Pitressin tannate	2.5–5 pressor units (IM) every 1–3 days
Desmopressin acetate	DDAVP	0.1 ml t.i.d. (intranasally)
Lypressin	Diapid	Variable (intranasal spray) 3–4 times/day, with each spray containing 2 pressor units
Clofibrate	Atromid-S	1.5–2 g/day P.O.
Chlorpropamide	Diabinese	250–500 mg/day P.O.

[a] Representative adult regimens; children's doses are lower and are dependent on the particular agent.

metabolism characterized by polyuria, nocturia, low urine osmolality, polydipsia, and hypernatremia. Vasopressin is therapeutically effective only in diabetes insipidus of central origin. It is not effective in diabetes insipidus of primary nephrogenic vasopressin-resistant origin. In other words, vasopressin is not effective if there is a pathological defect in the kidney, since that is the site of action where the hormone exerts its antidiuretic effects. In primary nephrogenic diabetes insipidus, a rare hereditary disease, the epithelial cells of the renal collecting ducts do not respond to ADH even though levels of hormone may be normal. The etiology of most cases of central diabetes insipidus is either idiopathic or secondary to trauma. Sometimes central diabetes insipidus can be managed surgically, particularly if the etiology involves a pituitary tumor or a craniopharyngioma.

3.1.3.3a. Aqueous Vasopressin (Vasopressin Injection). This water-soluble posterior pituitary extract contains a mixture of arginine and lysine vasopressin. Commercially available as Pitressin, this preparation of vasopressin is perhaps most useful as a diagnostic agent in the so-called ACTH reserve test (see also Chapter 2); it is not the preparation of choice in the management of uncomplicated diabetes insipidus. Because it can be injected intramuscularly or subcutaneously, this preparation might be useful in a patient who is unconscious and cannot obtain the hormone by nasal insufflation. The usual dose of aqueous vasopressin ranges from 5 to 10 units (IM or SC) three to four times per day. This preparation has an onset of action of about 30–60 min, and its duration of action may extend to 6 hr. Dosages in children may range from 2.5 to 10 units three to four times per day.

3.1.3.3b. Vasopressin Tannate Injection. This preparation is suspended in an oil vehicle which gives it a longer duration of action. It can be injected by the intramuscular or subcutaneous route, with a usual dose of 2–5 units. Its most profound antidiuretic actions last for about 3 hr, but symptomatic relief may be achieved for upward of about 48 hr. Because of some moderate insolubilities between the hormone and the peanut oil vehicle, it is sometimes necessary not only to shake the ampule, but to immerse it in warm water before actual injection.

3.1.3.3c. Lypressin (8-Lysine Vasopressin) (Diapid). This is a synthetic vasopressin, the chemical structure of which is shown in Figure 3-4. This preparation is a nonirritating solution that can be sprayed deep into the nasal passages. Lypressin is rapidly absorbed from the nasal mucosa. It is most·effective if employed in the therapeutic management

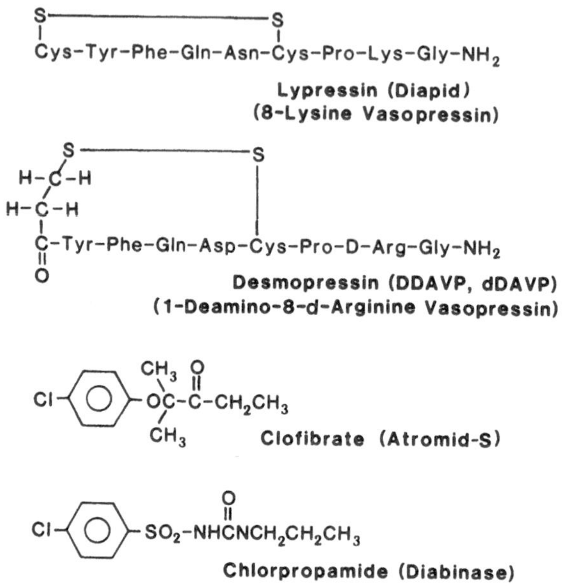

S————————————S
| |
Cys–Tyr–Phe–Gln–Asn–Cys–Pro–Lys–Gly–NH₂

Lypressin (Diapid)
(8-Lysine Vasopressin)

```
      S ———————————— S
      |                      |
 H–C–H                       |
 H–C–H                       |
      |                      |
      C–Tyr–Phe–Gln–Asp–Cys–Pro–D–Arg–Gly–NH₂
      ‖
      O
```

Desmopressin (DDAVP, dDAVP)
(1-Deamino-8-d-Arginine Vasopressin)

```
              CH₃  O
               \   ‖
Cl–⟨O⟩–OC–C–CH₂CH₃
               |
              CH₃        Clofibrate (Atromid-S)
```

```
                      O
                      ‖
Cl–⟨O⟩–SO₂–NHCNCH₂CH₂CH₃
```

Chlorpropamide (Diabinase)

Figure 3-4. Chemical structure of synthetic vasopressin and other drugs used in the therapeutic management of diabetes insipidus.

of mild to moderate diabetes insipidus. Because of its relatively brief duration of action, it is less effective than either vasopressin tannate or desmopressin in severe diabetes insipidus.

Desmopressin acetate (DDAVP) is an analogue of vasopressin, with a somewhat more specific and more prolonged antidiuretic action. It can be administered as a nasal spray and has a duration of action from between 10 to 20 hr. Desmopressin reduces urine volume, increases its osmolality, and relieves the symptoms of polyuria, nocturia, and polydipsia. Desmopressin is more advantageous than vasopressin tannate in the long-term therapy of severe central diabetes inisipidus, but its cost is greater. Desmopressin is not effective in nephrogenic diabetes insipidus.

In addition to vasopressin and vasopressin analogues, several non-hormonal drugs have been used in the therapeutic management of central diabetes insipidus. More specifically, chlorpropamide, clofibrate, and somewhat paradoxically, the thiazide diuretics, are also used in the treatment of diabetes insipidus. Chlorpropamide (Diabinase) is actually better known as an oral hypoglycemic agent (Chapter 10), although it is also capable of reducing polyuria in more than 50% of patients with central diabetes insipidus. Doses range from 250 to 500 mg/day, with onset of diuresis occurring within about 2 hr and a peak effect at about 2 days. Subsequently, urine flow may diminish as a result of a demonstrable elevation in urine osmolality. The modification in osmolarity by chlorpropamide leads to increased secretion of endogenous vasopressin. Should higher doses of chlorpropamide be required (e.g., 500–750 mg/kg), hypoglycemia can become a troublesome side effect in the management of the diabetes insipidus. The effectiveness of chlorpropamide in the treatment of central diabetes insipidus obviously depends on a certain amount of residual posterior pituitary vasopressin.

Clofibrate (Atromid-S) is best known as an oral hypolipidemic drug, yet oral doses of 1–2 g/day can be used to reduce urine flow in patients with central diabetes insipidus. Clofibrate is of no therapeutic value in nephrogenic diabetes insipidus. Clofibrate, like chlorpropamide, somehow brings about increased secretion of endogenous vasopressin. The duration of antidiuretic action of clofibrate is shorter than that of chlorpropamide, but this hypolipidemic agent does not possess the hypoglycemic side effect of the sulfonylurea agent. Like chlorpropamide, clofibrate is of no therapeutic value in the treatment of nephrogenic diabetes insipidus.

Thiazide diuretics (e.g., hydroflumethiazide) are effective in reducing urine flow in patients with both central and nephrogenic diabetes insipidus. The mechanism of action of these agents is related to their ability to cause negative salt balance. Sodium depletion and contraction of the extracellular fluid volume leads to increased reabsorption of glomerular filtrate in the proximal tubules. Frequently, when thiazides are employed in the therapeutic management of diabetes insipidus, they are used in combination with chlorpropamide. There appears to be an additive pharmacological action when thiazides are used concomitantly with chlorpropamide. Antidiuretic oral doses of hydroflumethiazide range from 25 to 100 mg, one or two times per day, once every other day, or once a day for 3–5 days of each week. The thiazide diuretics are not effective unless dietary sodium is restricted.

3.1.3.4. Adverse Effects

Vasopressin and its analogues may cause significant vasoconstriction of the coronary vessels; therefore, patients with concomitant ischemic heart disease (e.g., angina pectoris) should receive the minimal dose necessary to control polyuria. Desmopressin displays less vasoconstrictor action on the coronary artery than does vasopressin or lypressin. Vasopressin, particularly in large doses, can stimulate GI smooth muscle and produce nausea, cramping, and diarrhea. Uterine cramps are not uncommon. Desmopressin can sometimes cause transient headaches. Allergic reactions or hypersensitivities have occasionally been noted but occur with posterior pituitary extracts (e.g., Pitressin) and not usually with synthetic vasopressins.

Certain drugs are known to affect the secretion of ADH (Table 3-1), and this can sometimes affect the therapeutic management of diabetes insipidus. Furthermore, a number of pathological states can affect the secretion of ADH. Such aberrant production of ADH has been termed the syndrome of inappropriate secretion of ADH, or SIADH. SIADH may be associated with lesions of the CNS, as well as pain, trauma, and pulmonary disease. SIADH may also be associated with drugs such as barbiturates, diuretics, analgesics, certain tranquilizers, and some cancer chemotherapeutic agents. Lithium (see Chapter 4) and demeclocycline interfere with the action of ADH at the level of the nephron. In fact, both drugs have been indicated in the treatment of SIADH. Demeclocycline is more effective than lithium, but narcotic antagonists have also been demonstrated to be of value in the treatment of SIADH.

3.1.4. Oxytocin

3.1.4.1. Chemistry and Metabolism

Like vasopressin, oxytocin is a polypeptide. Oxytocin, however, differs from the vasopressins in the amino acid residues situated at positions 3 and 8 (see Figure 3-3). Vasotocin, a polypeptide obtained from most amphibians, is very similar in chemical structure to both mammalian oxytocin and vasopressin. Another polypeptide found in nonmammalian vertebrates that is similar in chemical structure to oxytocin is a hormone called oxypressin.

Oxytocin can be rapidly metabolized, and it has only a brief half-life in the blood. The liver and the kidney contain enzyme systems that can cleave oxytocin enzymatically. Plasma oxytocinase activity is affected by pregnancy and is higher during the first trimester than during later stages of gestation. Oxytocinase is a glycoprotein aminopeptidase; it is also present in placental and uterine tissue.

3.1.4.2. Mechanism of Action and Biological Effects

The existence of oxytocin (and of vasopressin) in the magnocellular neurons of the hypothalamus and neurohypophysis has long been known. Oxytocin is synthesized on large precursor molecules in hypothalamic neuronal perikarya and is packed into secretory granules (see Figure 3-2). During its transport from the paraventricular nuclei to the neurohypophysis, oxytocin is cleaved from its precursor through a series of processes. It is secreted from the neural lobe and into the bloodstream.

Once oxytocin is released into the blood, it can exert actions on several different organs or organ systems. Receptors, or at least specific binding sites, for oxytocin are present in the myometrium of the uterus of several species, including humans. Such binding sites are located on the plasma membrane of the uterine smooth muscle cells. Depending on species and dosage, vasopressin and oxytocin can often compete for the same receptor(s). Oxytocin may exert some of its biological actions by stimulating the formation of 3'5'-cAMP. Oxytocin-induced increases in glucose oxidation can be inhibited by puromycin, suggesting that this hormone stimulates protein synthesis, with carbohydrates providing the energy.

Oxytocin is capable of causing a number of biological effects (see Table 3-2). Its principal biological actions are upon the uterus and upon the process of lactation. Oxytocin is able to exert a profound stimulatory action upon the smooth muscles of the uterus. It also can stimulate the musculature of the G-U tract and the intestines.

One of the more important physiological actions of oxytocin in mammals is that of milk ejection. Suckling provides an important stimulus for a neuroendocrine reflex, which leads to the release of oxytocin. Oxytocin can stimulate the myoepithelial cells of the breast, thereby aiding the process of lactation. While oxytocin causes the ejection of milk, prolactin stimulates milk production (see Chapter 2).

There remains some confusion about the physiological role of oxytocin in the uterus during parturition. The sensitivity of uterine smooth muscle is enhanced by pregnancy. In other words, as pregnancy advances, the uterine myometrium becomes more sensitive to contractile stimulation. Several hormones, some acting together to cause stimulation and some actually inhibiting the contractility of the myometrium, can affect the uterus. Depending on the endocrine state, estrogens, prostaglandins, and oxytocin can all stimulate uterine contractility; progesterone can produce quiescence. Certain β-adrenergic drugs (e.g., isoxsuprine, ritodrine), perhaps acting partly through increased production of cAMP, can inhibit uterine contractility.

Since coitus can cause the release of oxytocin, it has been suggested that the resultant stimulation of the uterus and associated anatomical structures aids in the migration of spermatozoa in the female genital tract. Whether prostaglandins have a role in sperm activaiton or in their transport through the female reproductive tract remains to be established.

3.1.4.3. Therapeutic Uses and Preparations

There are a number of clinical indications for oxytocin (see Table 3-4). Oxytocin can be used as an abortifacient to enhance uterine contraction at term and during the postpartum period. When oxytocin is used to induce labor, it should be used only when continuation of pregnancy represents a risk to the mother or the fetus. Premature rupture of the membrane is the most common indication, but erythroblastosus fetalis, placental insufficiency, and antepartum bleeding may also warrant its use. Oxytocin has been used in prolonged pregnancies and sometimes to augment selected types of dysfunctional labor. There is no justification for the use of oxytocin in premature labor unless there is a clearly established medical indication. The preferred route of administration of oxytocin for inducing or augmenting labor is intravenously. Oxytocin should not be employed simultaneously by more than one route of administration. Table 3-5 presents selected dose regiments for the use of oxytocin.

When oxytocin is used in elective abortion, it should be used as early in pregnancy as possible because of the increasing incidence of morbidity and mortality associated with increasing length of gestation. The intra-amniotic administration of urea (50%), prostaglandins ($PGF_{2\alpha}$, dinoprost tromethamine) (30%), or hypertonic saline (20%) has also been used for elective abortions in the second trimester. Occasionally, and under selected conditions, oxytocin may be used with other abortifacients, but there may be increasing risk due to additive actions and side effects.

Oxytocin has been employed to stimulate expulsion of hydatidiform moles. As such an indication often requires high doses of oxytocin, the use of suction or prostaglandins may be preferred.

The oxytocin challenge test can be used to assess fetal well-being and may be indicated in selected high-risk obstetrical cases. The test might be useful in patients with diabetes mellitus, preeclampsia, and prolonged pregnancy.

Oxytocics are often used postpartum to cause firm uterine contrac-

Table 3-4. Therapeutic Indications for Oxytocin[a]

Induction of term labor
Elective abortion
Expulsion of hydatidiform moles??
Oxytocin challenge test
Management of postpartum uterine contraction
Check postpartum bleeding

[a] Commercial preparations include Pitocin and Syntocinon.

Table 3-5. Clinical Indications for Oxytocin

Indication/Use	Dose[a]
Induction of labor	1–2 mU/min, initially
Oxytocin challenge test	0.5 mU/min, initially; increasing rate to attain optimal uterine contractions
Postpartum bleeding	20–40 mU/ml at a rate of 40 mU/min
Postpartum bleeding	3–10 units, IM
Promote milk ejection	Nasal insufflation (one spray into one or both nostrils 2–3 min before nursing)

[a] Doses may vary, depending on the clinical state and the route of administration.

tions and to decrease uterine bleeding. Ordinarily, oxytocin is administered by slow intravenous infusion during the immediate postpartum interval. Because the ergot alkaloids have a more sustained action than that of oxytocin, they are sometimes preferred in the management of postpartum bleeding.

3.1.4.4. *Adverse Effects*

Oxytocin must be used with discretion, since it has the potential to harm both the mother and the fetus. Induction of labor ordinarily should not be attempted in obstetrical cases with cephalopelvic disproportion or malpresentation. There are a number of other complicating medical reasons for not attempting to induce labor with oxytocin. Hyperstimulation of uterine musculature during labor can sometimes lead to uterine tetany, resulting in an inhibition of uteroplacental blood flow, uterine rupture, and cervical laceration. Trauma to the infant can also occur.

A serious side effect of oxytocin is the development of water intoxication with convulsions, but this complication is seldom seen unless high doses and prolonged infusion regimens have been employed. Occasionally, oxytocin can cause allergic reactions and anaphylactic shock. It has also been known to cause sinus bradycardia, premature ventricular contractions, and certain other cardiac dysrhythmias in the fetus.

3.2. ERGOT ALKALOIDS

3.2.1. Chemistry

The chemical structure of various ergot alkaloids is depicted in Figure 3-5. The ergot alkaloids originate in a fungus that grows on rye; they

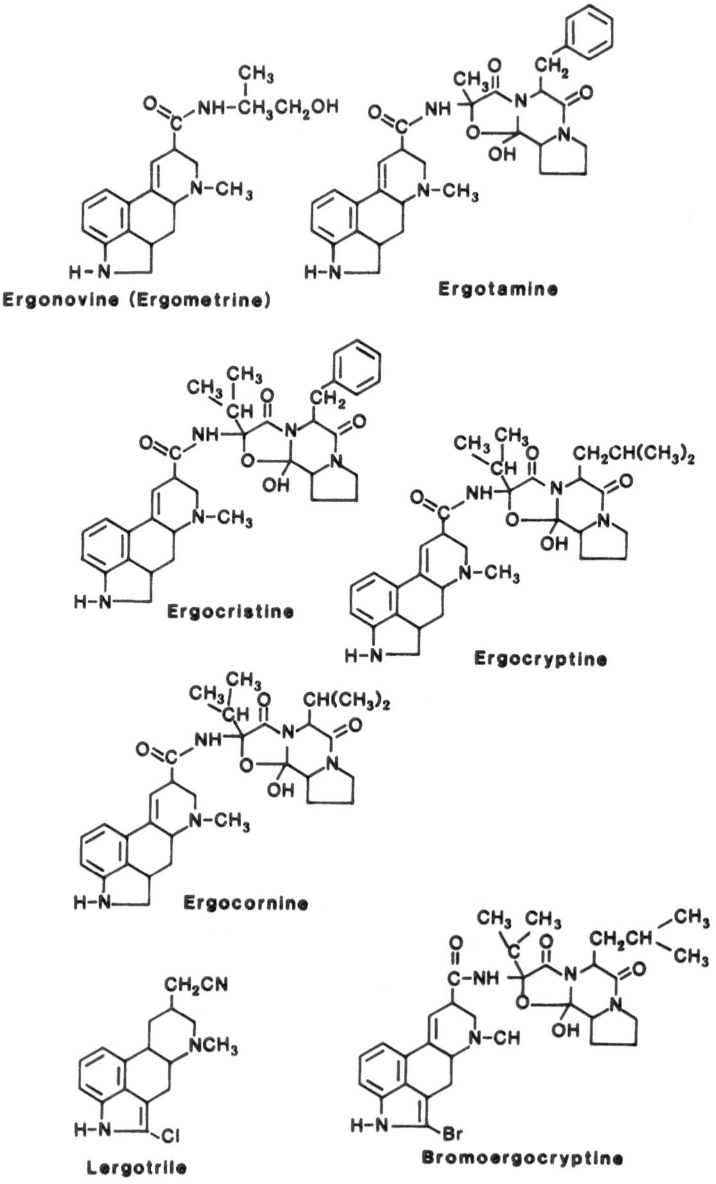

Figure 3-5. Chemical structure of various ergot compounds.

contain a variety of pharmacologically active substances, including histamine, tyramine ergosterol, and acetylcholine (Ach). There are three
basic chemical groups of ergot alkaloids: the ergotamine group, the ergotoxine group, and the ergonovine group. A structure common to all
ergot alkaloids is lysergic acid. The ergotoxine and ergotamine groups
are called amino acid alkaloids, since they contain an amide nitrogen
that bears the condensation product of amino acids. Ergonovine and
other alkaloids such as dihydroergotamine possess a saturation of the
double bond at C-9 to C-10, and this reduces the smooth muscle con-
tracting activity but enhances their vasodilating properties.

3.2.2. Mechanism of Action and Biochemical Effects

The pharmacology of the ergot alkaloids is very complex. The ergots
possess a direct vasoconstrictor property as well as an ability to stimulate
other smooth muscles, particularly the uterus. The ergots also possess
an α-adrenergic blocking activity. Thus, the ergots are able to block
certain of epinephine's effects on the vascular system. The fact that
certain of the ergots (*viz.* ergotamine) can effectively cause cerebral vasoconstriction has led to their clinical use in the treatment of migraine
headaches.

Some newer ergot alkaloid derivatives can also act as dopamine
receptor agonists (see Figure 3-5). Specifically, bromoergocriptine (CB-
154) and lergotrile are synthetic ergot alkaloids that act as dopamine
receptor agonists. Dopamine plays an important role in modulating neuronal and humoral functions of the hypothalamus. Prolactin inhibitory
factor (PIF) may itself be dopamine (see also Section 2.1.2, in Chapter
2). Thus agents like bromoergocriptine can mimic the actions of dopamine, causing an inhibition of the release of prolactin.

3.2.3. Therapeutic Uses and Preparations

While there are many ergot alkaloids and synthetic derivatives, those
agents used principally for their endocrine-inducing actions are ergonovine, methylergonovine, and bromocriptine.

Ergonovine maleate (Ergotrate Maleate) and methylergonovine maleate (Methergine) have been used after the delivery of the placenta to
induce firm uterine contractions and to diminish postpartum bleeding.
Either agent can be used for the same indication after suction abortion.
Both ergonovine and methylergonovine exhibit rapid onset of action,
depending on the route of administration. Intramuscularly, doses of 0.2
mg can be employed to control uterine bleeding. With uterine hemor-

rhage, an intravenous dose of 0.2 mg has been used. In nonemergency states, these drugs can also be administered orally in doses of 0.2–0.4 mg, two to four times per day.

Bromocriptine mesylate (Parlodel) is a dopamine agonist that has been indicated in several clinical conditions involving the endocrine system (see Table 3-6). Its use in the short-term treatment of amenorrhea and/or galactorrhea associated with hyperprolactinemia is related to its ability to cause a reduction in serum prolactin by directly inhibiting the release of prolactin from the adenohypophysis. Such actions lead to a restoration of ovarian function and the suppression of lactation. The mechanism of action of bromocriptine in the therapeutic management of acromegaly is not understood, but it is known to cause a suppression of secretion and a reduction in elevated levels of growth hormone (see Chapter 2). Bromocriptine is also used in the management of Parkinson's disease. In treating amenorrhea and/or galactorrhea, an initial oral dose of 1.25–2.5 mg/day is used with a maintenance dose of 2.5 mg, two to three times per day. To suppress postpartum lactation, an oral dose of 2.5 mg, two times per day for 14–21 days, may be required.

3.2.4. Adverse Effects

Ergonovine and methylergonovine are associated with similar side effects, but such complications are more severe after intravenous administration. Accordingly, adverse effects can be minimized if these ergots are given either orally or intramuscularly. Intravenously, these agents can produce transient hypertension. Neither agent should be used in pregnant patients or as an aid to induce labor. Some patients are allergic to the ergot alkaloids.

Bromocriptine has a number of side effects; interestingly, normal persons seem to be more sensitive to adverse effects than are patients with either hyperprolactinemia or acromegaly. Paradoxically, postpartum women treated with bromocriptine exhibit a lower incidence of adverse effects. Bromocriptine can cause postural hypotension, GI hem-

Table 3-6. Endocrine Indications for Bromocriptine

Galactorrhea
Amenorrhea/galactorrhea associated with hyperprolactinemia
Acromegaly
Prevention of postpartum lactation
Adjunct in treatment of breast cancer???
Adjunct in treatment of prostatic carcinoma???

orrhage, fainting, and hallucinations. Nausea, vomiting, anorexia, and intermittent claudications have also been reported.

3.3. PROSTAGLANDINS: REPRODUCTIVE ACTIONS

3.3.1. Chemistry

Prostaglandins (PGs) have been classified according to primary groups and consist of PGE_1, PGE_2, PGE_3, $PGF_{1\alpha}$, $PGF_{2\alpha}$, and $PGF_{3\alpha}$. Still other natural PGs include PGAs, PGBs, PGG_2 and PGH_2. PgI_2 (prostacylins) and thromboxane A_2 (TXA_2) are powerful regulators of blood clotting. From an endocrine standpoint, the PGEs and the PGFs, as well as their analogues, are particularly active on the reproductive system.

Prostanoic acid represents a hypothetical chemical molecule used in numbering the PG structure (see Figure 3-6). By convention, the chemical nomenclature uses PG to refer to the chemical structure of the five-membered ring. On the basis of early chemical separation procedures, PGE stood for ether, while F for phosphate buffer. The subscript numeral signifies how many double bonds or unsaturated groups are

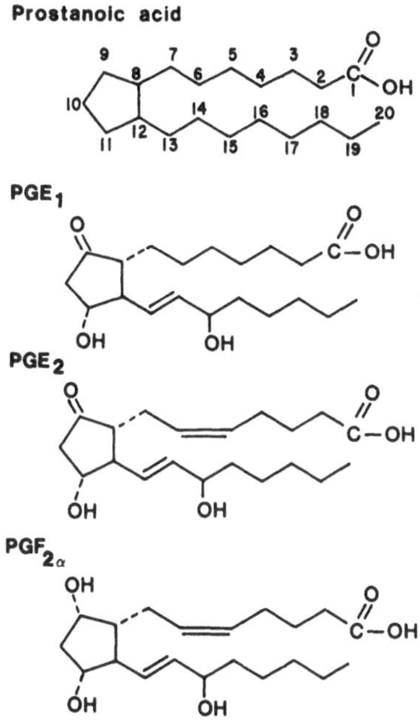

Figure 3-6. Basic chemical structures of selected prostaglandins (PGs).

present on the two side chains of the molecule. The Greek letter subscript, α or β denotes the spatial relationship of the hydroxyl groups on the side chains to the plane of the five-membered ring. PGE_1 and PGE_2 differ only in the number of double bonds present in the molecule (Figure 3-6); $PGE_{2\alpha}$ possesses a hydroxyl group at C-9, whereas the PGEs contain a keto group (Figure 3-6). Carboprost (15-methyl $PGF_{2\alpha}$) is a synthetic analogue of the naturally occurring $PGF_{2\alpha}$ (Figure 3-7).

PGs are biosynthesized from dihomo-α-linolenic acid (eicosatrienoic acid) and arachidonic acid (eicosatetranoic acid). Arachidonic acid, a derivative of the essential dietary fatty acid, linoleic acid, is relatively abundant in reproductive tissues (e.g., myometrium, placenta, umbilical cord, fetal plasma, fetal membranes). PGE_2 can be readily synthesized in several reproductive tissues.

3.3.2. Mechanism of Action and Biochemical Effects

The PGs function like hormones and are involved in modulating a host of physiological processes. Unlike hormones, however, the PGs are synthesized upon demand and are released by nonspecialized cells. The

Carboprost Tromethamine
(Prostin/M 15)

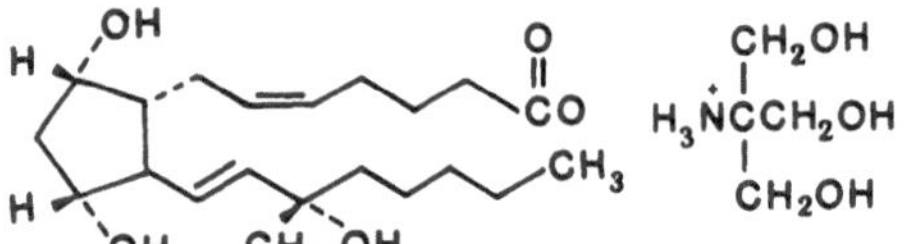

Dinoprostone
(Prostin E_2)

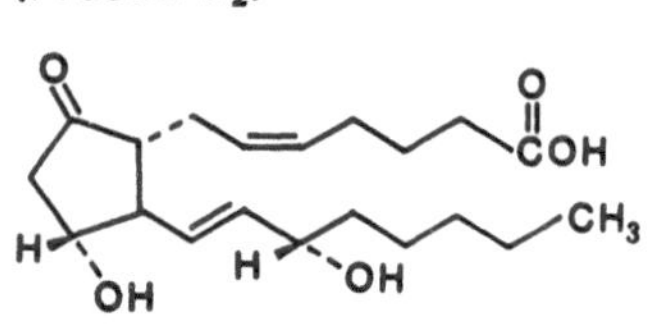

Dinoprost Tromethamine
(Prostin F_2 alpha)

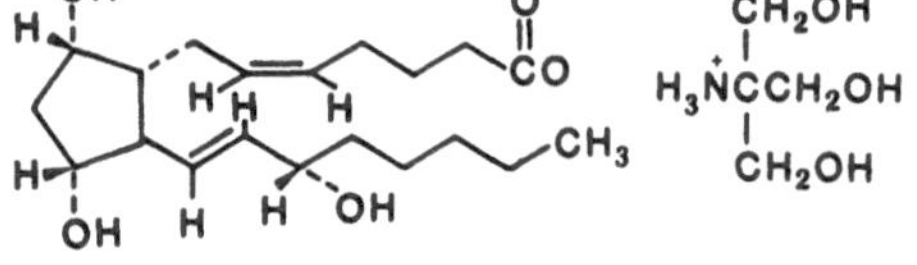

Figure 3-7. Clinically useful prostaglandins and prostaglandin analogues.

Table 3-7. Reproductive Processes Affected by Prostaglandins

Process	Effect of prostaglandin[a]
	Female
Ovulation	Rupture of follicles in some species
Ovum maturation	PGE_2 mimics action of LH
Follicular rupture	PGs generally required for follicular rupture
Luteinization	PGE_2-induced morphological luteinization and increased progesterone secretion???
Luteolysis	$PGF_{2\alpha}$ (or precursor) is probably uterine factor responsible for luteolysis in nonhuman species
Gonadotropin secretion	Modulate ovarian feedback; increase GnRH release
Tubal contractility	PGE inhibits tubal contractility; PGF stimulates
Implantation	Aid in implantation???
Uterine contractility	Stimulates but depends on endocrine state, species, and specific PG
	Male
Sperm penetration	$PGF_{2\alpha}$ may enhance???
Sperm transport	Increased???
Accessory sex glands	Affects smooth muscle tone???

[a] GnRH, gonadotropin-releasing hormone; LH, luteinizing hormone.

naturally occurring PGs ordinarily exert their actions within the cell (or organ) from whence they are released. PGs appear to function as an intracellular messenger like that of cAMP. PGs can act on cell membrane receptor molecules to cause an increase in intracellular cAMP. In certain cells (or organs), PGs can cause an increase in intracellular calcium ions. The precise role of PGs in mammalian reproduction remains to be elucidated, but they generally appear to be involved in several endocrine events (see Table 3-7). Specific classes of PGs vary in their specific influence on the various reproductive process. Indeed, there still remain many uncertainties regarding their physiological role. Furthermore, the role of endogenous PGs does not always parallel those pharmacological actions produced by exogenous PGs.

The PGs have perhaps three different, but crucial effects on the reproductive system. In pregnancy, PGs may act as (1) smooth muscle stimulants on the uterine myometrium; (2) cervical primers, leading to so-called cervical ripening; and (3) a luteolytic substance, inhibiting progesterone secretion by the corpus luteum. From a clinical standpoint, their uterine stimulating properties and their effect on the cervix seem to be important.

3.3.3. Therapeutic Uses and Preparations

3.3.3.1. Carboprost

Carboprost is a synthetic analogue of $PGF_{2\alpha}$, but it has a somewhat longer duration of action than that of $PGF_{2\alpha}$ (see Figure 3-7 and Table 3-8). Carboprost stimulates uterine contractions similar to those that occur during term labor. It is used to induce abortion between the 13th and 20th weeks of gestation. Carboprost seems to act directly on the myometrium. This agent stimulates, in the gravid uterus; contractions are usually sufficient to induce abortion.

Carboprost tromethamine can be administered by the intramuscular route in an initial dose of 250 µg, repeated every $1\frac{1}{2}$ to $3\frac{1}{2}$ hr, depending on the uterine response. The dose of carboprost may be increased to 500 µg when uterine contractility is insufficient, particularly after repeated doses of 250 µg. Sometimes an initial dose of only 100 µg might prove effective in stimulating uteine contractions. Commercial preparations of carboprost (Prostin/15M) are available in strengths of 250 µg/ml.

Table 3-8. Clinical Indications for PGE_2 and $PGF_{2\alpha}$ and Selected Analogues

Prostaglandin	Indications
PGE_2 (Dinoprostone)	Second-trimester abortion; intrauterine death and mole; induction of labor; cervical dilation before induction of labor
16,16-Dimethyl-PGE_2	First-trimester abortion; cervical dilation before first-trimester abortion
16-Phenoxy-ω-tetranor-PGE_2 methyl sulfonylamide (Sulprostone)	First- and second-trimester abortion; cervical dilation before first-trimester abortion
16,16-Dimethyl-trans-Δ^2-PGE, methyl ester	First- and second-trimester abortion
9-Deoxo-16,16-dimethyl-9-methylene-PGE_2	Second trimester
$PGF_{2\alpha}$	Second-trimester abortion; labor abortion
15-Methyl-$PGF_{2\alpha}$ tromethamine salt, Carboprost	First- and second trimester abortion; intrauterine death—Check postpartum bleeding
15-Methyl-$PGF_{2\alpha}$ methyl ester	First- and second-trimester abortion; cervical dilatation before first-trimester abortion

The fact that carboprost can be administered intramuscularly offers an advantage over other PG abortifacients because it avoids invasive intra-amniotic or extraoculatory procedures.

3.3.3.2. Dinoprostone

Dinoprostone is a naturally occurring PG found in several mammalian reproductive tissues and fluids (see Figure 3-7). Dinoprostone stimulates uterine contractility. It is indicated clinically to induce labor during the second trimester in cases of intrauterine fetal death and hydatidiform mole (see Table 3-8).

It has also been employed when uterine perforation has taken place at the time of curettage, but the uterus has not been evacuated.

Dinoprostone can be administered by several routes including i.v., IM and even intra-amniotically or extra-amniotically. In the United States, its route of administration is restricted to the intravaginal route. An intravaginal dose of 20 mg in the form of a suppository is used initially. This dose may be repeated every 3 to 5 hours until abortion occurs, but the total dosage should not exceed 240 mg.

Dinoprost tromethamine ($PGF_{2\alpha}$) is a potent stimulator of uterine smooth muscle (Figure 3-7). It is usually administered intra-amniotically to induce abortion during the second trimester. Dinoprost can pass across fetal membranes. It acts directly on the myometrium and is a very effective abortifacient.

The usual adult dose of dinoprost tromethamine, administered intra-amniotically, is 40 mg. In order to assess patient sensitivity, the initial 5-mg dose increment should be administered at a rate not to exceed 1 mg/min. Thereafter, the remaining 35 mg can be injected over a 5-min period, assuming no side effects have been observed. Dinoprost (Prostin E_2) is available in commercial strengths of 5 mg/ml.

3.3.4. Adverse Effects

Carboprost may produce several side effects, including nausea, vomiting, and diarrhea. Some patients experience wheezing and dyspnea. Fever and chills have been reported following the administration of carboprost. Carboprost is contraindicated in patients who are hypersensitive; it should not be used in patients with acute pelvic inflammation or pulmonary, renal, or liver dysfunction. Discretion should be used when administering carboprost in patients wih medical histories of asthma, anemia, jaundice, diabetes mellitus, and epilepsy.

Like carboprost, both dinoprostone and dinoprost tromethamine can produce nausea, vomiting, and GI disturbances. Similarly, fever, vasomotor reactions, bronchospasm, and convulsion can sometimes occur after the administration of dinoprost tromethamine or dinoprostone. Since PGs are metabolized rather rapidly, most adverse effects subside in about $\frac{1}{2}$ hr.

Dinoprostone should be used with considerable discretion in patients with cervicitis, asthma, renal/hepatic disease, diabetes mellitus, and epilepsy. Neither dinoprost tromethamine nor dinoprostone should be administered to patients with known hypersensitivity to PGs or to patients with acute pelvic inflammatory disease. Some PGs are teratogenic in animals; therefore, if PGs are unsuccessful as abortifacients, alternate methods should be undertaken to remove the conceptus.

The concurrent use of oxytocin and PGs may lead to uterine hypertonus, causing uterine rupture or cervical laceration, or both. Such a complication is more prevalent if cervical dilation is incomplete or absent.

3.3.5. Prostaglandin Inhibitors

While the PG inhibitors exhibit a wide spectrum of pharmacological activities, their principal endocrinological use is in the treatment of primary dysmenorrhea. Interestingly, many of the same signs and symptoms of primary dysmenorrhea (e.g., cramps, dizziness, flushing, headache) can be produced after the administration of PGs. PG synthesis inhibitors have therefore been used to alleviate the pain and cramping associated with primary dysmenorrhea. The PG inhibitory drugs act by interfering with the synthesis of PGs (see Table 3-9). These drugs inhibit the enzyme, cyclooxygenase, and thereby block the synthesis of PG. In addition, some PG inhibitors (e.g., fenamates) may actually block PG receptors, causing a reduction in the contraction of the myometrium.

PG inhibitors are currently undergoing clinical trials for the treatment of still other gynecological disorders in which excessive endogenous levels of PGs have been implicated. These drugs, particularly if they can be rendered more specific in action and possessing more extended duration of action(s), hold potential in the treatment of premature labor, dysmenorrhea due to intrauterine device (IUD) insertion, endometriosis, and postpartum pain.

3.3.6. Uterine Relaxants

Certain of the β-adrenergic agents have been used to delay premature labor. Such drugs can delay premature labor until term or until

Table 3-9. Prostaglandin-Inhibitory Drugs
Used in the Treatment of
Primary Dysmenorrhea

Drug	Representative dosage regimens[a]
Alclofenac	500 mg t.i.d.
Anaprox	Single dose: 1100 mg
Ibuprofen	400 mg ×2
Ketoprofen	500 mg q.i.d
Naproxen	250 mg up to 5×/day
Flufenamic acid	200 mg t.i.d.
Mefenamic acid	500 mg/8 hr
Tolfenamic acid	133 mg t.i.d.
Indomethacin	100 mg + 25 mg t.i.d.
Phenylbutazone	100 mg t.i.d.
Aspirin	500 mg t.i.d.

[a] Treatment is usually initiated on day 1 or 2 relative to the first day of menses.

additional time has passed to increase the chances of fetal survival. Perhaps the most widely used β-adrenergic agent employed for its tocolytic actions is ritodrine (Yutopar). Terbutaline (Brethine) may possess uterine-relaxant properties comparable to those of ritodrine.

RECOMMENDED READINGS

Posterior Pituitary Hormones

Brownstein, M. J., Biosynthesis of vasopressin and oxytocin, *Annu. Rev. Physiol.* **45**:129–135, 1983.

Brownstein, M. J., Russell, J. T., and Gainer, H., Synthesis, transport and release of posterior pituitary hormones, *Science* **207**:373–378, 1980.

Pauerstein, C. J., Use and abuse of oxytocic agents, *Clin. Obstet. Gynecol.* **16**:262–277, 1973.

Ergot Alkaloids

Lemberger, L., The pharmacology of ergots: Past and present, *Fed. Proc.* **37**:2176–2208, 1978.

Muller, E. E., Panerai, A. E., Cocchi, D., and Mantegazza, P., Endocrine profile of ergot alkaloids—Minireview, *Life Sci.* **21**:1545–1558, 1977.

Prostaglandins

Behrman, H. R., Prostaglandins in hypothalamo-pituitary and ovarian function, *Annu. Rev. Physiol.* **41:**685–700, 1979.

Chan, W. Y., Prostaglandins and nonsteroidal antiinflammatory drugs in dysmenorrhea, *Annu. Rev. Pharmacol. Toxicol.* **23:**131–149, 1983.

Karim, S. M. M., and Hillier, K., Prostaglandins in the control of animal and human reproduction, *Br. Med. Bull.* **35:**173–180, 1979.

Morrison, A. R., Biochemistry and pharmacology of renal arachidonic acid metabolism, *Am. J. Med.* **80:**3, 1986.

Richardson, D. W., and Robinson, A. G., Desmopressin, *Ann. Intern. Med.* **103:**228–239, 1985.

4

THYROID AND
ANTITHYROIDAL DRUGS

4.1. THYROID

4.1.1. History

Simple goiter has been recognized for centuries. In 1526, Paracelsus described goitrous cretinism. During the 1800s, several investigators described not only some of the clinical manifestations of hypothyroidal states, but surgical removal of the thyroid gland in laboratory animals led to further insight into hormone-deficient conditions. By the late 1800s, Bettancourt and Serrano reported on the relief of myxedematous symptoms in humans with the administration of sheep thyroid. Several other investigators established the usefulness of substitution therapy in the management of hypothyroidism during the latter part of the 1800s and the early 1900s. In 1896, Baumann discovered the presence of iodine in thyroid and identified diiodotyrosine. The efforts of Kendall in 1915 led to the isolation and crystallization of thyroid hormone. A decade later, Harrington and Barger actually determined the structure of thyroxin. A number of investigators, including Richter, Astwood, and McKenzie discovered chemicals that eventually became the first effective antithyroidal drugs to be used in the treatment of thyrotoxicosis or hyperthyroidism. While thyroxine was identified and characterized between 1915 and 1927, it was not until 1952 that Gross and Pitt-Rivers discovered triiodothyronine. The chemical structural requirements necessary for thyroidal activity were initially defined by Jorgensen in the 1960s, and subsequent groups of investigators, including Psychoyos and Pittman and their co-workers examined certain analogues and molecular configurations of this hormone.

4.1.2. Central Regulation of the Thyroid

The secretion of the thyroid hormones triiodothyronine (T_3) and thyroxine (T_4) from the thyroid gland is modulated by thyroid-stimulating hormone (TSH), which is secreted by the adenohypophysis (see Chapter 2 for the pharmacological use of TSH). The hormonal relationship between TSH and thyroid hormone synthesis and secretion is depicted in Figure 4-1. Hypothalamically secreted thyrotropin-releasing hormone (TRH) can enhance the secretion of TSH, in turn causing the increased synthesis and release of T_3 and T_4. The T_3 and/or T_4 released from the thyroid gland can inhibit the capcity of adenohypophyseal thyrotroph cells to respond to TRH. This property permits T_3 and/or T_4 feedback to the adenohypophysis to initiate decreased secretion of TSH; thus, these hormones regulate their own rate of synthesis and release.

A host of environmental stimuli (e.g., cold, heat, stress) can affect the hypothalamic–adenohypophyseal–thyroidal axis, resulting in changes

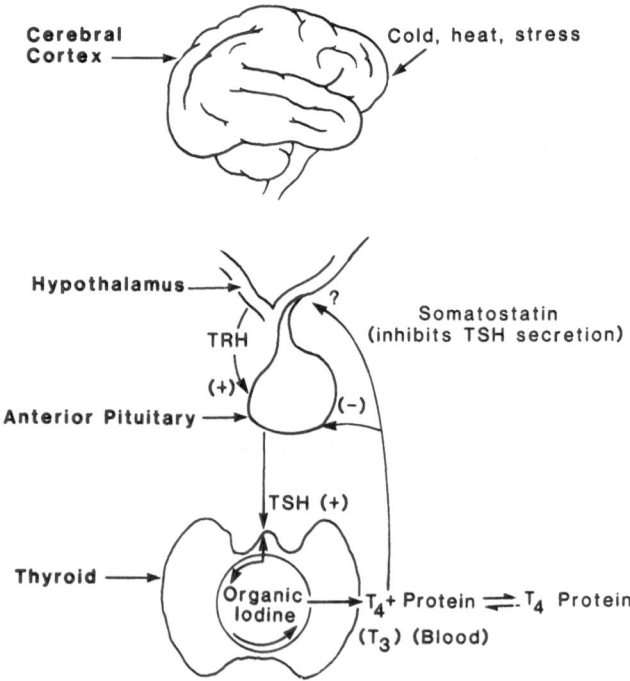

Figure 4-1. Factors regulating thyroid function. T_3, triiodothyronine; T_4, thyroxine; TRH, thyroid-releasing hormone; TSH, thyroid-stimulating hormone.

in the circulating blood levels of T_3 and/or T_4. Although it is generally agreed that TSH secretion is subject to negative feedback control by thyroid hormones, the molecular events at the level of the thyrotroph cells and the relative importance of T_3 and T_4 in suppressing TSH secretion remains unclear. The presence of a high-affinity, low-capacity receptor site(s) for T_3 located in the adenohypophysis suggests that T_3 causes a primary suppression of TSH release, but such a postulate fails to consider the possibility of intrapituitary bioconversion of T_4 to T_3. The adenohypophysis also contains specific receptors for T_4, but they are fewer in number than those of T_3.

4.1.3. Chemistry, Biosynthesis, Secretion, and Metabolism

The structural formulas of T_4 and T_3 are shown in Figure 4-2. The thyroid gland secretes a mixture of both T_3 and T_4. Both T_3 and T_4 are iodine-containing amino acids, both of which have the ability to affect the rate of cellular metabolism. The process of thyroid hormone formation involves the following steps:

Transport of iodide into the thyroid
Generation of an oxidizing agent such as peroxide
Synthesis of the receptor protein, thyroglobulin
Oxidation of iodide to a reactive higher valence state
Binding of iodine to tyrosine present in thyroglobulin
Formation of iodothyronines in thyroglobulin by coupling of iodotyrosyl
    residues
Storage and proteolysis of thyroglobulin
Deiodination of free iodotyrosines
Release of T_4 and T_3 into the blood

The bioxynthesis of T_3 and T_4 is shown in Figure 4-3. The synthesis requires the presence of peroxidase, iodide, and acceptor protein at a particular cellular locus. The peroxidase enzyme contains binding sites for both iodide and tyrosine.

The thyroid gland has an avidity for iodide. The gland contains a very effective trapping mechanism for removing iodide from the blood, the so-called anionic pump. This pump mechanism requires energy (e.g., ATP) to permit active transport of iodide into the thyroid gland and can be influenced by both physiological (e.g., TSH) and pharmacological factors. The gland usually concentrates iodide to an amount at least 25 times its concentration in the plasma.

Once iodide (I^-) has been trapped by the thyroid gland, it is oxidized

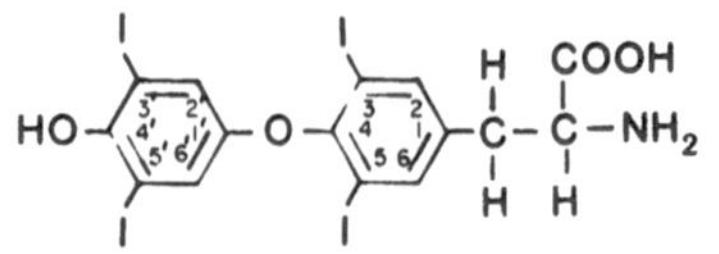

3,5,3',5'-tetraiodothyronine (Thyroxine, T_4)

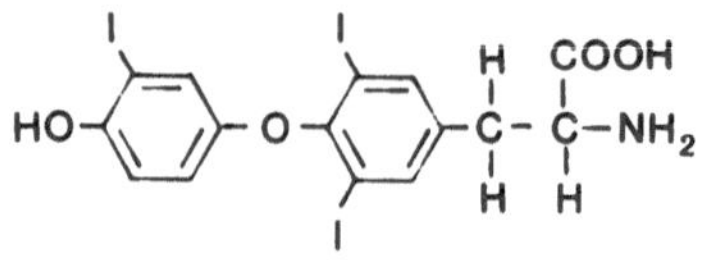

3,5,3'-triiodothyronine (T_3)

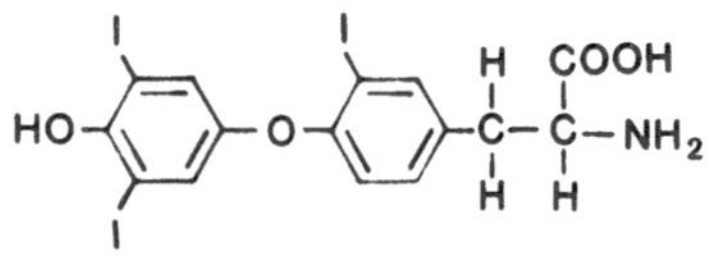

3,3',5'-triiodothyronine (reverse T_3; rT_3)

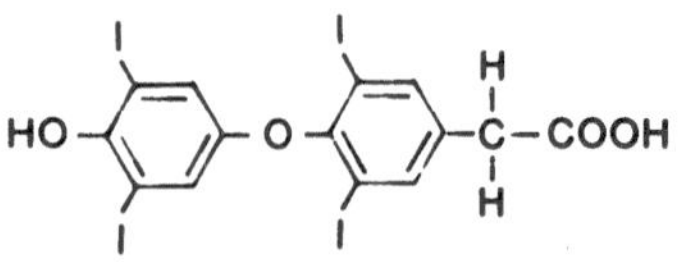

3,5,3',5'-tetraiodothyroacetic acid (Tetrac, TA_4)

Figure 4-2. Structural formulas of thyroxine and of several of its metabolites.

to iodine (I_2) (Figure 4-3). The conversion of iodide to iodine is mediated by thyroid peroxidase. Some antithyroidal agents, e.g., the thionamides, can inhibit thyroid peroxidase. Tyrosine iodinase can iodinate tyrosine to monoiodotyrosine (MIT) and to diiodotyrosine (DIT). The iodination of tyrosine occurs when this amino acid is bound to thyroglobulin. T_3 is formed by a coupling reaction between a molecule of MIT and DIT, while T_4 is formed by coupling two molecules of DIT (Figures 4-3 and 4-4). Thyroglobulin represents the storage form of thyroid hormones, and the actions of proteases cause the release of the different iodinated molecules. The synthesis of thyroglobulin is regulated by a hypotha-lamic–hypophyseal system. TRH controls the rate of secretion of TSH from the anterior pituitary gland. TSH modulates the synthesis of thy-roglobulin through increased synthesis of rRNA and mRNA.

   Thyroglobulin represents a highly specialized storage protein found in the thyroid gland. It occurs in the form of a colloid aggregate within the follicles of the gland. Thyroglobulin is composed of four polypeptide chains having a molecular weight of 600,000–700,000. Despite the fact that this protein contains more than 100 tyrosyl residues, only one to three thyronine molecules (e.g., T_3 or T_4) are produced when the molecule is hydrolyzed.

It is the action of proteases on thyroglobulin that leads to the release of MIT, DIT, T_3, and T_4. Amounts of T_3 and T_4 are secreted into the bloodstream, but MIT and DIT are deiodinated within the thyroid gland. Thyroidal deiodinase is quite specific for MIT and DIT. MIT and DIT possess no biological activity.

The thyroid gland of a healthy adult secretes about 75 μg of T_4 every 24 hr. Approximately 80% of this T_4 is deiodinated at extrathyroidal sites. The deiodination of T_4 can yield either T_3 (3,5,3'-triiodothyronine) or reverse T_3 (rT_3) (3,3',5'-triiodothyronine) (Figure 4-2). The peripheral conversion of T_4 to T_3 has been demonstrated in humans. T_3 and rT_3 can be further deiodinated to form di- and monoiodinated metabolites.

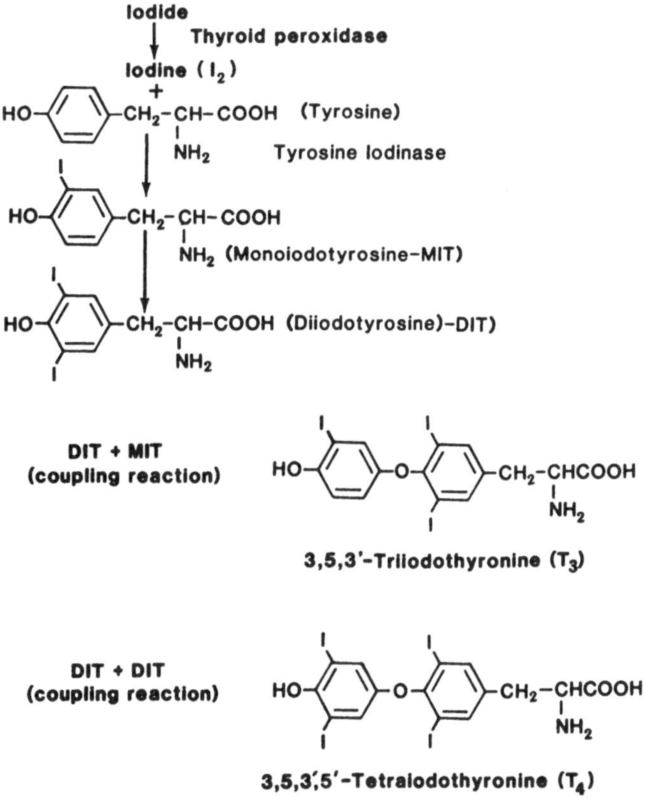

Figure 4-3. Biosynthesis of thyroid hormones.

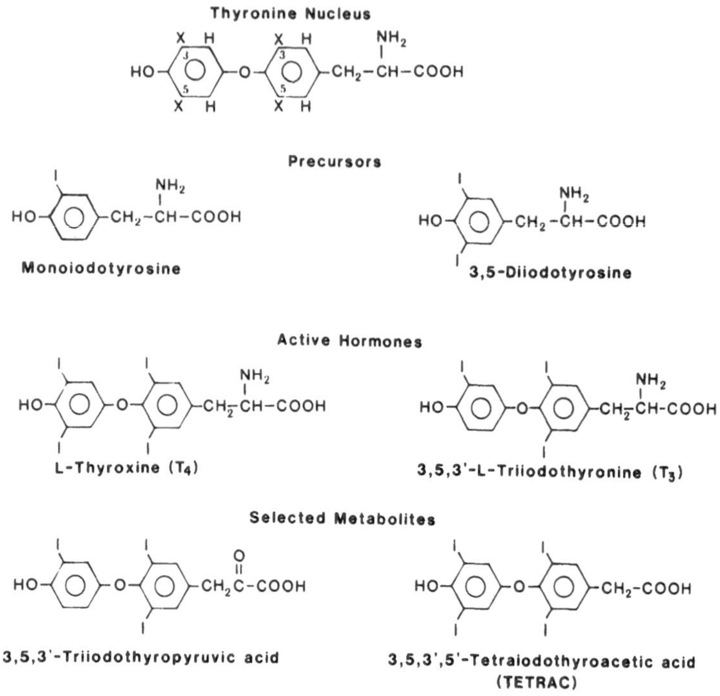

Figure 4-4. Chemical structure of thyroid hormones and related compounds.

Since T_3 is more potent than T_4, the conversion to T_3 represents a process of hormone activation.

Many tissues are able to metabolize T_3 and T_4, but the liver appears to be particularly important in conjugating thyroid hormone degradation products (e.g., glucuronide, sulfate). Such excretory products, e.g., tetraiodothyroacetic acid (TETRAC) (Figure 4-2) can be detected in the urine and feces. Renal mechanisms are effective in deiodinating these metabolites, and the iodide ions are recirculated to the thyroid, where they are retrapped and reutilized.

The biological half-life of T_4 is about 7 days, while that of T_3 is about 1 day. The difference in half-life is principally attributable to the fact that T_4 is more firmly bound to serum proteins. Once thyroid protease liberates T_3 or T_4 from its storage depot in the follicular colloid, the hormone enters the bloodstream, where it is selectively bound by one of several carrier proteins. Since there is no evidence that protein-bound T_3 or T_4 can enter cells, it is presumed that the hormone protein complex dissociates at the tissue sites, where the T_3 or T_4 can exert its biological effects.

Three serum proteins transport thyroxine: albumin, thyroxine-binding prealbumin (TBPA), and thyroxine-binding inter-α-globulin (TBG). About 60% of circulating T_4 is bound to TBG and about 30% to TBPA. Approximately 5% of the circulating T_4 is bound to albumin. T_3 has no affinity for TBPA, and it binds to TBG only to the extent of 3% of T_4. These hormones of the thyroid are bound to those transporting proteins by noncovalent interactions. Several factors can alter the concentration of TBG (see Table 4-1). Both physiological and pathological factors can alter the transport of thyroid hormones. Likewise a number of pharmacological agents can affect TBG levels (see Table 4-2). Drugs can also modify the binding capacity of TBG and TBPA.

4.1.4. Thyroid Hormone Receptors

Although the physiological importance of the thyroid gland has long been recognized, the mechanism of action of T_4 is not clearly understood at the molecular level. The relatively slow progress in elucidating the molecular basis of thyroid hormone action is partly attributed to the lack of well-defined target tissues and the absence of a universally recognized model for the *in vitro* study of this hormone's action(s). Recent efforts, however, have revealed the presence of specific nuclear binding sites for iodothyronines. Accumulating evidence indicates that thyroid hor-

Table 4.1 Factors Associated with Alterations in the Concentration of Thyroid-Binding Globulin[a]

Increased concentration of TBG
   Pregnancy
   Neonatal period
   Estrogens and hyperestrogenic states
   Oral contraceptives
   Acute intermittent porphyria
   Infectious hepatitis
   Genetic factors
Decreased concentration of TBG
   Androgenic or anabolic steroids
   Glucocorticoids (high doses)
   Active acromegaly
   Nephrotic syndrome
   Major illnesses
   Genetic factors

[a] TBG, thyroid-binding globulin.

Table 4-2. Pharmacologically Induced
Changes in Thyroxine-Binding Globulin
and Thyroxine-Binding Prealbumin[a]

Drug/Hormone	TBG	TBPA
Drugs Interfering with Thyroxine Binding		
Salicylates	—	+[b]
Phenytoin (DPH)	+[b]	—
Drugs Affecting Thyroxine-Binding Capacity		
Anabolic steroids	↓	↑
Corticosteroids	↓	↑
Testosterone	↓	↑
Progestogens	↑	—
Estrogens	↑	—

[a] ↑, Increased; ↓, decreased.
[b] (+) Interferes with binding.

mones initiate their actions by enhancement of the transcription of genetic information. It has been proposed that the early actions of thyroid
hormone are due principally to protein synthesis brought about by increased transcription of DNA. While this concept of thyroid hormone
action involving early increases in protein synthesis has been supported
by some experimental evidence, it has also been proposed that the hor-
mone(s) acts directly on intracellular organelles. *In vitro* experimental
models have provided evidence of interactions between the iodothyronines and the mitochondria. Still other evidence points to the existence
of specific T_3-binding sites in the nuclei of liver and kidney. Cytosolic
fractions obtained from liver and kidney also contain proteins that bind
T_3 and T_4. These proteins appear to have a higher capacity and lower
affinity than is demonstrated by proteins found in the nuclei. The affinity
for different iodothyronines exhibited by cytoplasmic sites varies from
the affinity exhibited by nuclear sites for T_3 and T_4. Specific nuclear
binding for T_3 and T_4 can be demonstrated in the absence of cytosol
protein, hence differs markedly from steroid protein–cellular interactions. Although extranuclear events cannot by excluded from some of
the early biological actions of T_4 (and T_3), increasing evidence suggests
that nuclear sites are important in initiating the hormone's action. While
there is a growing belief that T_4 interacts with nuclear sites, resulting in
a series of biochemical effects, little is known about the molecular mech-
anism(s) by which such an interaction might lead to enhanced transcription of DNA.

4.1.5. Biochemical Actions

A multiplicity of physiological effects are exerted by thyroid hormones. Overall, the physiological effects of T_3 and T_4 are similar, but T_3 has a more rapid onset of action than does T_4. T_3 generally causes a greater stimulatory response than does T_4. Relative to other hormones, thyroid hormones act more slowly. The physiological (or pathological) effects (or lack thereof) of the thyroid hormones are readily apparent in either hypothyroidism (e.g., myxedema) or hyperthyroidism (e.g., thyrotoxicosis) (see Table 4-3).

Perhaps the most classic action of the thyroid hormones is their ability to stimulate oxygen consumption—they are calorigenic. Thyroid hormones can affect protein, carbohydrate, and lipid metabolism. Depending on the hormonal status and the particular organ involved, T_4 generally exerts a stimulatory effect on protein metabolism and glycogenolysis. Generally, lipid metabolism is enhanced by the thyroid hormones. Among the metabolic effects produced by thyroid hormones on lipid metabolism is their ability to cause hypocholesterolemia. Thyroxine stimulates cholesterol synthesis and increases its clearance through increased bile acid excretion. The D-form of T_4, dextrothyroxine sodium (Choloxin) as well as its acetic acid derivatives, triiodoacetic acid (TRIAC) and tetraiodoacetic acid (TETRAC) (Figure 4-4), because of their less potent effects on metabolism, have been used as pharmacological agents to lower blood cholesterol.

At supraphysiological levels, T_4 affects mitochondrial activity and

Table 4-3. Actions of Thyroid Hormone in Hyperthyroidal and Hypothyroidal States[a,b]

Organ system	Hyperthyroidism (thyrotoxicosis)	Hypothyroidism (myxedema)
Cardiovascular system	↑ Cardiac output, hypertension, tachycardia	↓ Cardiac output, bradycardia
CNS	Restlessness, wakefulness, nervousness	Sluggishness, somnolence, mental retardation
Muscle	Weakness	Weakness, tremor, twitching
Metabolic	↑ BMR, hyperglycemia, ↓ cholesterol	Hypoglycemia, ↑ cholesterol, low body temperature

[a] ↑, Increased; ↓, decreased.
[b] Magnitude of effect depends on the relative excess or deficiency of the hormone.

leads to an uncoupling of oxidative phosphorylation. There are a large number of enzymes whose synthesis is affected by thyroid hormone. Many of these enzymes, such as α-glycerophosphate dehydrogenase, succinic dehydrogenase, and cytochrome oxidase, are associated with the mitochondrion. All the biochemical effects of T_3 and T_4 can be blocked by the RNA-synthesis inhibitor, actinomycin D, as well as by the protein-synthesis inhibitor, puromycin.

4.1.6. Management of Hypothyroidal States

Thyroid hormone preparations have been used with considerable effectiveness and can cause a striking and complete reversal of the clinical signs and symptoms myxedematous patients. Myxedema, or Gull's disease, is generally an adult disorder resulting from deficient functioning of the thyroid gland. The clinical symptoms are manifested in a large variety of ways, including a cold, dry, puffy appearance of the face in particular and of the skin in general, deepening of the voice, possible hearing and mental impairment, diminished appetite, and impairment of both smooth and skeletal muscle function. Optimal replacement therapy of T_3 and/or T_4 in hypothyroidal states can effectively reverse those manifestations listed in Table 4-3. The therapy of hypothyroidism entails the careful selection of dose regimens of one of the several commercially available thyroid preparations (see Table 4-4). Thyroxine is used in the routine management of myxedema. Severe hypothyroidism with an onset in infancy is called cretinism (clinically characterized by most of the symptoms described for myxedema plus dwarfism, diminished heart rate, lowered body temperature, and severe mental retardation), whereas hypothyroidism with an onset in childhood is called juvenile hypothyroidism. The indications for thyroid hormone therapy are listed in Table 4-5.

4.1.7. Therapeutic Uses and Preparations

4.1.7.1. Thyroid USP

Thyroid USP, (dessicated thyroid, thyroxine fraction, thyroxine cytosol) is derived from dried and defatted thyroid glands of domestic animals (bovine, ovine, or porcine). The thyroid hormone content varies somewhat among species. For example, the $T_4 : T_3$ ratio of bovine preparations may range from about 3 to nearly 5. Porcine $T_4 : T_3$ ratios are somewhat lower, ranging from 2.5 to 3.6. Thyroid preparations are therefore standardized on the basis of their iodine content because of variations in the actual ratio of $T_4 : T_3$. There are also some differences in the

Table 4-4. Thyroidal Agents Used in the Treatment of Hypothyroidism

Agent	Trade name(s)	Relative potency[a]	Average daily dose[b] (mg)
Thyroid USP	Thyrar	65	150
Thyroglobulin	Proloid	65	150
Sodium levothyroxine	Levothroid, Levoid, Synthroid	0.100–0.125	0.150
Sodium liothyronine	Cytomel	0.025–0.035	0.075
Liotrix	Euthroid (4 : 1) Thyrolar (4 : 1) Novothyral (5 : 1)		

[a] Metabolically calorigenically equivalent to 65 mg of thyroid USP.
[b] Representative dose only, depending on the degree of myxedema.

rates of absorption among animal thyroid preparations, since some contaminating thyroglobulin may be present as well. In the latter compound, T_4 and T_3 are incorporated into the molecule by peptide bonds. Proteolytic enzymes of the gastrointestinal (GI) tract act to liberate iodothyronines and iodotyrosines. As a result, thyroid USP is orally active and is relatively inexpensive.

Thyroid hormone therapy should not be administered until hypothyroidism has been confirmed by laboratory testing. Dosage must be adjusted to the individual requirements of the patient and on the basis of clinical response and thyroid function tests. The suppression of THS should not be used as the sole index of adequacy of dose in congenital hypothyroidism, since TSH levels may remain elevated despite adequate or even excessive doses of thyroid hormone. Blood levels of T_4 are a more accurate predictor of optimal therapy in the infant or child. Lower replacement dose therapy may be required for the elderly patient. The clinical effects of replacement therapy may not be evident for 1–3 weeks. If no therapeutic response is evident after prolonged therapy (e.g., approximately 3 months), particularly with progressively increasing doses of T_4, the diagnosis should be reevaluated. Conversely, if symptoms of hyperthyroidism occur during replacement therapy, thyroid hormone therapy should be withdrawn for 2–6 days and subsequently resumed at a lower dose.

4.1.7.2. Thyroglobulin

Thyroglobulin (Proloid) is a partially purified preparation of thyroid glands obtained from domestic animals. It is active orally. Thyroglobulin

Table 4-5. Therapeutic Indications
for Thyroid Hormone Preparations

Myxedema
Myxedema coma
Nontoxic goiter
Thyroiditis
Thyroid-suppression test
Thyroid cancer
Graves' disease (adjunct)
Other?

is standardized by iodine content and is assayed for metabolic potency. The $T_4 : T_3$ ratio is also somewhat variable in animal preparations of thyroglobulin. Thyroglobulin is slightly more expensive than is dessicated thyroid and offers no particular therapeutic advantage over thyroid USP. The approximate equivalent dosage, based on clinical response, is 60 mg for thyroid USP and for thyroglobulin. Thyroglobulin tablets are available for oral administration and come in several strengths, i.e., 16, 32, 54, 100, 130, 200, and 325 mg. The usual oral dose in the adult patient with hypothyroidism without myxedema is 32 mg/day initially, with increments every 1 or 2 weeks until the desired therapeutic results are achieved. An oral maintenance dose may range from 32 to 200 mg/day. In myxedema or hypothyroidism with concomitant cardiovascular disease, the initial oral dose may be 16–32 mg/day, with increments of a comparable amount every 2 weeks until the desired therapeutic results are obtained.

4.1.7.3. Sodium Levothyroxine

Sodium levothyroxine (Levothroid, Synthroid, Levoid) was introduced for the management of hypothyroidism during the 1950s. This synthetic preparation of T_4 can be administered orally or intravenously. The onset of action and the duration of action are comparable to either thyroid USP or thyroglobulin. L-Thyroxine, on a milligram basis, is more potent than either thyroid USP or thyroglobulin. T_4 may be the drug of choice in the treatment of myxedema. Levothyroxine is available in several oral dosage forms, i.e., 25, 50, 75, 100, 125, 150, 175, 200, or 300 μg, and in injectable formulations of 100, 200, or 300 and 500 μg. Initial oral doses will vary with the degree of the hypothyroidism but may vary from 25 to 100 μg/day. Oral maintenance doses range from 100 to 150 μg/day. However, oral absorption is variable among different commercial preparations, and hence there is a need to titrate thyroxine levels very closely when switching from one formulation to another. In elderly patients or in patients with concomitant cardiovascular disease, initial doses and maintenance doses may be lower than in the young adult patient. In myxedema coma or stupor, intravenous doses ranging between 200 and 500 μg may be required with a possible additional 100–300-μg dose on the second day if improvement has not occurred. Levothyroxine is considered the drug of choice in the treatment of congenital hypothyroidism.

4.1.7.4. Sodium Liothyronine

Sodium liothyronine (Cytomel) is the sodium salt of synthetic T_3. It has a relatively rapid onset of action, but its peak effect and its duration of action are shorter than that of T_4. T_3 is active orally, and about 90% is absorbed. While it may be useful in emergency states, the expense of sodium liothyronine cannot be justified for therapy of hypothyroidism. The calorigenic actions of liothyronine are difficult to compare with those of thyroid USP, T_4, or Liotrix since it has such a rapid action. In mild hypothyroidism, an initial oral dose of 25 μg/day is given with increments of 12.5 or 25 μg every 1 or 2 weeks until the desired therapeutic results are obtained. An oral maintenance dose may range from 25 to 100 μg/day. In simple (nontoxic) goiter, an initial oral dose of 5 μg/day with increments of 5–10 μg every 1 or 2 weeks is recommended. When a dosage of 25 μg/day is reached, increments may be increased by 12.5 or 25 μg every week.

4.1.7.5. Liotrix

Liotrix (Euthroid, Thyrolar) is a 4 : 1 mixture of the sodium salts of T_4 and T_3. This preparation has the advantage of having a constant ratio of T_4 : T_3 from batch to batch, accounting for more consistent and reliable physiological responses to its administration as compared with those produced by either thyroid USP or thyroglobulin. However, the ratio of levothyroxine to liothyronine is 4 : 1, while the normal ratio in human thyroid gland secretion is 20 : 1, so thyrotoxic symptoms due to excess T_3 are common. Liotrix does not offer any particular therapeutic advantage over T_4, especially when considering that it is also more expensive than T_4.

The initial adult dose in hypothyroidism without myxedema is usually 50 μg of levothyroxine and 12.5 μg of liothyronine or 60 μg of levothyroxine and 15 μg of liothyronine a day, with increments of comparable amounts at monthly intervals until the desired therapeutic results are achieved. In myxedema, in hypothyroidism with cardiovascular disease, and in elderly patients with thyroidal disorders, both initial doses and maintenance doses may be considerably lower.

4.1.8. Adverse Effects

All the various thyroid preparations are capable of producing toxicity. In many respects, excessive thyroid hormone therapy can mimic the physiological (or pathological) actions listed in Table 4-3. Nervousness, hyperirritability, insomnia, cardiac dysrhythmias, and hypertension are all toxic manifestations of excessive thyroid hormone therapy. Adverse effects are dose related; their incidence may begin to increase after the initial dose. Skin rash and hypersensitivity reactions are rare. Chest pain, shortness of breath, changes in appetite, vomiting, diarrhea, weight loss, profuse sweating, sensitivity to heat, fever, and changes in menstrual periods may also be side effects associated with hormone therapy.

Thyroid hormone therapy should be used with caution in patients who have the following medical problems:

Adrenocortical insufficiency
Arteriosclerosis
Cardiac disease (including angina pectoris)
Diabetes mellitus
Hypertension
Hyperthyroidism (history of)
Myocardial infarction
Panhypopituitarism
Renal function impairment
Thyrotoxicosis

4.2. ANTITHYROIDAL AGENTS

4.2.1. Thyrotoxicosis (Hyperthyroidism)

Once the diagnosis of hyperthyroidism (thyrotoxicosis) has been established (see Table 4-3 for selected signs and symptoms), several therapeutic approaches can be undertaken. Thyrotoxicosis can be managed clinically through the use of antithyroid drugs, radioactive iodine (^{131}I), and/or surgery. Unfortunately, the etiology of the thyrotoxicosis often remains obscure; it is only in rare instances that elevated levels of TSH can be detected. Thyroid hyperfunction is characterized by an abnormally elevated rate of metabolism. The basal metabolic rate (BMR) may be 30–60% above normal or euthyroidal states. A particular clinical syndrome characterized by excessive thyroid activity is Graves' disease. It has also been called exophthalmic goiter because thyroid gland enlargement and exophthalmos are frequent clinical manifestations. Graves' disease has been classically defined as a triad of a diffuse goiter, hyperthyroidism, and infiltrative ophthalmopathy.

The blood of patients with Graves' disease contains a substance referred to as long-acting thyroid stimulator (LATS). LATS is an immunoglobulin of the class IgG; thyroid-stimulating immunoglobulin (TSI), possessing certain actions similar to those of TSH. However, unlike TSH, LATS can traverse the placental barrier and stimulate the fetal thyroid and it is not suppressed by exogenously administered thyroid hormone. The clinical indications for antithyroidal drugs are listed in Table 4-6.

4.2.2. Drugs Used in the Management of Thyrotoxicosis

It is possible to interfere pharmacologically with varous metabolic steps in the synthesis, release, and/or transport of thyroid hormone(s). Ordinarily, antithyroid drugs that interfere with the organification process are most widely used. Iodides, lithium, and β-adrenergic blocking drugs are also employed. Because of their associated toxicity, such as the complication of aplastic anemia, compounds that inhibit the anionic pump (e.g., potassium perchlorate) have become therapeutically obsolete. In some instances, the mechanism of antithyroidal agents is generally understood; for example, it is known that monovalent anions competitively inhibit iodide transport. In other instances, such as antidiabetic drugs, diethyl ether, and dimercaprol (BAL), the mechanism(s) of action remain unclear.

The term antithyroidal agent ordinarily applies to those substances that inhibit thyroid function. Such agents include those that prevent the release of hormone from the thyroid by a feedback mechanism. Other agents interfere with the synthesis of thyroid hormone. Still other substances inhibit the utilization of thyroid hormones. Radioactive iodide

Table 4-6. Therapeutic Indications for Antithyroidal Agents

Graves' disease (initial therapy)
Neonatal Graves' disease
Thyroid storm
Preoperative for thyroidectomy
Preparation for radioiodine therapy
Pregnancy complicated by thyrotoxicosis
Iodine-induced thyrotoxicosis

in high doses can depress thyroid gland activity. Finally, certain agents without any inherent hormonal activity (e.g., lithium, propranolol) can suppress certain of the clinical manifestations of thyrotoxicosis. The site(s) of action of some of these antithyroidal agents are depicted in Figure 4-5. The antithyroidal drugs commonly in use throughout the world are generically thionamides. Perhaps the two most commonly used anti-thyroidal agents used in the United States are propylthiouracil and meth-imazole (Figure 4-6). Aminoheterocylic agents, including the antidiabetic agent tolbutamide, as well as certain substituted phenol compounds, can suppress thyroid gland activity. These latter chemical classes of compounds play no major therapeutic role in the management of thy-rotoxicosis but, when used for other nonthyroid indications, can exert suppressive side effects.

4.2.2.1. Thiocarbamides (Thionamides)

Undoubtedly the major group of antithyroidal agents used in clinical medicine are the thiocarbamides. The general formula for this compound is as follows:

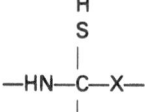

where X is either carbon or nitrogen. The most active of these compounds possess the thiourethylene group

$$S = C \underset{\diagdown N}{\overset{\diagup N}{}}$$

In the United States, methimazole (Tapazole) is widely used, while in England carbimazole (Neomercazole) is commonly prescribed. The pro-pyl- and methylthiouracil preparations are also effective antithyroid drugs.

The antithyroid mechanism of action of the thionamides involves their ability to interfere with the organification process; they inhibit the organic binding of iodine. The thionamides have little or no effect on T_4 that has already been synthesized. The thionamides act primarily by inhibiting thyroid peroxidase (TPO), an enzyme that catalyzes both the oxidation of iodide ion to a form in which it can be covalently bound into the tyrosyl residues in thyroglobulin, and the so-called coupling reaction of iodotyrosyl residues in thyroglobulin to form T_4 and T_3. The action of thiocarbamide on TPO may involve competitive inhibition with

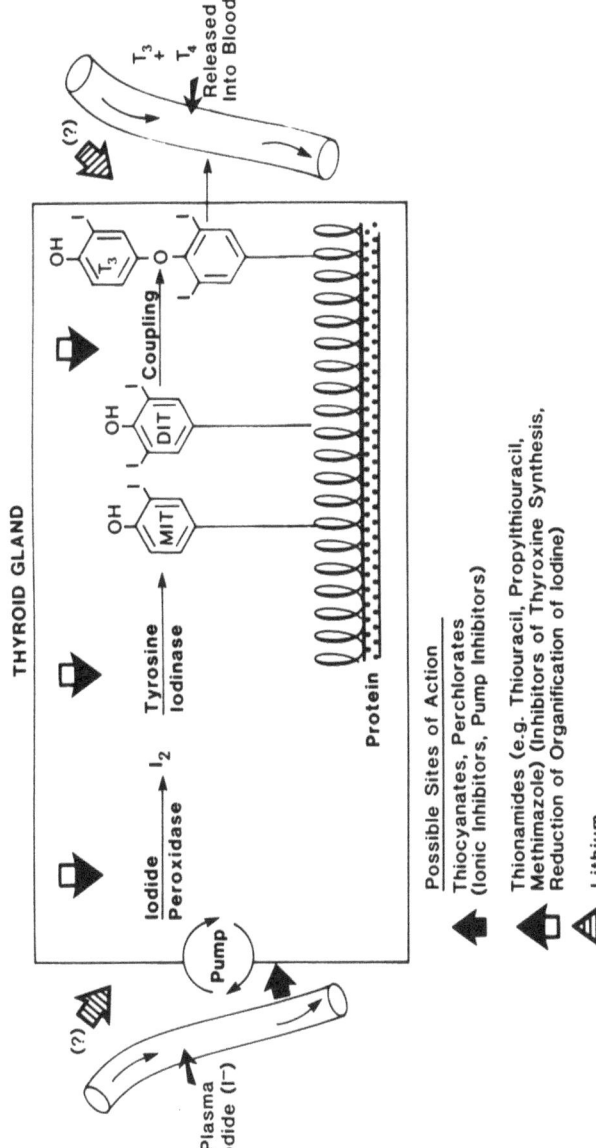

Figure 4-5. Site of action of antithyroidal agents. DIT, diiodotyrosine; MIT, monoiodotyrosine; T₃, triiodothyronine; T₄, thyroxine.

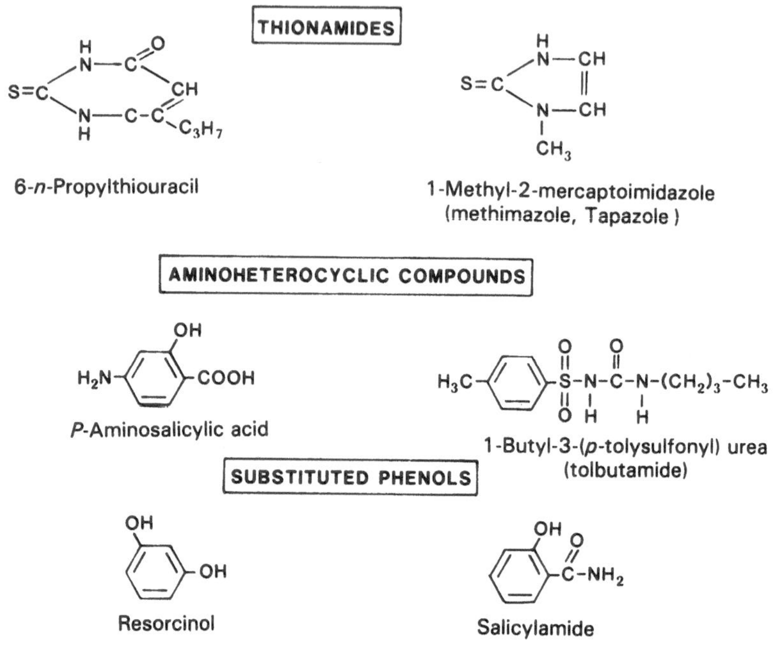

Figure 4-6. Chemical formulas of representative antithyroid compounds.

the hydrogen donor for the active site on the enzyme. The coupling reaction appears to be particularly sensitive to inhibition by thionamides. While the thionamide agents inhibit the iodination of thyroglobulin as well as the synthesis of thyroid hormone, they have no effect on the anionic pump of the thyroid gland. Propylthiouracil may inhibit the peripheral monodeiodination of T_4, but it is doubtful that this action results in any significant therapeutic benefit. Propylthiouracil, but not methimazole, is a potent inhibitor of the 5'-deiodinase enzyme system that converts T_4 and T_3 in peripheral tissue. Since the thionamides exert their actions by inhibiting T_4 formation, and since this process may take at least 1–2 weeks, the onset of action may not occur until about 1–2 weeks after the initiation of therapy. There is usually a large store of hormone within the thyroid gland, enough in a normal person with a normal rate of secretion to maintain a euthyroid state for about 6 months even if all synthesis of thyroid hormone is abolished.

The thionamides are usually well absorbed from the GI tract. The specific drugs within this class of antithyroidal agents undergo varying degrees of metabolism. These agents are rapidly excreted by the kidney, and very little additional drug can be detected in the urine after 24 hr. While the tissue distribution varies with the particular thionamide, high concentrations can be detected in the thyroid and kidney.

Methimazole (Tapazole) is a thionamide derivative indicated in varying degrees of hyperthyroidism. The usual oral adult dose in mild hyperthyroidism is 15 mg/day divided into three doses at 8-hr intervals. In moderately severe hyperthyroidism and in severe hyperthyroidism, the usual initial oral adult dose is 30 mg and 60 mg, respectively. Maintenance oral doses of methimazole range from 5 to 30 mg/day in two to three divided doses. Pediatric doses are considerably lower.

The duration of treatment necessary to produce a prolonged remission varies from 6 months to several years, with an average duration of about 1 year with either methimazole or propylthiouracil. Premature cessation of antithyroidal therapy with either methimazole or propylthiouracil may lead to exacerbation of hyperthyroidism, but sometimes withdrawal of agents once a euthyroid state is achieved can also result in problems of thyroid rebound.

Propylthiouracil and methimazole cross the placental barrier and can be excreted in breast milk. Initial oral doses of propylthiouracil range from 300 to 1200 mg/day divided into three doses at 8-hr intervals or four doses at 6-hr intervals until the patient becomes euthyroid. Patients with severe hyperthyroidism may require daily doses upward to 2 g. Maintenance doses may range from 50 to 800 mg/day in two to four divided doses. In neonatal thyrotoxicosis, an oral dose of 10 mg/kg per day in divided doses may be prescribed.

Carbimazole is administered initially in a dose of 15 mg three times daily, after which the dosage is reduced gradually to a maintenance level of 5 to 15 mg/day in divided doses.

The most frequently observed side effect during thionamide therapy is the development of a skin rash. Arthralgia, myalgia, cholestatic jaundice, lymphadenopathy, drug fever, ototoxicity, psychosis, and a lupuslike syndrome also have been reported after the use of thionamides. However, the most serious complication is agranulocytosis. In addition, prolonged drug administration can actually result in goiter formation, since an increased secretion of TSH will occur secondary to an inhibition of the synthesis of T_3 and/or T_4. This goitrogenic action is usually the result of overtreatment, necessitating an adjustment in the dosage regimen. Therapeutic failures or remissions are not uncommon and may necessitate the institution of other measures, including thyroidectomy. Propylthiouracil is bound to protein to a greater extent than is methimazole and therefore does not cross the placenta as readily. However, propylthiouracil can cause goiter in about 10% of exposed infants.

4.2.2.2. *Anionic Inhibitors*

Potassium perchlorate is an agent that interferes with iodide transport into the thyroid gland; it is an inhibitor of the anionic pump. Because this drug can cause fatal aplastic anemia, it is no longer considered therapeutically useful, although at one time it was considered an alternative form of therapy for those patients in whom a hypersensitivity to the thionamides had developed . Thiocyanate and certain other anions, particularly perchlorate and nitrate, exert a thyroid-inhibiting effect by interfering with iodide uptake by the thyroid gland. Thiocyanate is widely distributed in nature; consumption of large amounts of foodstuffs containing this substance can lead to an increased incidence of endemic goiter in certain regions of the world. Potassium perchlorate at high concentrations can also inhibit TPO.

4.2.2.3. *Radioactive Iodine*

^{131}I is a safe and effective compound for the management of thyrotoxicosis. The β-emissions of this isotope are responsible for most thyroidal radiation. There is no evidence that radioactive iodine increases the incidence of leukemia or thyroid carcinoma. A primary disadvantage associated with radioactive iodine therapy is the possibility of an increased incidence of hypothyroidism. Microcurie (μCi) amounts ^{131}I are used for diagnostic evaluation of thyroid function, while millicurie (mCi) quantities are used for the selective destruction of thyroid cells.

Administration of ^{131}I is contraindicated during pregnancy in order to avoid fetal injury. Any genetic hazard associated with ^{131}I therapy for hyperthyroidism is so minimal that it should not constitute a major reason for avoiding radioiodine therapy.

4.2.2.4. *Iodides*

The effects of iodides on the thyroid gland are complex and poorly understood. The use of iodides as a means of preparing a patient for a thyroidectomy is being replaced by thionamide and thyroxine administration. Management of thyrotoxicosis with iodine alone frequently results in a phenomenon of iodine escape, which leads to an exacerbation of the hyperthyroidism. Iodide in the form of potassium iodide tablets or as Lugol's iodine solution was once extensively used in the management of thyrotoxicosis. ^{131}I therapy is not possible in a patient who is receiving iodide because the marked increase in the body iodide pool prevents effective concentration of ^{131}I by the thyroid. Increasing the intraglandular stores of thyroid hormone by iodide administration increases the time required for the onset of subsequent thioamide therapy. The short-term use of iodide therapy has been largely replaced by propranolol.

4.2.2.5. Lithium Carbonate

Lithium carbonate was used for many years in the treatment of manic-depressive states before it was realized that it suppresses thyroid gland activity. Lithium seems to act by preventing the release of both hormonal and nonhormonal iodine from the thyroid gland. In addition, lithium somehow interferes with the interaction of TSH and the adenyl cyclase–cAMP system. Lithium offers no advantage over drugs of the thionamide class (e.g., methimazole) insofar as the rate at which thyroid hormone levels are reduced. It may be useful in patients who are allergic to other antithyroid drugs. Since lithium causes an accumulation of thyroidal iodide, which leads to eventual iodine escape, there is probably no therapeutic place for this agent in the long-term management of thyrotoxicosis. Lithium administration is occasionally accompanied by the appearance of tremors, depersonalization, nephrogenic diabetes insipidus, hyperaldosteronism, and a possbile increased risk of cardiac failure. Because lithium has a very narrow therapeutic ratio, lithium therapy in hyperthyroidism requires careful monitoring of serum lithium levels and of the patient's clinical status. Effective serum concentrations of lithium range from 0.5 to 1.2 mEq/liter, with toxic manifestations occurring at or above 1.5 mEq/liter (8 mEq of lithium is equivalent to approximately 300 mg of lithium carbonate).

4.2.2.6. Propranolol

It has long been recognized that many of the cardiovascular, metabolic, and neuromuscular characteristics of thyrotoxicosis resemble those features due to catecholamine excess. Propranolol (Inderal) is a β-adrenergic blocking agent effective in alleviating many of the signs and symptoms of thyrotoxicosis. Propranolol (and perhaps chlorpromazine) appears to block the increase in intracellular colloidal droplet produced by TSH (and LATS). Propranolol also seems to block the stimulation of the adenyl cyclase–cAMP system by TSH (and prostaglandin). Propranolol may therefore act on the thyroid plasma membrane. The antithyroidal oral dose of propranolol ranges from 10 to 40 mg three to four times per day, the dosage being adjusted as needed and tolerated.

Propranolol may reduce hyperthyroid-induced tachycardia, tremor, sweating, heat intolerance, and anxiety. However, propranolol is less effective in the treatment of such hyperthyroid-induced symptoms as myopathy of the limbs and bulbar muscles, periodic paralysis, and steatorrhea. In the short term, propranolol has proved useful in the management of selected neonatal thyrotoxicosis and thyrotoxic crises, but for long-term management of hyperthyroidal states it is inferior to the thionamides. Propranolol is contraindicated in the thyrotoxic patient with obstructive airway disease, since it impairs bronchodilation. The hyperglycemia resulting from propranolol administration would also limit its usefulness in diabetic patients with thyrotoxicosis.

4.3. DRUG INTERACTIONS AND THYROID FUNCTION TESTS

Several drugs have been found to interfere with thyroid gland activity. Table 4-7 lists a wide variety of drugs, hormones, and diagnostic dyes that can alter thyroid function tests and produce changes in the circulating levels of T_4 and its carrier proteins, e.g., TBG. The nature of the various drug–hormone interactions differs among the various agents. Some agents produce alterations in the circulating levels of TBG, while others may compete with T_4 for binding sites on serum proteins.

A variety of classes of drugs can interfere with thyroid function. The hydrazines (e.g., isoniazid) can inhibit the iodination of thyroid hormone by competing with iodide for thyroid peroxidase (TPO). TPO

Table 4-7. Effects of Selected Pharmacological Agents on Thyroid Activity[a]

Drug/hormone	T_3 uptake	^{131}I uptake	Thyroid-binding globulin levels
Aminosalicylic acid	—	↓	—
Anabolic steroids	↑	—	↓
Anticoagulants (Dicumarol and heparin)	↑	—	—
Anti-inflammatory agents (phenylbutazone)	↑	↓	—
Indocyanine Green (Cardio-Green)	—	↓	—
Corticosteroids	—	↓	↓
Phenytoin (DPH)	↑	—	—
Oral contraceptives	↓	—	↑
Lithium carbonate	—	↑	—
Phenothiazines	—	↓	↓
Salicylates	↓	—	—
Sulfonamides	—	↓	—

[a] ↑, Increased; ↓, decreased.

is irreversibly inhibited by iproniazid, which is covalently bound to enzyme. The inhibitory effects of p-aminobenzoate and p-aminosalicylic acid (PAS) (see Figure 4-6) on thyroid gland activity are related to their suppressive actions on TPO. Both cyanide and thiocyanate effectively inhibit TPO. Cyanide forms dissociable covalent complexes with protohematin proteins. Cyanide also inhibits the iodination of tyrosine.

α-Methyldopa (AMD) is a potent inhibitor of the iodination of soluble tyrosine. α-Methylparatyrosine (AMPT) competes with tyrosine for iodination and is itself iodinated. 3-Amino-1,2,4'triazole (ATD), sodium azide (NaN$_3$), and tranylcypromine sulfate, a monoamine oxidase inhibitor, can effectively inhibit TPO. Similarly, resorcinol (Figure 4-6) and sulfathiazole are potent inhibitors of TPO.

It is evident that numerous classes of drugs, many without any inherent thyroid hormone activity, can affect the hypophyseal–thyroidal axis. Furthermore, many thyroid diagnostic tests can be altered by prior or coadministration of various agents (see also Chapter 11). It should be evident that a knowledge of the patient's past medication history is crucial before a diagnosis of thyroid dysfunction can be established.

RECOMMENDED READINGS

Brennan, M. D., Thyroid hormone, *Mayo Clin. Proc.* **55**:33–44, 1980.

Cobb, A. E., and Jackson, I. M. D., Management of hypothyroidism, *Forum N. Engl. Med. Ctr. Hosp.* **7**(1):1978.

Cooper, D. S., Antithyroid drugs. *N. Engl. J. Med.* **311**:1353, 1984.

Degroot, L. G., and Niepomniszicze, H., Biosynthesis of thyroid hormone: Basic and clinical aspects, *Metabolism* **26**:665, 1977.

Gardner, D. F., Cruikshank, D. P., Hays, P. M. and Cooper, D. S., Pharmacology of propylthiouracil (PTU) in pregnant hyperthyroid women: Correlation of maternal PTU concentrations with cord serum thyroid function tests, *J. Clin. Endocrinol. Metab.* **62**:217, 1986.

Giles, H. G., Long, J. P., Orrego, H., and Sellers, E. M., Mechanism of alterations in propylthiouracil disposition after long-term therapy, *Clin. Pharmacol. Ther.* **31**:559, 1982.

Kampmann, J. P., Hansen, J. M., Clinical pharmacokinetics of antithyroid drugs, *Clin. Pharmacokinet.* **6**:401–428, 1981.

Larsen, P. R., Thyroid–pituitary interaction: Feedback regulation of thyrotropin secretion by thyroid hormone, *N. Engl. J. Med.* **306**:23–32, 1982.

Liberti, P., and Stanbury, J. B., The pharmacology of substances affecting the thyroid gland, *Annu. Rev. Pharmacol.* **11**:113, 1971.

McClung, M. P., and Greer, M. A., Treatment of hyperthyroidism, *Annu. Rev. Med.* **31**:385, 1980.

Nimalasuriya, A., Spencer, C. A., Lin, S. C., Tse, J. K., and Nicoloff, J. T., Studies on the diurnal pattern of serum 3,5,3'-triiodothyronine, *J. Clin. Endocrinol. Metab.* **62**:153, 1986.

Selenkow, H. A., and Rose, L. I., Comparative clinical pharmacology of thyroid hormones, *Pharmacol. Ther. C.* **1**:331, 1976.

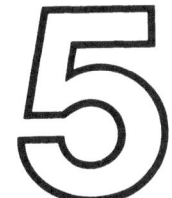

PARATHYROID HORMONE AND CALCITONIN

5.1. INTRODUCTION

The balance of endogenous calcium is maintained by the interaction of several intrinsic factors that control the remodeling of bone as well as the absorption and excretion of calcium. In general, hormonal regulation of calcium homeostasis is particularly important. Parathyroid hormone (PTH), vitamin D, and calcitonin are the principal hormones involved in modulating the distribution of endogenous calcium.

Serum calcium levels must be maintained within a narrow range (8.6–10.5 mg/dl) for the support of neuromuscular transmission, muscle cell contraction, blood coagulation, cardiac function, cell membrane integrity, enzyme function, and cellular secretory activity. It should be appreciated that calcium ion is involved in crucial metabolic and structural roles. The metabolic requirements for calcium are of paramount importance, and calcium levels are maintained at the expense of the structural element (i.e., bone), if necessary.

Approximately 98% of endogenous calcium is present in skeletal tissue. An additional 1% of calcium is sequestered in soft tissues and 1% is found in the extracellular fluid. Serum calcium exists in its ionized form (50%) and is complexed with either serum proteins, principally albumin (40%), or with other ions, such as phosphate, carbonate, citrate, and sulfate (10%). Ionized calcium is biologically active, and the levels of serum calcium are primarily regulated by PTH and metabolites of vitamin D and to a lesser extent by calcitonin (see Figure 5-1).

A fall in serum ionized calcium levels provokes the secretion of PTH, leading to enhanced renal tubular reabsorption of calcium, in-

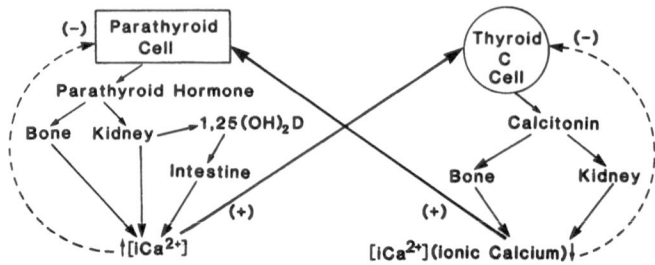

Figure 5-1.   Hormonal regulation of calcium in the extracellular fluid.

creased renal excretion of phosphate, and mobilization of calcium from bone. PTH also stimulates the renal production of 1,25-dihydroxycholecalciferol (1,25-dihydroxy vitamin D_3), the biologically active metabolite of vitamin D that enhances absorption of calcium and phosphate ions from the intestine.

By contrast, a rise in serum levels of ionized calcium stimulates the release of calcitonin, which inhibits calcium mobilization from bone and increases the renal excretion of calcium, phosphate, sodium, chloride, potassium, and magnesium (Figure 5-1).

PTH and calcitonin are currently of limited therapeutic use in the management of calcium imbalance. PTH is utilized in diagnosing end-organ insensitivity to PTH. States of abnormal bone remodeling (Paget's disease) and emergency states associated with hypercalcemia are sometimes managed by calcitonin therapy. Hypocalcemia is more easily managed by calcium replacement therapy or by administration of vitamin D.

5.2. HISTORY

The anatomical description of the parathyroid glands as entities distinct from the surrounding thyroid tissue was made by Sandström in 1880. Eleven years later, von Recklinghausen described hyperparathyroidism and Gley demonstrated that the removal of the parathyroid glands in addition to the thyroid gland was required to produce tetany. Vasale and Generali demonstrated in 1900 that removal of only the parathyroid glands was sufficient to produce convulsions and tetany. The effectiveness of calcium salts in preventing the tetany produced by parathyroidectomy was revealed by MacCallum and Voegtlin in 1909.

By 1911 Greenwald had shown that parathyroidectomy decreased the renal excretion of phosphate. Hanson and Collip (1924–1925) prepared the first active extracts of parathyroid tissue. This led Albright to propose the renal theory of PTH action in 1929. Five years later, Collip and associates described the direct effects of PTH extracts on bone. The importance of the calcium content of the blood as a signal in the regulation of PTH secretion was recognized by Patt and Luckhardt in 1942.

Barnicot (1948) grafted parathyroid tissue adjacent to bone and observed a local decalcifying action, providing further support for the direct actions of PTH on bone. The tissue culture studies by Gaillard (1955) confirmed the observations of Barnicot. Pure preparations of PTH became available in 1959 as a result of separate studies by Rasmussen and Aurbach. By 1970, several groups (Brewer, Ronan, Niall, and Potts) had established the amino acid sequence of PTH.

The hypocalcemic hormone, calcitonin, was identified by Copp in 1962, who further concluded that the parathyroid glands secrete calcitonin in response to hypercalcemia, thereby reducing elevated calcium levels to the normal range. Hirsh proposed in 1963 that the thyroid gland is the source of a hypocalcemic substance, which he called thyrocalcitonin. Calcitonin and thyrocalcitonin are now recognized as identical entities. Calcitonin is the preferred name for the hypocalcemic peptide hormone.

Foster established in 1964 that the parafollicular C cells of the thyroid gland are the source of calcitonin. The direct effects of calcitonin in preventing bone resorption were established by MacIntyre in 1967, and Foster demonstrated (1969) that this effect is attributable to the inhibition of osteoclast activity. Gudmundson demonstrated in 1967 that calcitonin reduces serum phosphate content; Robinson revealed 1 year later that this effect requires the presence of the kidneys. The stimulatory effects of calcitonin on the renal excretion of calcium, sodium, potassium, and magnesium as well as phosphate were described by Hass in 1971. The amino acid sequence of calcitonin was elucidated by a number of investigators, including Potts, Neher, Bell, and Beesley, in 1968.

5.3. PARATHYROID HORMONE

5.3.1. Chemistry

PTH is a linear polypeptide consisting of 84 amino acids with a molecular weight of 9500 (see Figure 5-2). The amino acid sequences of bovine, porcine, and human PTH have been elucidated, and significant differences in primary structure exist. Biological activity resides in the

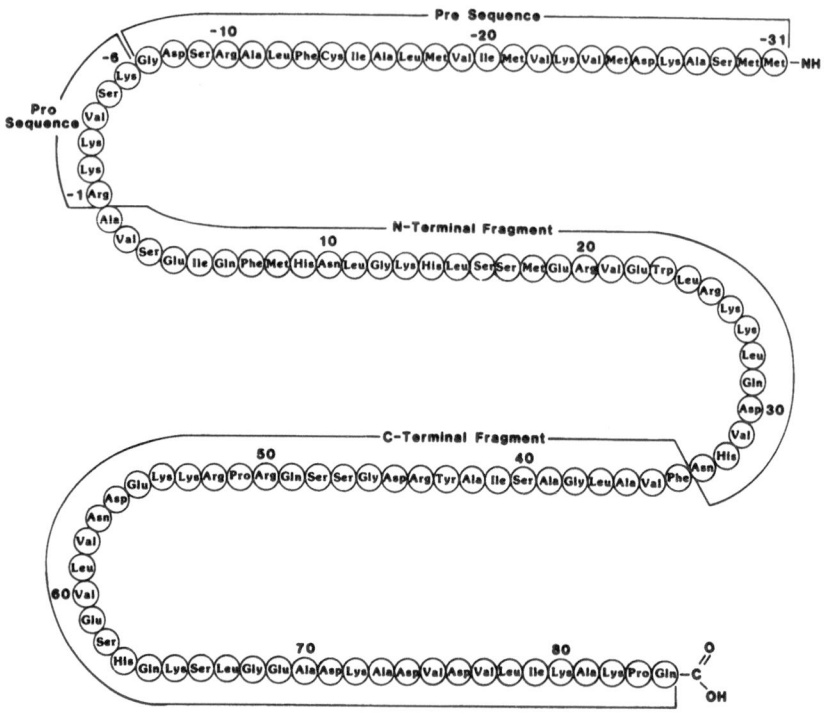

Figure 5-2. Amino acid sequence of parathyroid hormone and precursor forms.

amino-terminal region of the PTH molecule, and the receptor binding and activating domains within the PTH structure have been defined.

Receptor activation requires the amino terminus consisting of the 1–34-amino acid sequence. Deletion of the amino-terminal dipeptide resulting in the 3–34-amino acid fragment markedly reduces the PTH receptor activating capacity of this fragment but does not diminish its ability to associate with the PTH receptor. Thus, the 3–34-amino acid sequence is an antagonist of PTH action. Complete loss of receptor binding capacity occurs after the removal of the 28–34-amino acid sequence. Consequently, the structural requirements for receptor activation reside in the amino-terminal portion of 1–34-PTH, while the receptor recognition component of the PTH molecule resides in the carboxy-terminus of this PTH fragment.

5.3.2. Biosynthesis, Secretion, and Metabolism

Synthesis of PTH occurs in the chief cells of the parathyroid glands. These cells possess the characteristics of active secretory cells with prominent Golgi apparatus and rough endoplasmic reticulum (RER) and many secretory granules. The process of PTH synthesis is complex and involves the sequential enzymatic cleavage of a precursor molecule as outlined in Figure 5-3.

The initial gene product is referred to as prepro-PTH; it consists of 115 amino acids with a molecular weight of 13,000 (see Figure 5-2). This PTH precursor is short-lived, and the 25-amino acid leader sequence is cleaved within a few minutes after translation. The leader sequence is particularly rich in hydrophobic amino acids, which probably play a role in the transport of prepro-PTH across the membranes of the RER. Cleavage of the leader sequence from prepro-PTH yields pro-PTH, a peptide consisting of 90 amino acids with a molecular weight of 10,200. This PTH precursor represents the 84-amino acid structure of intact PTH and a highly charged hexapeptide extension at the amino terminus of the molecule (see Figure 5-2). Pro-PTH is transported through the endoplasmic reticulum to the Golgi apparatus, where the hexapeptide extension is cleaved to form PTH. The conversion of pro-PTH to intact PTH occurs about 15 min after the translation of the PTH gene product. Subsequently, PTH is sequestered within secretory granules for storage and secretion.

In addition to storage and secretion, PTH is also subject to lysosomal-mediated degradation (see Figure 5-3). When serum calcium levels are low, approximately 60% of PTH is degraded and 40% is available for secretion. High levels of calcium result in increased degradation of PTH, leaving only about 20% of the newly synthesized PTH available for secretion. The rate of PTH synthesis is only slowly influenced by the

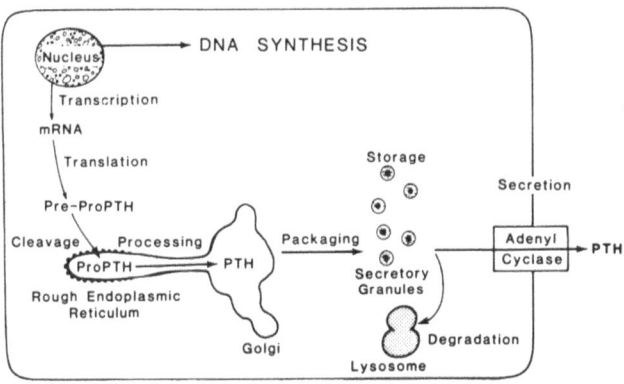

Figure 5-3. Schematic representation of the pathway of parathyroid (PTH) hormone synthesis and secretion.

concentration of extracellular calcium ion, while PTH secretion is exquisitely responsive to fluctuations in serum levels of ionized calcium. Total synthesis of PTH is more closely related to the mass of parathyroid tissue such that the rate of DNA synthesis or proliferation of parathyroid chief cells regulates the amount of PTH produced.

The major regulator of PTH secretion is the level of ionized calcium in the serum (see Figure 5-4). Dips in the serum levels of calcium below 9.0 mg/dl produce sharp increases in PTH secretion that are maximal (fivefold increase) at serum calcium levels of 8.0 mg/dl. Chronic hypocalcemia results in hyperplasia of the parathyroid glands and maximal production of PTH up to 50 times the basal rate. Increases in serum calcium concentration above 10.5 mg/dl reduce the rate of PTH secretion to basal levels, which are about 15% of normal. The basal secretion of PTH probably represents a calcium-independent component of PTH release. The actual process of PTH secretion is dependent on adenyl cyclase and the production of cAMP.

Circulating PTH is heterogeneous, consisting of intact PTH (84 amino acids), an amino-terminal fragment with a molecular weight of 3000–4000, and a larger carboxy-terminal fragment of 6000–7000 molecular weight (see Table 5-1). Intact PTH represents 10% of the total plasma immunoreactive PTH and exhibits a short half-life ($t_{\frac{1}{2}}$) of approximately 10 min. Similar amounts of the N-terminal fragments are found in the peripheral circulation and these also are short-lived. Both intact and N-terminal PTH possess biological activity. The majority (80%) of the immunoreactive PTH in plasma consists of carboxy-terminal fragments that are biologically inactive and cleared slowly ($t_{\frac{1}{2}}$ = 60 min).

The organs involved in the peripheral metabolism of PTH include

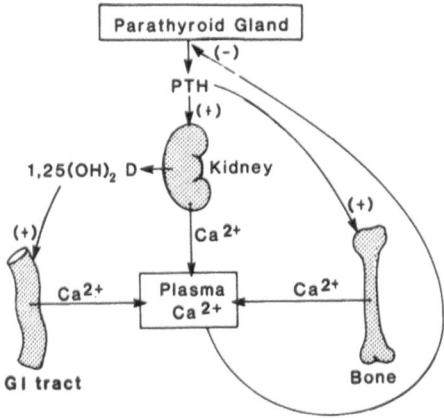

Figure 5-4. Regulation of parathyroid hormone (PTH) secretion.

Table 5-1. Characteristics of the Immunoreactive Fragments of Parathyroid Hormone

Fragment	Molecular weight	Total immunoreactivity (%)	Biological activity	Plasma half-life (min)
Intact PTH	9500	10	Yes	10
N-terminal	3000–4000	10	Yes	10
C-terminal	6000–7000	80	No	~60

the liver and kidneys (see Figure 5-5). Glomerular filtration is the primary route of elimination of the carboxy-terminal fragments, which are subsequently reabsorbed and degraded by the renal tubules. Intact PTH as well as the amino-terminal fragments are also eliminated by glomerular filtration.

5.3.3. Mechanism of Action

PTH effects are initiated after the interaction of the hormone with its receptors localized in the plasma membranes of target cells from bone and kidney (see Figure 5-6). The PTH receptor complex probably consists of three proteins: a receptor or recognition subunit, a guanine regulatory or coupling protein, and a catalytic or activating subunit, namely, adenyl cyclase. Increased levels of cAMP lead to the activation of cAMP-dependent protein kinases that phosphorylate key proteins involved in the regulation of calcium balance in bone and the kidneys.

The significance of the PTH receptor complex in mediating the actions of PTH is supported by studies of resistance to PTH. Pseudohypoparathyroidism is characterized by a hypoparathyroid state (i.e., hypocalcemia and hyperphosphatemia) despite adequate circulating levels of PTH. It is now apparent that patients with pseudohypoparathyroidism demonstrate insensitivity to PTH due to a deficiency of guanine regulatory protein or the coupling subunit in the PTH receptor system. In addition, chronically elevated levels of PTH can produce end-organ resistance to PTH by decreasing the number of PTH recognition (receptor) subunits in the plasma membranes of target cells. Presumably, chronically elevated PTH induces the internalization of its receptor by a homologous regulatory pathway without commensurate replacement of PTH receptors. The depletion of PTH receptors underlies the insensitivity of target cells to PTH after exposure to chronically elevated levels of the hormone.

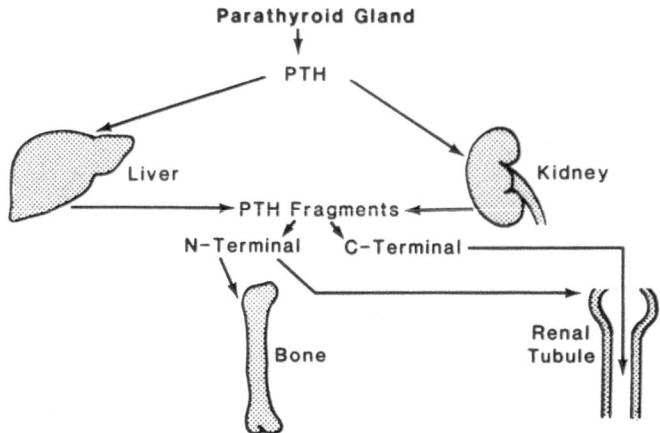

Figure 5-5. Peripheral metabolism of parathyroid hormone (PTH).

5.3.4. Physiological and Pharmacological Actions

The primary function of PTH is to prevent hypocalcemia. This is achieved by stimulating release of calcium from bone, increasing the reabsorption of calcium and the elimination of phosphate by the kidney, and indirectly enhancing the absorption of calcium by the intestine (see Table 5-2).

Mobilization of calcium from bone results from several actions of PTH, including stimulation of osteocytic osteolysis and resorption of

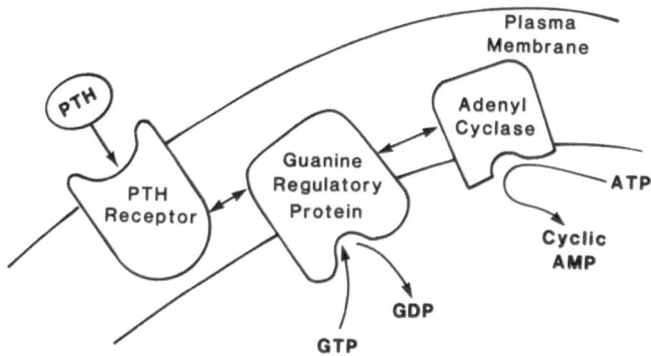

Figure 5-6. Schematic representation of the mechanism of parathyroid hormone action. GDP, guanine diphosphate; GTP, guanine triphosphate; PTH, parathyroid hormone.

Table 5-2. Physiological and Pharmacological Effects of Parathyroid Hormone

Organ	Effect
Bone	Increased resorption of calcium and phosphate
Kidney	Decreased calcium excretion; increased phosphate excretion; decreased reabsorption of bicarbonate; increased conversion of 25(OH) vitamin D to 1,25(OH)$_2$ vitamin D
Intestine	Increased calcium and phosphate absorption [*via* increased production of 1,25(OH)$_2$ vitamin D]

bone by existing osteoclasts, formation of new osteoclasts, and acute inhibition of osteoblast function and collagen synthesis (see Figure 5-4).

PTH acts on the kidney to stimulate renal tubular reabsorption of calcium and magnesium and to inhibit reabsorption of phosphate and bicarbonate in the proximal renal tubule. These actions are associated with the production of cAMP and an increase in urinary excretion of cyclic AMP is an indirect measure of PTH secretion and responnse. PTH also enhances the conversion of 25-hydroxy vitamin D to 1,25-dihydroxy vitamin D by stimulating 1-hydroxylase activity in the kidney. Increased levels of 1,25-dihydroxy vitamin D lead to enhanced reabsorption of calcium and phosphate by the intestine (see Figure 5-4).

5.3.5. Preparations

Parathyroid injection USP (Paroidin) is an extract prepared from bovine parathyroid tissue. PTH is administered by the subcutaneous, intramuscular, or intravenous routes. The oral route of administration is precluded due to the peptide nature of the hormone and its degradation in the gastrointestinal (GI) tract. The usual dose of PTH for diagnostic purposes in the assessment of pseudohypoparathyroidism is 200 units administered intravenously. One unit of PTH is 1/100 of the amount needed to elevate plasma calcium levels by 1 mg/dl within 16–18 hr after subcutaneous injection. Maximal effects are observed about 16 hr after subcutaneous injection and considerably sooner (usually within 30–60 min) after intravenous infusion. The duration of response varies from up to 36 hr after subcutaneous injection to a few hours after intravenous infusion of PTH.

5.3.6. Therapeutic Uses

PTH is not used in the treatment of hypocalcemia. Rather, hypo-calcemia is more appropriately managed by the administration of calcium and/or vitamin D. PTH is used in the diagnosis of pseudohypo-parathyroidism. Since these patients exhibit end-organ insensitivity to PTH, administration of PTH fails to alter plasma levels of calcium and fails to stimulate urinary excretion of phosphate or cAMP. PTH is also useful in preventing the hypocalcemic tetany that initially follows surgical parathyroidectomy.

5.3.7. Adverse Effects

Untoward actions of PTH are uncommon, since it is not used ther-apeutically in the management of chronic hypocalcemia.

5.4. CALCITONIN

5.4.1. Chemistry

Calcitonin is a 32-amino acid peptide with a molecular weight of 3500. A disulfide bond exists between amino acid residues 1 and 7 and forms a ring at the amino-terminus (see Figure 5-7). The amino acid sequences of human, rat, cow, pig, sheep, and salmon calcitonins are different. Rat differs from salmon calcitonin by only two amino acids. Salmon calcitonin is available in the United States for therapeutic pur-poses and differs from human calcitonin in 16 amino acids. Not sur-

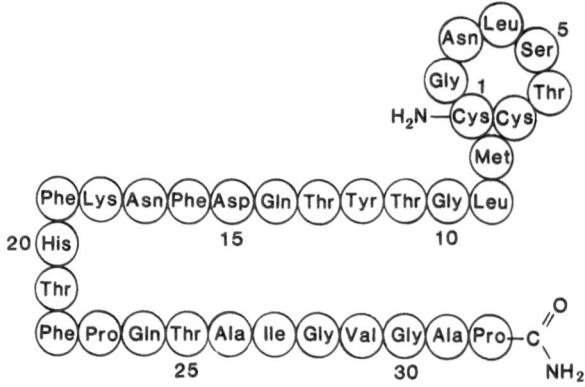

Figure 5-7.   Amino acid sequence of human calcitonin.

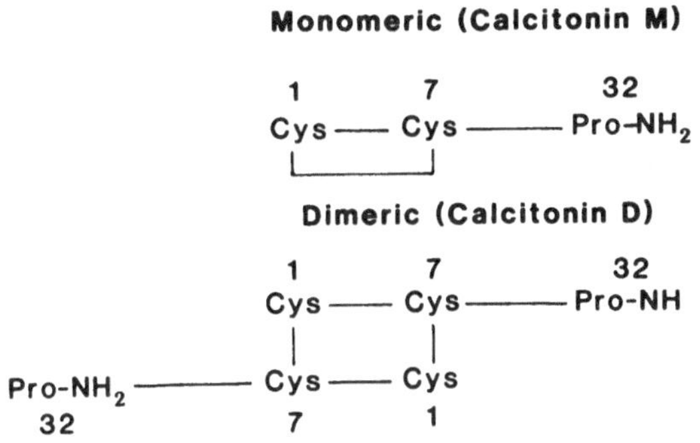

Monomeric (Calcitonin M)

```
   1       7        32
 Cys —— Cys ——————— Pro-NH₂
 |_____|
```

Dimeric (Calcitonin D)

```
          1       7        32
        Cys —— Cys ——————— Pro-NH
         |       |
Pro-NH₂ ——————— Cys —— Cys
  32              7      1
```

Figure 5-8. Monomeric and dimeric forms of calcitonin.

prisingly, salmon calcitonin is immunogenic in humans. Salmon calcitonin is, however, significantly more potent than most mammalian calcitonins. The increased potency of salmon calcitonin is largely attributable to a slower rate of degradation and a higher affinity for the calcitonin receptor. The entire 32-amino acid sequence of calcitonin is required for biological activity.

The reactivity of the disulfide bridge leads to the formation of dimeric and polymeric forms of calcitonin (see Figure 5-8). Dimeric calcitonin consists of two monomers associated in an antiparallel fashion. Polymeric forms of calcitonin are biologically inactive and constitute the major fraction of calcitonin produced by thyroid medullary carcinomas.

5.4.2. Biosynthesis, Secretion, and Metabolism

Calcitonin is synthesized in the parafollicular or C cells located in the middle third of the lateral lobes of the thyroid gland. These cells are distinct from thyroid follicular cells and contain well-defined nuclei, prominent mitochondria and Golgi apparatus, and secretory granules containing calcitonin.

Newly synthesized calcitonin exists in a larger precursor form. This calcitoninlike peptide has a molecular weight of 15,000. The amino-terminal leader sequence is cleaved producing a 12,000-M_r procalcitonin molecule that *in vivo* appears as a 17,000-M_r precursor due to glycosylation. Subsequent post-translational processing results in the calcitonin monomer, wth a molecular weight of 3500. Calcitonin is probably formed following the cleavage of both amino- and carboxy-terminal peptide sequences of procalcitonin.

Secretion of calcitonin is modulated by changes in serum levels of ionized calcium (see Figure 5-1). Small increases in the calcium concentration of the extracellular fluid above 9.0 mg/dl provoke the release of

calcitonin. Hypocalcemia reduces the plasma calcitonin to undetectable
levels. The process of calcitonin secretion is dependent on the generation
of cAMP. Gastrin, a GI hormone, and β-adrenergic agents also stimulate
the release of calcitonin.

The plasma half-life of human calcitonin is approximately 10 min;
however, salmon calcitonin is cleared more slowly. Clearance and metabolism of calcitonin occur in both the liver and kidneys, with the latter
playing a predominant role. Calcitonin is both filtered and metabolized
by the kidneys, since immunoreactive calcitonin is present in the urine
in only minor amounts. In patients with medullary thyroid cancer, the
calcitonin levels are elevated, and heterogeneous forms of the hormone
are present. Approximately 20–50% of the calcitonin in these patients is
monomeric. Circulating calcitonin in normal subjects is also probably
heterogeneous, but the low levels of hormone present make the degree
of heterogeneity difficult to resolve. Normal plasma levels of calcitonin
fluctuate between 5 and 100 pg/ml.

5.4.3. Mechanism of Action

Calcitonin binds selectively to plasma membrane-associated receptors in target tissues; this interaction leads to the production of cAMP.
It appears that cAMP is the second messenger mediating the actions of
calcitonin. Since both PTH and calcitonin increase cellular levels of cAMP,
the transfer of hormonal information must involve additional, more specific, factors. Alternatively, these hormones may interact with different
target cells. Calcitonin response cells in the renal tubules are localized
in the thick region of the loop of Henle and in the distal convoluted
tubule. These areas of the renal tubule respond poorly to PTH. Although
calcitonin antagonizes the effects of PTH, it does not prevent PTH-
induced actions. Therefore, calcitonin is a physiological antagonist of
PTH.

5.4.4. Physiological and Pharmacological Actions

The precise physiological role of calcitonin is unknown. There exist
no definitive clinical consequences of calcitonin deficiency or excess.
Removal of the thyroid gland is not associated with a tendancy toward
hypercalcemia. Similarly, the high levels of calcitonin produced by medullary thyroid carcinomas do not produce significant abnormalities in
calcium and phosphate balance. The observation that gastrin stimulates
calcitonin secretion before any alteration occurs in the plasma levels of

calcium suggests that calcitonin may be involved in preventing post-prandial hypercalcemia and in conserving calcium after feeding. Calci-tonin may also play an important role in calcium conservation during physiological states associated with high demands for calcium, such as during skeletal growth and lactation (see Table 5-3).

Inhibition of bone resorption is the most important pharmacological action produced by calcitonin. Osteoclastic bone resorption is almost com-pletely inhibited by sufficient doses of calcitonin. Loss of the resorbing surfaces of the osteoclasts occurs within 15 min after administration and is clearly apparent after 60 min. Osteocyclic osteolysis is also impaired by calcitonin but not to the extent of osteoclastic bone resorption. Diffusable levels of cytosolic calcium in bone cells are also reduced by calcitonin. Uri-nary excretion of hydroxyproline is reduced due to the decreased resorp-tion of the organic phase of the skeletal structure. Calcitonin does not stimulate bone formation. The most pronounced effects of calcitonin are seen under conditions of increased bone resorption, such as during growth, after PTH or vitamin D stimulation of bone metabolism, or in disease states characterized by an increase in bone resorption and turnover (e.g., Pa-get's disease, primary hyperparathyroidism).

The decreases in serum calcium and phosphate concentrations pro-duced by calcitonin are probably also related to the hormone-induced increases in the renal clearance of these ions. Renal tubular reab-sorption of calcium, phosphate, sodium, potassium, and magnesium is impaired by calcitonin action on the proximal tubular ion-transport systems. Unlike PTH, calcitonin does not stimulate urinary excretion of cAMP.

Calcitonin also influences the GI tract. Secretion of gastrin and gas-tric acid is decreased by calcitonin. As discussed previously, gastrin is capable of stimulating the secretion of calcitonin. It is likely that calci-tonin does not exert a major influence on the absorption of calcium by the intestine.

Table 5-3. Physiological and Pharmacological Effects of Calcitonin

Conservation of calcium after feeding and during lactation or
    skeletal growth (?)
Inhibition of osteoclastic bone resorption
Reduction of serum phosphate levels
Inhibition of gastrin and gastric acid secretion

5.4.5. Preparations

Calcitonin (Calcimar) is a synthetic 32-amino acid polypeptide that is identical to salmon calcitonin is provided in sterile solution containing 200 units/ml. One unit of activity is equivalent to approximately 4 μg of pure procine calcitonin. The hormone is administered subcutaneously or intramuscularly. Subcutaneous administration is more convenient for patients, and the intramuscular route is reserved for administering calcitonin doses in volumes greater than 2 ml. Synthetic human calcitonin (Cibacalcin) will soon be available for the treatment of Paget's disease.

The recommended dosage for the management of Paget's disease is 50–100 units/day or three times per week until a response is obtained. Maintenance therapy consists of 50 units of calcitonin administered three times per week. For hypercalcemia, 4 units/kg every 12 hr is indicated. If the response is not satisfactory after 1–2 days, dosage may be increased to 8 units every 12 hr.

Calcitonin (Calcimar) has been indicated for postmenopausal osteoporosis. Similarly, calcitrol (Rocaltrol) will soon be available for the treatment of senile osteoporosis.

5.4.6. Therapeutic Uses

There are two therapeutic indications for the use of calcitonin: Paget's disease of bone and hypercalcemic states (see Table 5-4). Bone pain is a common problem in Paget's disease, and approximately 70–80% of patients respond within 2–8 weeks of therapy. Patients who fail to benefit from calcitonin therapy may also be suffering from osteoarthritis. Neurological symptoms such as deafness and other cranial nerve palsies, and ataxia, paresis, and paraplegia may occur in as many as 40% of patients with Paget's disease. Calcitonin can reverse or halt the progression of neurological complications.

Table 5-4. Therapeutic Uses of Calcitonin

Paget's disease
Emergency treatment of hypercalcemia
   Hyperparathyroidism
   Idiopathic hypercalcemia of infancy
   Vitamin D intoxication
   Osteolytic bone metastases
Osteoporosis (?)

The effectiveness of calcitonin therapy is monitored by following decreases in urinary hydroxyproline and in serum alkaline phosphatase activity. After a year of therapy, a partial loss of responsiveness to calcitonin is seen in about 20% of those patients with Paget's disease who initially responded well to calcitonin. The loss of responsiveness may be related to the generation of neutralizing antibodies, since salmon calcitonin is immunogenic. Some of these patients subsequently respond to human calcitonin. It should be noted that approximately two-thirds of patients receiving salmon calcitonin develop neutralizing antibodies, yet most of these individuals do not become resistant to the drug. Downregulation of calcitonin receptors may also be involved in end-organ resistance to calcitonin.

Calcitonin is also widely used in the management of hypercalcemia, particularly cases produced by malignant disease. Approximately 75–90% of patients respond to treatment. Lowering of serum calcium occurs within a few hours after administration, decreasing further between 12 and 24 hr. Serum calcium levels may return to an elevated state in many patients despite continued calcitonin therapy. Therefore, calcitonin therapy should be considered for short adjunctive purposes in severe hypercalcemia, particularly if cardiac, hepatic, or renal disease limits other forms of therapy.

The effectiveness of calcitonin in the management of osteoporosis is unclear. If the osteoporosis is related to increased bone resorption, calcitonin therapy may be beneficial. The combination of calcium supplementation and calcitonin appears to be more effective in the management of osteoporosis associated with increased bone resorption. Osteoporosis resulting from reduced bone formation is not likely to respond to calcitonin therapy.

5.4.7. Adverse Effects

Chronic administration of calcitonin usually produces only mild untoward effects (see Table 5-5). The most common problem is nausea, which may occur in as many as 50% of patients but usually disappears with continued therapy. Facial flushing occurs in 20–30% of patients and usually lasts for 1–2 hr after administration. Less common problems include skin rash, swelling, and tenderness of the hands, as well as itching and frequent urination.

Clinical resistance to calcitonin occurs in up to 10% of cases. The molecular basis for this resistance is poorly understood but may be partially attributable to down-regulation of calcitonin receptors in target cells. Development of secondary hyperparathyroidism may also be in-

Table 5-5. Adverse Effects Associated with Calcitonin

Nausea
Facial flushing
Swelling and tenderness of hands
Inflammatory reaction at injection site
Urticaria (nonhuman calcitonin)
Antibody neutralization (nonhuman calcitonin)
Clinical resistance

volved in the development of clinical resistance to calcitonin. The generation of neutralizing antibodies to nonhuman calcitonin is not well correlated with the emergence of calcitonin insensitivity, but such a phenomenon may be a factor in diminishing the efficacy of calcitonin in some patients.

RECOMMENDED READINGS

Parathyroid Hormone

Arnaud, C. D., Calcium homeostasis: Regulatory elements and their integration, *Fed. Proc.* **37**:2557, 1978.

Habener, J. F., Recent advances in parathyroid hormone research, *Clin. Biochem.* **14**:223, 1981.

Habener, J. F., Regulation of parathyroid hormone secretion and biosynthesis, *Annu. Rev. Physiol.* **43**:211, 1981.

Habener, J. F., and Potts, J. T., Biosynthesis of parathyroid hormone, *N. Engl. J. Med.* **299**:580, 1978.

Habener, J. F., Rosenblatt, M., and Potts, J. T., Parathyroid hormone: Biochemical aspects of biosynthesis, secretion, action and metabolism, *Physiol. Rev.* **64**:985, 1984.

Martin, K. J., Hruska, K. A., Fretag, J. J., Klahr, S., and Slatopolsky, E., The peripheral metabolism of parathyroid hormone, *N. Engl. J. Med.* **301**:1092, 1979.

Raisz, L. G., Calcium regulation, *Clin. Biochem.* **14**:209, 1981.

Raisz, L. G., Mundy, G. R., Dietrich, J. W., and Canalis, E. M., Hormonal regulation of mineral metabolism, *Int. Rev. Physiol.* **16**:199, 1977.

Slatopolsky, E., Martin, K., Morrissey, J., and Hruska, K., Current concepts of the metabolism and radioimmunoassay of parathyroid hormone, *J. Lab. Clin. Med.* **99**:309, 1982.

Spiegel, A. M., and Marx, S. J., Parathyroid hormone and vitamin D receptors, *Clin. Endocrinol. Metab.* **12**:221, 1983.

Spiegel, A. M., Levine, M. A., Aurback, G. D., Downs, R. W., Marx, S. J., Lasker, R. D., Moses, A. M., and Breslau, N. A., Deficiency of hormone receptor adenylate cyclase coupling protein: Basis for hormone resistance in pseudo hypoparathyroidism, *Am. J. Physiol.* **243**:E37, 1982.

Calcitonin

Austin, L. A., and Heath, H., Calcitonin: Physiology and pathophysiology, *N. Engl. J. Med.* **304**:269, 1981.

Aviolo, L. B., Calcitonin therapy for bone disease and hypercalcemia, *Arch. Intern. Med.* **142**:2076, 1982.

Baba, H., Kishihara, M., Tohmon, M., Fukase, M., Kizaki, T., Okada, S., Matsuzuka, F., Kobayashi, A., Kuma, K., and Fujita, T., Identification of parathyroid homone messenger ribonucleic acid in an apparently nonfunctioning parathyroid carcinoma transformed from a parathyroid carcinoma with hyperparathyroidism, *J. Endocrinol. Metab.* **62**:247, 1986.

Deftos, L. S., and First, B. P., Calcitonin as a drug, *Ann. Intern. Med.* **95**:192, 1981.

Hoekman, K., Papapoulos, S. E., Peters, A. C. B., and Bijvoet, O. L. M., Characteristics and bisphosphonate treatment of a patient with juvenile osteoporosis, *J. Clin. Endocrinol. Metab.* **61**:952, 1985.

Martin, T. J., The therapeutic uses of calcitonin, *Scott. Med. J.* **23**:161, 1978.

Queener, S. F., and Bell, N. H., Calcitonin: A general survey, *Metabolism* **24**:555, 1975.

Stevens, J. C., and Evans, I. M. A., Pharmacology and therapeutic use of calcitonin, *Drugs* **21**:257, 1981.

Ziegler, R., Deutschle, U., and Raue, F., Calcitonin in human pathophysiology, *Horm. Res.* **20**:65, 1984.

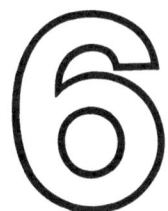

ANDROGENIC AND ANABOLIC STEROIDS

6.1. INTRODUCTION

Androgens are steroid hormones that possess virilizing actions and, consequently, serve to stimulate differentiation and maintenance of the androgen-dependent tissues of the male reproductive system. These hormones also play an important role in facilitating protein synthesis in androgen-sensitive tissues such as skeletal muscle, bone, and the kidneys. Both the androgenic and anabolic actions of the androgens are exploited therapeutically. The principal clinical uses of the androgens include replacement therapy in hypogonadism and anabolic stimulation in states of negative nitrogen balance. Significant interest has also been devoted to the development of androgen antagonists. These compounds hold great potential usefulness in the management of prostatic hyperplasia and carcinoma. Both conditions represent abnormal growth patterns that often exhibit a significant degree of androgen dependence, which could be antagonized by antiandrogens.

6.2. HISTORY

The relationship between castration and regression of male accessory sex organs was first characterized by Hunter during the late 1700s. Approximately a half-century later, the German physiologist Berthold demonstrated that the effects of castration in birds could be prevented by testicular implants. He concluded that the testes are responsible for the secretion of hormonelike substances that reverse the influences of castration. It was not until the 1930s that significant progress was made in the understanding of androgen physiology. In 1935, David and associates isolated testosterone from the testes; the same year, testosterone was successfully synthesized. The androgenic and anabolic actions of androgens were soon recognized, and efforts were devoted to the development of androgens devoid of virilizing (androgenic) actions. The steroids with the greatest ratio of anabolic-to-virilizing efficacy to be developed were 19-nortestosterone and its derivatives.

Before 1940, castration was utilized in the palliative management of androgen-dependent prostatic neoplasms. Huggins and colleagues developed a nonsurgical approach to the treatment of prostatic cancer by administering estrogens. The estrogenic hormones were capable of lowering plasma androgen levels and thereby limiting the growth of this androgen-dependent malignancy. The adverse effects of large doses of estrogen as well as incomplete suppression of androgen biosynthesis prompted investigations into the development of effective androgen antagonists. These drugs were designed to block the effects of androgens directly within target cells and limit their growth. Progestational compounds such as cyproterone acetate were recognized as effective antiandrogens. This area continues to be one of significant interest for the development of therapeutically effective compounds.

6.3. CHEMISTRY

Testosterone is a 19-carbon steroid molecule derived from cholesterol (Figure 6-1). The presence of angular methyl groups at positions 18 and 19 provides the fundamental structural formulation of the androgenic steroids. Substitution of a hydrogen atom at position 5 provides for the reduced series of androgens, the androstanes, of which 5α-dihydrotestosterone is a significant member. Like most steroid hormones, the androgens are highly lipid soluble, a property that markedly influ-

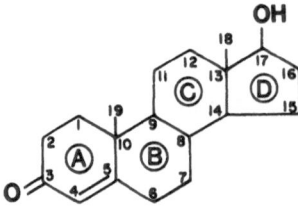

Figure 6-1. Molecular structure of testosterone, showing the numbering of the molecule.

ences their pharmacological use. Because of its chemical characteristics, testosterone is poorly absorbed from the gastrointestinal (GI) tract, and that which is absorbed is readily metabolized by hepatic oxidative enzyme systems. Chemical modification of the testosterone molecule has increased the therapeutic usefulness of the androgenic steroids. For example, alkylation at the C-17 position conveys significant efficacy *via* the oral route due to reduced susceptibility to hepatic metabolism. The 19-nortestosterone derivatives represent compounds that exhibit significantly greater anabolic actions than virilizing androgenic effects. In addition, members of this group are effective as antiandrogens and represent important constituents of oral contraceptive preparations (see Chapter 8).

6.4. BIOSYNTHESIS, SECRETION, AND METABOLISM

The biosynthesis of androgens occurs in several organs, including the testes, ovaries, adrenal cortex, and placenta. Conversion of precursors to androgens occurs in the liver, adipose tissue, and skin. In fact, in males two-thirds of the testosterone precursors (17-ketosteroids) are secreted by the adrenal cortex. The adrenocortical proandrogens are androstenedione and dehydroepiandrosterone. Importantly, the peripheral conversion of the proandrogens in males is limited; thus the androgens synthesized and secreted by the Leydig cells of the testes are the physiologically important androgens in the male.

Regulation of testicular androgen biosynthesis involves an intricate balance among the hypothalamus, adenohypophysis, and the testes (see Figure 6-2). Gonadotropin-releasing hormone (GnRH) is released by the hypothalamus and traverses the hypothalamic–adenohypophyseal portal vasculature to interact with specific receptor sites incorporated into the plasma membranes of gonadotrophs. GnRH stimulates the release of luteinizing hormone (LH) and follicle-stimulating hormone (FSH) from the anterior pituitary gland into the systemic circulation. Subsequently, LH stimulates the biosynthesis of testosterone by the testicular Leydig cells. FSH is responsible for regulating Sertoli cell function and spermatogenesis, which are dependent on androgens. The steroidogenic activity produced by LH is mediated by the induction of cAMP production and occurs following the association of LH with its specific receptors. Circulating androgens, principally testosterone, have a negative feedback on the adenohypophysis and the hypothalamus, suppressing LH and GnRH release and thereby modulating peripheral levels of androgens (see Figure 6-2).

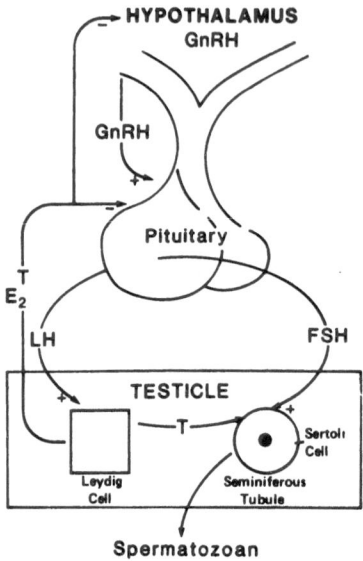

Figure 6-2. Regulation of testicular androgen biosynthesis. E_2 estradiol; FSH, follicle-stimulating hormone; GnRH, gonadotropin-releasing hormone; T, testosterone.

The pathways of testicular androgen biosynthesis are shown in Figure 6-3. Cholesterol derived from acetate by a series of reactions occurring in the endoplasmic reticulum is the required substrate for androgen synthesis. Transport of cholesterol to the mitochondria is followed by enzyme-mediated side-chain cleavage resulting in the production of pregnenolone. This reaction is the rate-limiting step in testicular androgen synthesis and is stimulated by LH. Pregnenolone serves as the principle precursor for testosterone synthesis, and the cytosolic metabolism of pregnenolone proceeds by two potential pathways.

The metabolic routes are identified as the Δ^4 and Δ^5 pathways, which refer to the position in the steroid molecule where unsaturation is maintained (see Figure 6-3). In the Δ^4 pathway, the bond between C-4 and C-5 (A ring) remains unsaturated (see Figure 6-1) whereas in the Δ^5 pathway the bond between C-5 and C-6 (B ring) remains unsaturated. In the testes, testosterone is primarily synthesized *via* the Δ^5 pathway. Therefore, pregnenolone is converted to 17α-hydroxyprogesterone, dehydroepiandrosterone, androstenediol and subsequently to testosterone.

Approximately 2.5–10 mg of testosterone is produced daily by the testes of normal men. Plasma levels usually range from 350 to 1000 ng/dl and fluctuate in a circadian pattern, with highest levels in the early morning. Levels of testosterone in the castrated adult are approximately 45 ng/dl and about 6–7 ng/dl in prepubertal males.

The ovaries and adrenal cortex in women normally secrete very little testosterone. However, these organs do secrete the testosterone precursors, androstenedione and dehydroepiandrosterone. These 17-ketosteroids are converted to testosterone by peripheral tissues such as the liver, adipose tissue, and skin. The daily production of androgens in women is about 0.23 mg, and normal plasma levels range from 15 to 65 ng/dl. Various pathological conditions (e.g., hyperplasia or carcinoma) of the ovaries and the adrenal cortex can markedly increase the

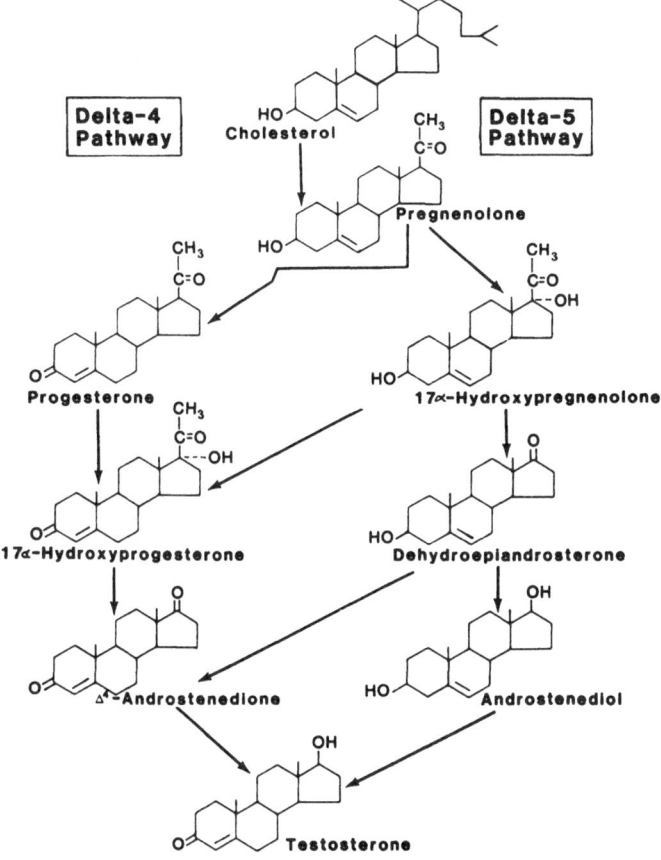

Figure 6-3. Pathways of testicular androgen biosynthesis.

production of testosterone and its precursors. If overproduction is marked and prolonged, precocious puberty, virilism, or amenorrhea may result. Hirsutism generally does not develop as a response to elevated total levels of androgens but rather to increased levels of free or unbound androgens.

Unexplained (idiopathic) failure of the Leydig cells in males occurs only rarely with aging. In addition, total plasma levels of testosterone change very little with age. Although the rate of secretion of testosterone declines after the fifth decade of life, a commensurate reduction in clearance of the androgens occurs, resulting in relatively stable age-related blood levels of testosterone. It does appear that the concentration of unbound (i.e., free) testosterone declines with age.

In men approximately 98% of peripheral testosterone is bound to plasma proteins, primarily to sex hormone-binding globulin (SHBG) and to albumin (see Figure 6-4). The binding to albumin is relatively non-specific, demonstrates low affinity, and is of high capacity, while the association of testosterone with SHBG is specific, demonstrates high affinity, and is of limited capacity. Approximately 58% of plasma testosterone is bound to SHBG, 40% is bound to albumin, and the remaining

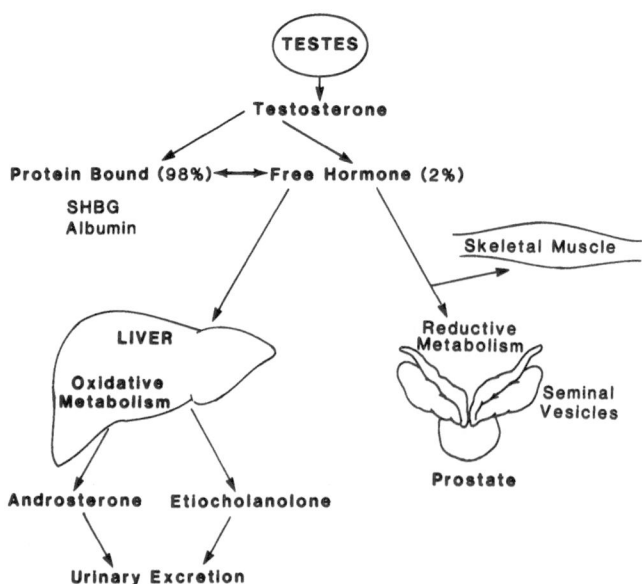

Figure 6-4. Dynamics of androgen assimilation. SHBG, sex hormone-binding globulin.

2% is unbound (free) and is therefore available for assimilation by peripheral target and nontarget tissues. SHBG levels are elevated by estrogens, explaining the rise in SHBG levels observed in cirrhotic patients, aging males, pregnant women, and women consuming combination-type oral contraceptives. Estrogens also compete with testosterone for the limited number of steroid-binding sites associated with SHBG.

The unbound testosterone is available either for oxidative metabolism by the liver and subsequent renal excretion or for assimilation by androgen-dependent tissues (e.g., prostate, seminal vesicles, epididymis) and by androgen-sensitive tissues (e.g., kidney, skeletal muscle, bone). Reductive metabolism of testosterone predominates in androgen-dependent tissues such as the male accessory sex organs. Testosterone is reduced to 5α-dihydrotestosterone (DHT) and subsequently to androstanediol (see Figure 6-5). The plasma half-life of testosterone is approximately 10–20 min; its short half-life largely limits the therapeutic use of the natural androgen testosterone.

The hepatic metabolism of testosterone is depicted in Figure 6-6. In addition to the primary metabolites, etiocholanolone and androsterone, small amounts of testosterone glucuronides and sulfates are also eliminated *via* the kidney. Only 6% of the testosterone is excreted unchanged, usually *via* the bile. The effect of hepatic metabolism is to increase the water solubility of the testosterone metabolites, thus increasing their rate of urinary elimination.

Free testosterone entering androgen-dependent tissues such as the prostate gland and related male accessory organs is readily metabolized to 5α-reduced derivatives of testosterone. Androgen-sensitive tissues such as the kidneys are organs that do not grow in response to testosterone but that are otherwise influenced by testosterone. In general, these tissues do not readily convert testosterone to 5α-reduced metabolites, and testosterone itself represents the active androgen. The reductive pathways of testosterone metabolism are represented in Figure 6-5. DHT is formed from testosterone by the enzyme 5α-reductase, which irreversibly reduces the Δ^4 double bond in the testosterone molecule. This reaction occurs in both the endoplasmic reticulum and the nuclear membrane. DHT is about 1.5–2.5 times more potent than testosterone as an androgenic steroid. Very little DHT enters the systemic circulation, where concentrations range from 35 to 75 ng/dl. Most DHT is localized within androgen-dependent target cells, where it modulates cell growth and function. In these tissues, DHT is subsequently converted, primarily to 3α,17β-androstanediol and to a lesser extent to 3β,17β-androstanediol. The 3α-derivative is readily converted back to DHT (see Figure 6-5). It

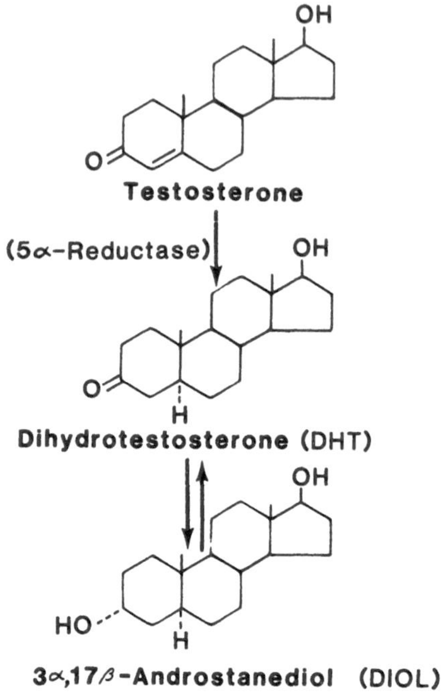

Figure 6-5. Metabolism of testosterone in androgen-dependent tissues.

is not certain whether 3α,17β-androstanediol possesses independent androgenic activity or whether it must be converted to DHT. Androstane 3β,17β-diol is not appreciably converted back to DHT and exhibits very low androgenic potency.

6.5. MECHANISM OF ACTION

Androgens, like all steroid hormones, produce their effects in target cells by associating with specific receptor proteins that exhibit both a high degree of specificity and a high affinity for androgenic steroids and related derivatives (see Figure 6-7). Androgen-dependent and -sensitive tissues contain cytosolic receptor proteins that recognize both testosterone and dihydrotestosterone. The affinity of these receptors for these androgens as reflected by the equilibrium dissociation constant (K_D) is approximately 1 nM. *In vitro* studies of the androgen receptor indicate that it is a protein of 8S molecular conformation as characterized by sucrose density gradient analysis. A smaller 3–4S-receptor protein also exists. Molybdate ion, a phosphatase enzyme inhibitor, stabilizes the androgen receptor in the large-molecular-weight form, suggesting that phosphorylation/dephosphorylation reactions are possibly involved in the activation of the androgen receptor. A similar phenomenon is postulated for the progesterone receptor (see Chapter 8). Little is known concerning the actual activation process for androgen receptors or the precise nature of the molecular events that mediate androgen effects. However, the importance of androgen receptors in mediating the actions of androgens is well recognized and is supported by the existence of complete or partial androgen insensitivity syndromes in humans that result from androgen receptor absence or the presence of abnormal androgen receptor proteins.

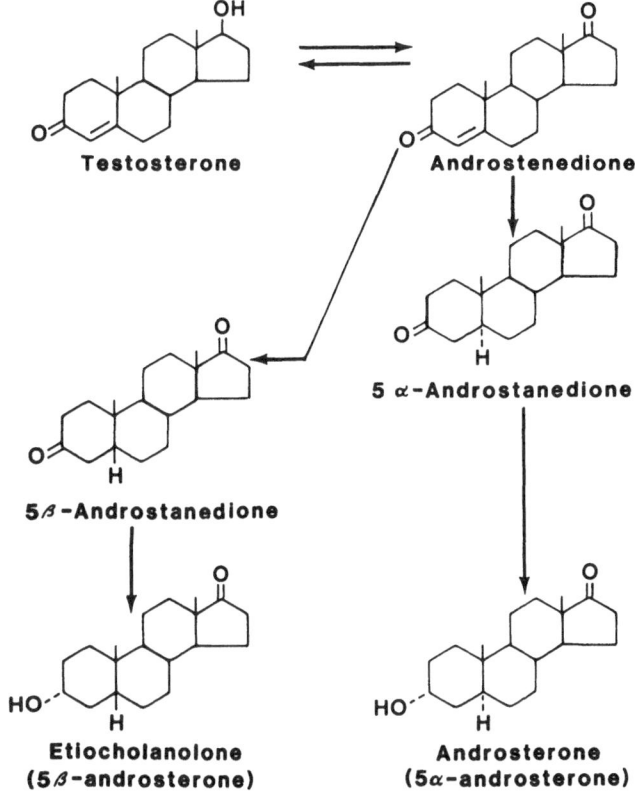

Figure 6-6. Pathways of hepatic catabolism of testosterone.

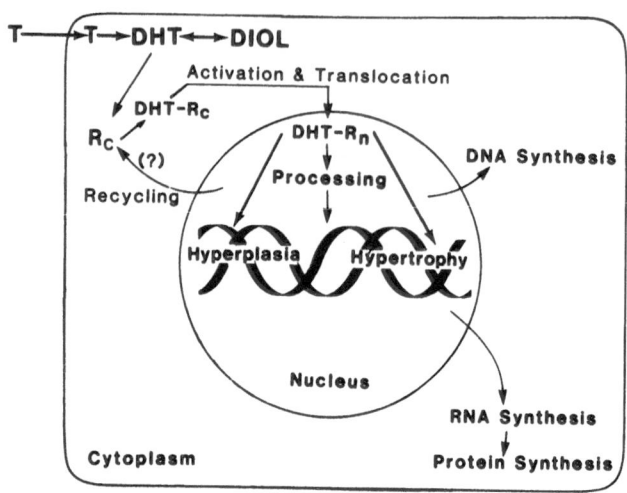

Figure 6-7. Schematic representation of the mechanism of androgen action. DHT, dihydrotesterone; Diol, androstanediol; R$_c$, cytoplasmic receptor; R$_n$, nuclear receptor; T, testosterone.

Normally, the majority (70–80%) of androgen receptors are localized in the nuclear compartment. The predominance of androgen receptors in the nucleus is a reflection of the relatively stable circulating levels of testosterone and of the significant availability of DHT in target tissues. Concentrations of DHT in male accessory sex organs are generally higher than the number of androgenic receptors. Association of testosterone, or more usually DHT, with the androgen receptor results in the translocation of this molecular complex to the nucleus (see Figure 6-7). Consequently, a significant proportion of cellular androgen receptors reside intranucularly. In the nucleus, the androgen receptor complexes associate with select sites on DNA, resulting in the stimulation of RNA synthesis, protein synthesis, and, at the appropriate periods of development, the proliferation of androgen-dependent target cells (see Figure 6-7).

The nature of the intranuclear actions of androgen receptor complexes is poorly understood. It is believed that at least a portion of these complexes associate with the nuclear matrix, the fundamental and dynamic proteinacious skeleton of the nucleus. A schematic representation of the interaction between androgen receptors and the nuclear matrix is outlined in Figure 6-8. The nuclear matrix is probably involved in a number of important nuclear events. Gene sequences, which are linked to the nuclear matrix, are those portions of the DNA molecule that are expressed. Processing of mRNA before transport to the cytoplasm apparently occurs on the matrix of the nucleus. Newly synthesized DNA is attached to the nuclear matrix and is then processed in supercoiled loops off the nuclear matrix (see Figure 6-8). Finally, the nuclear matrix changes appreciably in size during DNA synthesis and may be responsible for the increases in nuclear volume required for the initiation of cell proliferation. In view of the important role of androgens in regulating RNA and DNA synthesis, it is not surprising that androgen receptor complexes would be localized to, or associated with, the nuclear matrix, where critical portions of the genome are expressed. Although the localization of androgen receptors to nuclear matrix sites has been demonstrated, the precise biological role of androgen receptors and the nuclear matrix remains to be developed.

Androgen receptors represent important sites for interfering with androgen action. Indeed, the androgen antagonists or antiandrogens block androgen action by associating with androgen receptors, but these complexes fail to convey androgen efficacy. Access of testosterone or DHT to the androgen receptors is prevented by antiandrogens, and induction of androgen effects does not occur.

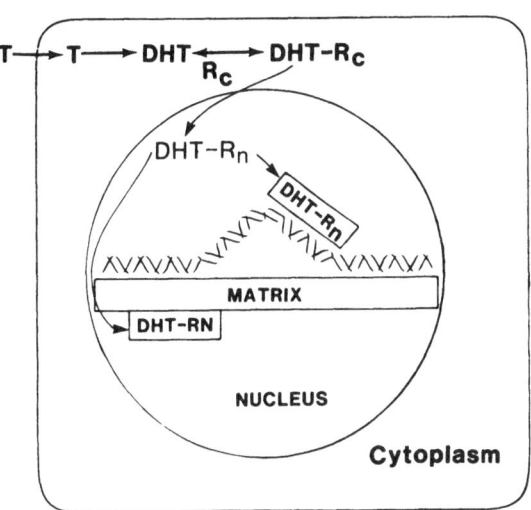

Figure 6-8. Schematic representation of the association of androgen receptors with the nuclear matrix. DHT, dihydrotesterone; Diol, androstanediol; R_c, cytoplasmic receptor; R_n, nuclear receptor; T, testosterone.

6.6. PHYSIOLOGICAL AND PHARMACOLOGICAL ACTIONS OF ANDROGENS

The androgens in males are responsible for the development and maintenance of the secondary sexual characteristics, normal reproductive function, and sexual performance. Androgens also stimulate growth and development of the skeleton and skeletal muscles during puberty (see Table 6-1). These hormones induce increases in long bone growth and subsequently terminate growth by initiating closure of the epiphyseal plates.

Growth of pubic hair and probably stimulation of libido are functions of androgens in women. Excessive production of androgens in women results in virilization characterized by acne, hirsutism, hoarseness, baldness, clitoromegaly, and menstrual irregularities.

The role of androgens in mediating aggressive male behavior is poorly understood, probably due to the complexity of factors influencing expression of behavior. It is likely that not only peripheral levels of androgens, but also the androgen-mediated imprinting of behavior, combine to constitute the male behavioral pattern. Additional factors are no doubt involved.

The physiological and pharmacological actions of androgens are classified as either morphogenic or excitatory, i.e., maintenance activity. The morphogenetic actions occur during embryogenesis and involve differentiation of the CNS and male reproductive system. The excitatory or maintenance actions consist of the pubertal and postpubertal effects of androgens on the male reproductive system. These effects are generally reversible, while the *in utero* effects of androgens are irreversible. Androgens are not involved in gonadal differentiation, but they do stim-

Table 6-1. Physiological and Pharmacological Actions of the Androgens

Androgenic Actions
Stimulate development of male reproductive tract *in utero*
Stimulate growth of male accessory sex organs, penis, and scrotum at puberty
Stimulate long bone growth and subsequent induction of epiphyseal plate closure at puberty
Maintain male secondary sex characteristics
Increase libido
Mediate aggressive behavior (?)
Anabolic Actions
Stimulate muscle development
Stimulate erythropoiesis

Table 6-2. The Androgenic Steroid Drugs

Drug	Trade name
Natural and Esterified Derivatives	
Testosterone	Oreton, Neo-Hombreo
Testosterone propionate	
Testosterone cypionate	Andro-Cyp, Depo-Testosterone, T-Ionate-PA
Testosterone enanthate	Andryl, Delatestryl, Generic
17 α-Aklylated Derivatives	
Methyltestosterone	Metandren, Oreton Methyl, Testred
Fluoxymesterone	Halotestin

ulate differentiation of the wolffian ducts into seminal vesicles, epididymus, and vas deferens. Androgens also stimulate the development of the labioscrotal swellings into the scrotum, the genital tubercle into the penis, and the urogenital sinus into the prostate gland. In addition to the protein anabolic actions of androgens, these steroids stimulate erythropoiesis by increasing renal production of erythropoietin and by exerting direct effects on bone marrow stem cell division.

6.7. PREPARATIONS

The androgens are classified broadly as either androgenic or anabolic in terms of biologic activity. It should be emphasized that no androgen exhibits solely androgenic or anabolic effects. The androgenic steroid drugs are listed in Table 6-2. These agents are further delineated as either natural and esterified androgens or as 17α-alkylated derivatives (see Figure 6-9). Esterification of testosterone extends its duration of action by delaying systemic absorption from intramuscular sites. In general, the longer the carbon chain of the ester substituent, the slower the release of the hormone into the circulation from intramuscular depot sites. Testosterone propionate is administered intramuscularly two to three times per week, while the longer-acting cypionate and enanthate derivatives are injected at 2–4-week intervals. Alkylation at the 17α-position retards the hepatic oxidative metabolism of testosterone. Therefore, methyltestosterone and fluoxymesterone are orally active androgenic steroid drugs. In contrast to the esterified derivatives, these an-

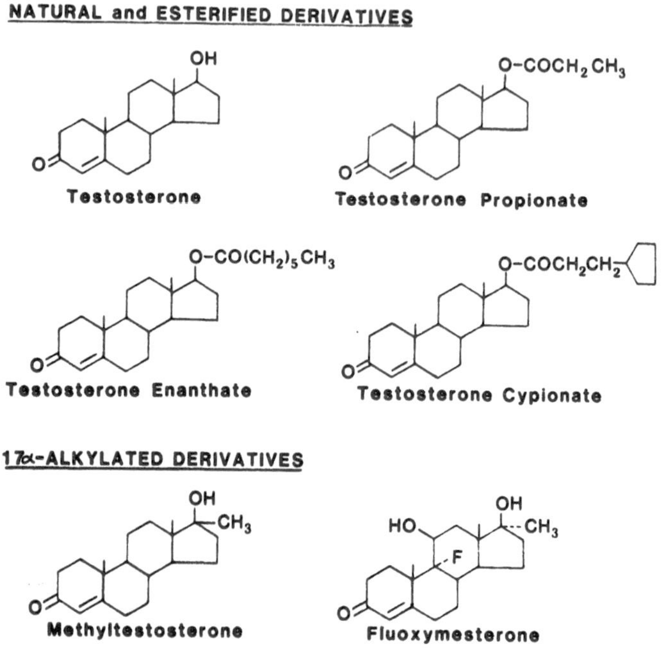

NATURAL and ESTERIFIED DERIVATIVES

Testosterone

Testosterone Propionate

Testosterone Enanthate

Testosterone Cypionate

17α-ALKYLATED DERIVATIVES

Methyltestosterone

Fluoxymesterone

Figure 6-9. Chemical structure of the androgenic steroid drugs.

drogenic hormones must be administered daily. The half-lives of the orally active androgenic steroids are brief, 10 hr for fluoxymesterone and 2.5 hr for methyltestosterone. Alkylation of the 17α-position conveys the potential for inducing hepatotoxicity.

The androgens that predominantly produce anabolic activity are listed in Table 6-3, and their molecular structures are detailed in Figure 6-10. It can be seen that these drugs are 19-nortestosterone derivatives. Anabolic androgens can be administered either orally or parenterally (see Table 6-3). Ethylestrenol, methandrostenolone, oxandrolone, oxymetholone, and stanozolol are orally active as a result of alkylation at C-17 of the androgen steroid nucleus. The anabolic steroids suitable for intramuscular injection are nandrolone phenpropionate, nandrolone decanoate, and methandriol. Among this group of anabolic drugs, only methandriol contains a 17α-alkyl group (see Figure 6-10).

The anabolic actions of these steroid drugs are largely a reflection of dose. When administered in high doses, even the anabolic androgens will produce virilizing side effects.

6.8. THERAPEUTIC USES

The androgenic steroids are used primarily for the induction of puberty in hypogonadism and in replacement or maintenance therapy of hypogonadism resulting from pre- or postpubertal failure of the testes (see Table 6-4). The longer-acting esterified derivatives of testosterone, the cypionate and enanthate esters, are preferred for induction of full sexual development when normal pubertal development fails. For induction of puberty, a dose of 25–50 mg/m^2 per month closely simulates the initial year of puberty. A dose of 100–150 mg/m^2 per month provides for normal mid-pubertal sexual development and for the growth spurt. Administration of 100–200 mg every 2 weeks will establish normal adult male plasma levels of testosterone. Large doses (200 mg) administered weekly will produce full sexual development in 2–3 years. The use of the long-acting esters is both convenient and also avoids the potential hepatotoxicity associated with the 17α-alkylated derivatives.

Testosterone propionate, the short-acting ester form, must be administered parenterally several times per week and is therefore not convenient for long-term replacement therapy. In older patients requiring androgenic steroids, the initial administration of a short-acting androgenic steroid is sometimes beneficial. If such therapy induces hypertrophy of the prostate gland and urethral obstruction, it can be readily reversed by cessation of therapy.

The short-acting orally active androgenic steroids with 17α-alkyl substitutions, such as fluoxymesterone and methyltestosterone, are generally less effective in replacement therapy than are the testosterone

Table 6-3. The Anabolic Steroid Drugs

Drug	Trade name
Oral Administration	
Ethylestrenol	Maxibolin
Methandrostenolone	Dianabol
Oxandrolone	Anavar
Oxymetholone	Anadrol-50
Stanozolol	Winstrol
Parenteral Administration	
Nandrolone phenpropionate	Androlone, Durabolin, Nandrolin
Nandrolone decanoate	Androlone-D, Deca-Durabolin
Methandriol	Anabol, Durabolic, Methabolic, Methydiol, Steribolic

ORALLY EFFECTIVE
_____

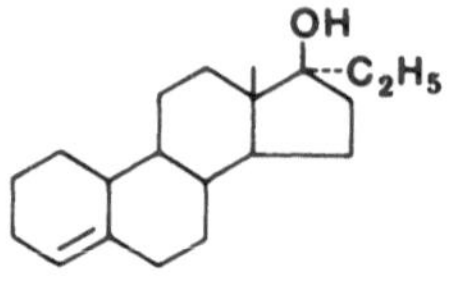

Ethylestrenol

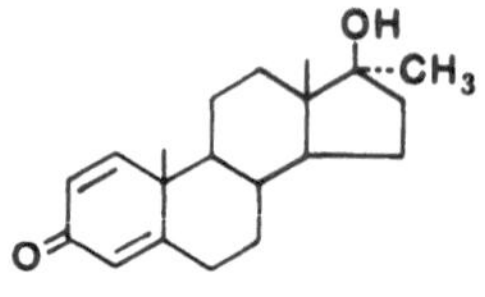

Methandrostenolone

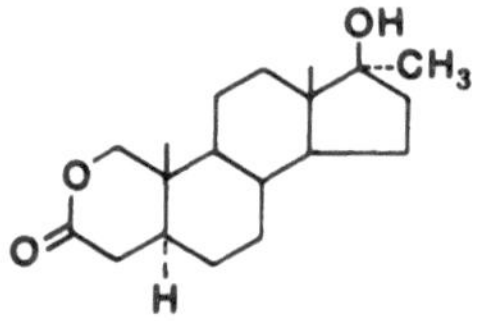

Oxandrolone

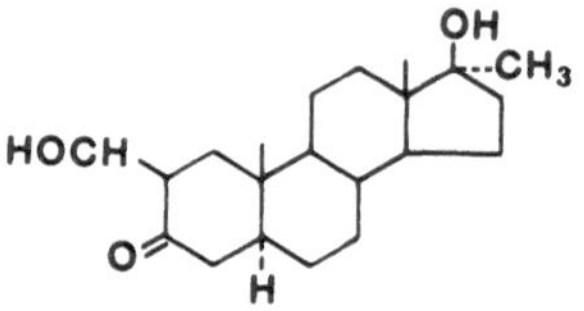

Oxymetholone

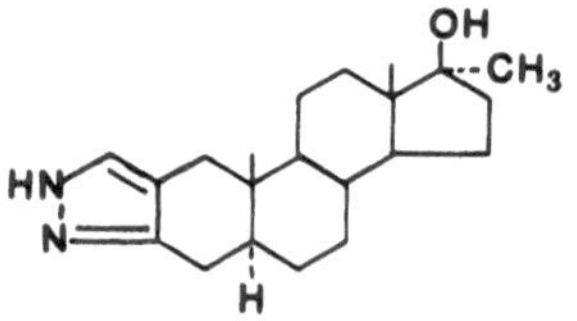

Stanozolol

PARENTERALLY EFFECTIVE
_____

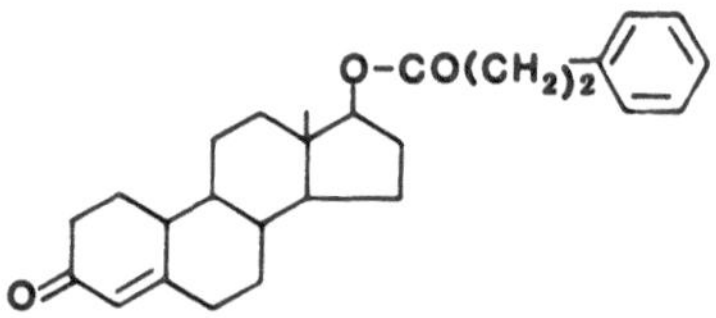

Nandrolone Phenpropionate

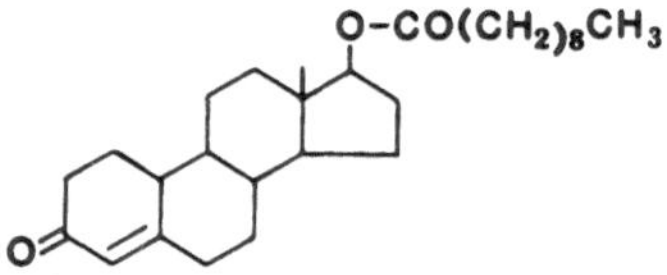

Nandrolone Decanoate

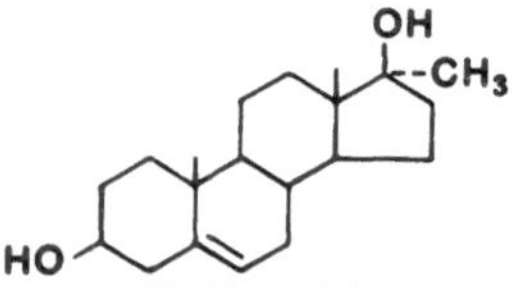

Methandriol

Figure 6-10. Chemical structure of the anabolic steroid drugs.

Table 6-4. Therapeutic Uses of the Androgenic and
Anabolic Steroids

Induction of puberty
Replacement therapy in hypogonadism
Maintenance of secondary sex characteristics
Stimulation of libido (females)
Stimulation of erythropoiesis (severe anemia)
Catabolic states (reverse negative nitrogen balance)

esters. However, they are useful in maintenance therapy when hypogonadism occurs in adulthood or after the development of secondary sexual characteristics. Doses ranging from 10 to 40 mg/day are usually employed in the management of androgen deficiency.

Anabolic steroids are usually utilized to reverse the negative nitrogen balance associated with certain catabolic states and to stimulate erythropoiesis in severe anemias (see Table 6-4). These drugs are sometimes used controversially for stimulation of growth in children. An anabolic steroid with a favorable anabolic : androgenic ratio is usually chosen for promoting growth. Oxandrolone with an anabolic : androgenic ratio of between 3 : 1 and 13 : 1 is such an agent. The choice of drug requires consideration for the balance between growth and stimulation of sexual maturation. Children should be 12 years or older with a bone age at least 2 years behind chronological age. The objective is to stimulate long bone growth without initiating premature closure of the epiphyseal plates, thereby limiting adult height. Therapy with oxandrolone (0.1–0.25 mg/kg per day) is usually pursued for 3–6 months, followed by a 6-month observation period without hormone administration.

Refractory anemias are sometimes managed with anabolic steroids. However, fewer than 50% of patients usually respond to this therapeutic approach. Three months of therapy are required. Anabolic steroids with low androgenic potency are usually used in women and children to minimize masculinization. Esterified androgenic steroids are reserved for long-term, high-dose therapy to avoid hepatic dysfunction.

Administration of high doses of glucocorticosteroids produces a negative nitrogen balance, which can be reversed by anabolic steroids. The use of anabolic steroids prevents corticosteroid side effects such as muscle wasting and demineralization of bone. Patients with chronic debilitating illnesses and those recovering from severe infections, surgery, burns, trauma, irradiation, or cytotoxic drug therapy often demonstrate defective protein synthesis, resulting in a negative nitrogen balance. Anabolic steroids are effective in decreasing or reversing this clinical condition, but the efficacy of these drugs requires adequate protein and caloric intake.

Athletes will occasionally use anabolic steroids to improve athletic performance, particularly in those events requiring acute muscular exertion. Such use of anabolic steroids is trivial and in some instances ineffective. In well-conditioned males there is little evidence to support the efficacy of these drugs. The weight gain associated with the use of anabolic steroids by these individuals is most likely related to fluid retention. Furthermore, large doses of anabolic steroids with 17α-alkyl groups may produce altered hepatic function, reduced serum gonadotropin and testosterone levels, and azospermia. Greater stimulatory effects of anabolic steroids on skeletal muscular development are observed in female athletes. However, the virilizing actions and menstrual irregularities associated with the use of these drugs underscore the inappropriateness of such use of the anabolic steroids.

Small doses of androgens are sometimes useful in increasing libido in women. Weak or impeded androgens are employed in the management of gynecological problems such as fibrocystic breast disease and endometriosis (see Section 6.10). The use of androgens in the palliative management of breast cancer is limited. These drugs are not particularly efficacious, and their use is superseded by endocrine ablative therapy and the administration of estrogen antagonists (see Chapter 7).

6.9. ADVERSE EFFECTS

Relative to other classes of steroid hormones, particularly the estrogens and glucocorticoids, the androgens are seldom capable of producing serious toxic side effects. The side effects associated with androgen therapy usually result from chronic administration (see Table 6-5). An excessive degree of virilization can occur in children and in women. In children this will be evidenced by signs of precocious puberty; in women signs of hirsutism, deepening of the voice, acne, alopecia, clitoral enlargement, and menstrual irregularities will indicate excessive androgenic stimulation. Acne and facial hair will usually be the earliest signs indicating a need for dose adjustment. Androgens may stimulate benign enlargement of the prostate gland in aging men, resulting in urethral obstruction. Paradoxically, androgens may cause gynecomastia in men and in boys as a result of the peripheral conversion of testosterone to estrogenic substances. This is more likely to occur after prolonged high-dose therapy or in men with liver disease.

Table 6-5. Adverse Effects of the Androgenic and
Anabolic Steroid Drugs

Excessive virilization in children and women
Stimulation of prostatic hyperplasia
Azoospermia
Gynecomastia
Salt and water retention
Jaundice (17 α-alkylated derivatives)
Masculinization of the female fetus

The alkylated androgenic and anabolic steroids have also been noted to produce hepatic dysfunction. Clinical jaundice occurs rarely, but the incidence suggests caution in the use of these drugs by patients with preexisting liver disease. Long-term, high-dose therapy with 17α-alkylated derivatives has been associated with hepatocellular and endothelial malignancy and intrahepatic hemorrhage. The testosterone esters and other parenteral androgens lacking the 17α-alkyl substitution do not alter hepatic function.

Androgens may produce fluid and salt retention, but this is rarely a serious problem except for elderly patients with congestive heart failure. These drugs will also suppress gonadotropin secretion. The fall in FSH impairs spermatogenesis (azoospermia), and the decline in LH levels reduces the rate of testicular androgen synthesis.

Pregnant women should not be treated with androgenic or anabolic steroids, since these agents can potentially masculinize the female fetus. Likewise, the androgens should not be administered to patients with prostatic carcinoma, since these cancers often exhibit androgen dependence, and administration of the androgens may exacerbate the disease.

The risk of hemorrhage in patients receiving coumarin and indandione anticoagulants is increased when 17α-alkylated androgens are administered. The androgens appear to enhance the potency of the anticoagulants. Methandrostenolone may inhibit the metabolism of oxyphenbutazone, producing a longer and more variable degree of antiinflammatory activity. Anabolic steroid use may require decreasing dosage of antidiabetic medication.

6.10. WEAK OR IMPEDED ANDROGENS

Danazol (Danocrine) is a synthetic derivative of 17α-ethinyl testosterone (ethisterone) that exhibits mild androgenic activity and is devoid of estrogenic or progestational activity. This drug is capable of suppressing the ovulatory surge in LH and FSH during the menstrual cycle. The molecular structure of danazol is given in Figure 6-11.

Peak blood levels of danazol are produced approximately 1–2 hr after oral administration. The plasma half-life of danazol is approximately 4.5 hr, and the drug is metabolized by the liver and excreted as sulfate and glucuronide conjugates. Danazol binds to androgen receptors and is capable of translocating cytosolic drug–receptor complexes to the nucleus. Data from clinical studies indicate that danazol directly inhibits gonadal and adrenal steroidogenesis.

Danazol is clinically useful when suppression of gonadal function in women is needed. Table 6-6 lists the therapeutic uses of danazol. In women this impeded androgen is employed in the management of fibrocystic breast disease and endometriosis.

The breast pain and tenderness associated with fibrocystic breast disease may be reduced during the initial month of danazol therapy, and the nodularity may disappear after 4–6 months of daily therapy. Approximately 80% of patients benefit from danazol administration. Symptoms may recur in 50% of patients within 1–2 years after the cessation of therapy. Another course of therapy can then be initiated. Irregular menses or amenorrhea is common during danazol therapy. The usual dosage of danazol for control of fibrocystic breast disease is 100–400 mg/day.

Danazol also produces atrophy of the endometrium in the uterus and at ectopic sites and, as such, is useful in the management of endometriosis. Amenorrhea results during therapy, but ovulation and menstruation are reestablished upon termination of danazol administration. Consequently, danazol is capable of restoring fertility in some women. Mild cases of endometriosis respond to danazol therapy in dosages of 200 mg/day. However, most women require 400–600 mg/day, and severe endometriosis may necessitate daily dosages of 800 mg/day.

Combined with testosterone therapy, danazol is being evaluated as a potential orally active male contraceptive. Danazol is the drug of choice in the treatement of hereditary angioedema, for which it is preferred because of its efficacy and low androgenic potency.

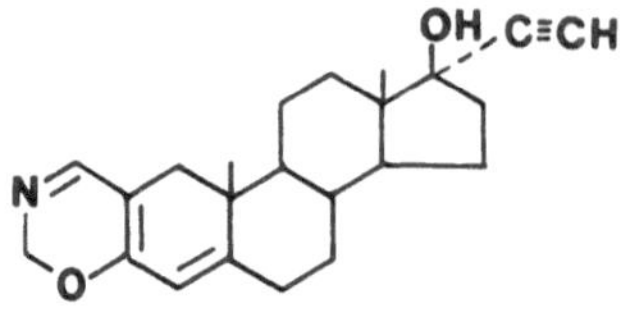

Figure 6-11. Chemical structure of danazol (Danocrine).

Table 6-6. Therapeutic Uses
of Danazol

Fibrocystic breast disease
Endometriosis
Hereditary angioedema
Male contraception (experimental)
Hemophilia A (classic hemophilia)

The adverse effects produced by danazol are attributable to its weak androgenic and anabolic actions. These effects include weight gain, edema, acne, decreased breast size, and hirsutism. Hypoestrogenic effects such as hot flushes and vaginitis occur in women. The safety of danazol during pregnancy is not known, but it may impair sexual development of the fetus. Danazol can produce hepatotoxicity and is not recommended for patients with impaired liver function.

6.11. ANDROGEN ANTAGONISTS

Antiandrogens are substances that prevent or depress the actions of testosterone and related androgens within target cells. Androgen antagonists would be of great benefit in the management of androgen excess, precocious puberty, acne, and hirsutism, as well as benign prostatic hyperplasia (BPH) and androgen-dependent carcinoma of the prostate gland.

Progesterone produces antiandrogenic activity, and other progesterone derivatives have been developed as antiandrogens as well. Two potential androgen antagonists are cyproterone acetate and flutamide, the molecular structures of which are presented in Figure 6-12. These drugs block androgen action by impeding androgen receptors. Flutamide consists of a nonsteroidal structure but acts in the same manner as cyproterone acetate. The antiandrogens produce fewer feminizing side effects as compared with estrogenic drugs, which minimize androgen action by suppressing testicular androgen biosynthesis. Primary side effects produced by the antiandrogens include inhibition of spermatogenesis, decreased libido, and occasionally gynecomastia. The effectiveness of cyproterone acetate in the management of BPH and prostatic cancer is being investigated. However, the antiandrogens are not formally established therapeutic agents.

Spironolactone is an exception (see Figure 6-12). Although spironolactone is an aldosterone antagonist (see Chapter 9), it also produces

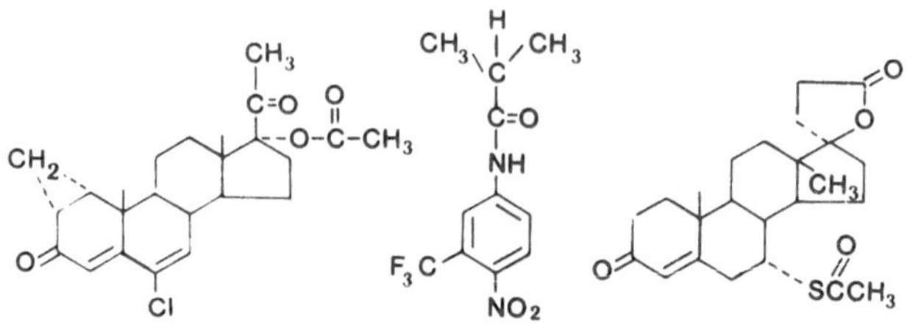

Figure 6-12. Chemical structure of the antiandrogenic drugs.

significant antiandrogenic activity. Spironolactone is therefore employed clinically in the management of hirsutism. Daily doses of 200 mg will usually reduce the density, diameter, and rate of hair growth in hirsute patients within 2 months. A maximal effect requires 6 months of therapy. As an aldosterone antagonist, spironolactone is utilized as a low-potency, potassium-sparing diuretic drug. Side effects of spironolactone include hyperkalemia, menstrual abnormalities, gynecomastia, sedation, headache, GI distress, and skin rashes.

Leuprolide acetate, an LH-RH analogue (see also Chapter 2) while not strictly considered an antiandrogen, will soon be available for the treatment of prostatic cancer. This agent represents a nonsteroidal approach to the therapy of adenocarcinoma of the prostate gland.

RECOMMENDED READINGS

Physiology of the Androgens

Brooks, R. V., Androgens, *Clin. Endocrinol. Metab.* **4**:503, 1975.

Bruchovsky, N., and Lesser, B., Proliferative growth by androgens, *Recent Prog. Horm. Res.* **32**:1, 1976.

deGroat, W. C., and Booth, A. M., Physiology of male sexual function, *Ann. Int. Med.* **92**:329, 1980.

Givens, J. R., Normal and abnormal androgen metabolism, *Clin. Obstet. Gynecol.* **21**:115, 1978.

Griffin, J. E., Leshin, M., and Wilson, J. D., Androgen resistance syndromes, *Am. J. Physiol.* **243**:E81, 1982.

Grody, W. W., Schrader, W. T., and O'Malley, B. W., Activation, transformation and subunit structure of steroid hormone receptors, *Endocrine Rev.* **3**:141, 1982.

Hammond, M. G., Talbert, L. M., and Groff, T. R., Hyperandrogenism, *Postgrad. Med.* **79**:107, 1986.

Janne, P. A., and Bardin, C. W., Androgen and antiandrogen receptor binding, *Ann. Rev. Physiol.* **46**:107, 1984.

Lipsett, M. B., Physiology and pathology of the Leydig cell, *N. Engl. J. Med.* **303**:682, 1980.

Lipsett, M. B., Physiology and pathology of the Leydig cell, *N. Engl. J. Med.* **303**:682, 1980.

Mawhinney, M. G., and Neubauer, B. L., Actions of estrogen in the male, *Invest. Urol.* **16**:409, 1979.

Penney, R., The testis, *Pediatr. Clin. North Am.* **26**:107, 1979.

Steinberger, E., Etiology and pathophysiology of testicular dysfunction in man, *Fertil. Steril.* **29**:481, 1978.

Wilson, J. D., Pathogenesis of benign prostatic hyperplasia, *Am. J. Med.* **68**:745, 1980.

Wilson, J. D., George, F. W., and Griffin, J. E., The hormonal control of sexual development, *Science,* **211**:1278, 1981.

Pharmacology of the Androgens

Kelley, V. C., and Ruvalcaba, R. H. A., Use of anabolic agents in treatment of short children, *Clin. Endocrinol. Metab.* **11**:25, 1982.

Lipsett, M. B., Use and abuse of androgens, *Consultant* **20**:146, 1980.

London, D. R., Medical aspects of hypogonadism, *Clin. Endocrinol. Metab.* **4**:597, 1975.

Ryan, A. J., Anabolic steroids are fool's gold, *Fed. Proc.* **40**:2682, 1981.

Snyder, P. J., Clinical use of androgens, *Annu. Rev. Med.* **35**:207, 1984.

Wilson, J. D., and Griffin, J. E., Use and misuse of androgens, *Metabolism* **29**:1278, 1980.

Pharmacology of Weak Androgens and Antiandrogens

Barbieri, R. L., and Ryan, K. J., Danazol: Endocrine pharmacology and therapeutic applications, *Am. J. Obstet. Gynecol.* **141**:453, 1981.

Chalmers, J. A., Danazol in the treatment of endometriosis, *Drugs* **19**:331, 1980.

Cumming, D. C., Treatment of hirsutism with spironolactone, *JAMA* **247**:1295, 1982.

Dowski, W. P., Endocrine properties and clinical application of danazol. *Fertil. Steril.* **31**:237, 1979.

Neumann, F. Pharmacology and potential use of cyproterone acetate, *Horm. Metabol. Res.* **9**:1, 1977.

Potts, G. O., Schane, H. P., and Edelson, J., Pharmacology and pharmacokinetics of danazol, *Drugs* **19**:321, 1980.

Smith, J. A., Luteinizing hormone-releasing hormone (LH-RH) analogs in treatment of prostatic cancer, *Urology* **27**:9, 1986.

Tindall, D. J., Chang, C. H., Lobl, T. J., and Cunningham, G. R., Androgen antagonists in androgen target tissues, *Pharmacol. Ther.* **24**:367, 1984.

7

ESTROGENS AND ANTIESTROGENIC DRUGS

7.1. ESTROGENS

7.1.1. Introduction

The estrogens acting in concert with progesterone are the ovarian hormones responsible for the regulation of female reproductive function. Importantly, the estrogens are required for the development and maintenance of the secondary sexual characteristics and the reproductive tract in females. These actions constitute the basis for the principal clinical uses of the estrogens. It is estimated that approximately 5–10 million women in the United States utilize estrogens in managing the symptoms secondary to the estrogen deficiency of menopause. Likewise, as many as 15–20% of women in their childbearing years employ combinations of estrogens and progestins for fertility control. Thus, the estrogens represent an important class of widely used drugs. However, the use of estrogens requires careful consideration of their pharmacological characteristics and their potential adverse effects.

7.1.2. History

Initial understandings of the estrogens and their actions developed in the early 1900s. Knauer in 1900 established the endocrine function of the ovaries by transplanting these glands into animals and preventing the symptoms associated with ovariectomy. At the same time, Halban demonstrated that sexual development and function were normal in castrated, immature animals that had been transplanted with ovaries. By 1923, Allen and Doisey had revealed that secretions from the ovarian follicle (graafian) were capable of stimulating growth of vaginal epithelium in ovariectomized rats.

In 1929 Doisey reported the isolation of estrone from the urine of pregnant women. Butenandt subsequently identified the structure of estrone in 1930, and MacCorquodale isolated estradiol-17β in 1935. Three years later, Dodd and associates prepared diethylstilbestrol (DES), the first orally active estrogen. Also in 1938, Inhoffen demonstrated that estradiol-17β could be made orally active by addition of an ethinyl substituent at the 17α-position. These early observations led subsequently to the development of a variety of standardized estrogenic preparations for clinical use.

During the past 20 years, emphasis has been focused on the molecular mechanism by which estrogenic drugs exert their effects in target cells. These studies were propelled largely by the development of radiolabeled estrogens that were essential for characterizing the molecular biology of estrogen action. During the early 1960s, Jensen and colleagues demonstrated the presence of receptors for estrogen in the cytoplasm and nuclei of uterine cells. Numerous investigators have subsequently revealed the significance of these specific receptor proteins in mediating estrogen action in normal and neoplastic target cells.

Studies of the estrogen receptor eventually led to the development of an additional group of drugs referred to as antiestrogens. These agents effectively block the receptor-mediated actions of the estrogens. Drugs in this class have an important role in the regulation of fertility and in the palliative management of estrogen-dependent neoplasms.

7.1.3. Chemistry

The estrogenic drugs are categorized according to their molecular structure as steroid hormones or as nonsteroidal compounds. Estradiol-17β, estrone, and estriol are naturally occurring estrogenic steroids in mammalian species (see Figure 7-1). DES and related drugs are examples of nonsteroidal estrogens and represent substituted stilbene derivatives. Methallenestril is a naphthylene derivative belonging to the nonsteroidal estrogen class.

Naturally occurring estrogens possess a cyclopentanophenanthrene nucleus and are characterized as 18-carbon molecules with an aromatic or phenolic A ring that is essential for estrogenic activity. Unlike the androgens and the progestins, the estrogens lack the angular methyl group at C-19. Chemical alteration of natural estrogens increases their

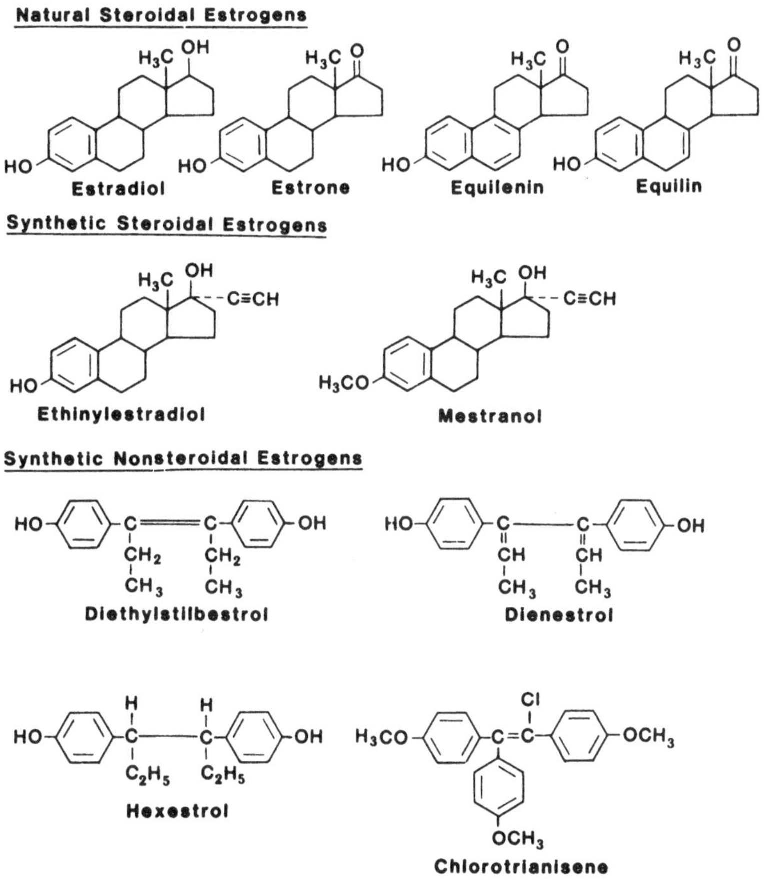

Natural Steroidal Estrogens

Estradiol   Estrone   Equilenin   Equilin

Synthetic Steroidal Estrogens

Ethinylestradiol   Mestranol

Synthetic Nonsteroidal Estrogens

Diethylstilbestrol   Dienestrol

Hexestrol

Chlorotrianisene

Figure 7-1. Molecular structure of the estrogenic drugs.

potency and affords oral efficacy by protecting the molecules from hepatic inactivation. Ethinyl estradiol is an example of a highly potent and synthetic (steroidal) estrogen to which an acetylene group has been added at C-17. The 3-methyl ether of ethinyl estradiol is mestranol, which must be demethylated in order to be biologically active (see Figure 7-1).

7.1.4. Biosynthesis, Secretion, and Metabolism

Estradiol-17β is the principal estrogen secreted by the ovary. Estrone, although secreted in small amounts by the ovary, is produced in the liver and muscle and in adipose tissue by oxidation of estradiol-17β. Estriol is produced by hydration of estrone.

Estrogen biosynthesis involves the conversion of cholesterol *via* intermediate products to estradiol-17β (see Figure 7-2). Cholesterol is either taken up by ovarian tissue or is synthesized as 2-carbon structures from acetate through acetyl coenzymes *via* mevalonic acid, squalene, lanosterol, and related substances.

Following the production of pregnenolone from cholesterol, estrogen biosynthesis in the ovary proceeds by either the Δ^5-3,β-hydroxysteroid pathway or *via* the Δ^4-3 ketone pathway. The first pathway is characteristic of steroidogenesis in the follicular phase of the menstrual cycle, reflecting the function of the thecal cells (see Figure 7-3). The Δ^5-3,β-hydroxysteroid pathway involves the production of 17α-hydroxypregnenolone and dehydroepiandrosterone en route to the synthesis of androstenedione, testosterone, and estradiol-17β. By the Δ^4-3 ketone pathway, androstenedione production occurs *via* intermediates, progesterone and 17α-hydroxyprogesterone. This pathway of steroidogenesis predominates in the luteal phase as a result of vascularization of the granulosa cells and of development of the corpus luteum (see Figure 7-3). Consequently, the elevated levels of estrogen in the follicular phase of the cycle are dependent on the limited development of luteal tissue, whereas postovulatory levels of both estrogen and particularly progesterone occur in the systemic circulation (see Figure 7-4).

Conversion of androstenedione to testosterone is followed by aromatization of the A ring of the steroid molecule, loss of C-19, and the production of estradiol-17β (see Figure 7-2). Metabolism of estradiol-17β to estrone occurs to a limited extent in ovarian tissue but occurs extensively in peripheral tissues such as liver, fat, skin, muscle, and endometrium and in the hypothalamus. Similar metabolism of androstenedione by these tissues also results in estrone production. The peripheral conversion of androstenedione to estrone can account for 20–30% of the daily estrogen production in premenopausal women.

A total of 100–600 μg of estradiol-17β is secreted daily by the ovaries of premenopausal women. Plasma levels of estradiol-17β vary during the menstrual cycle from a low of 50 pg/ml to as high as 200–300 pg/ml at the time of the preovulatory surge in gonadotropin secretion (Figure 7-4). During the initial portion of the follicular phase of the menstrual cycle, plasma estrogen levels rise slowly as the ovarian follicle grows in response to increasing levels of follicle-stimulating hormone (FSH). FSH interacts with receptors on the granulosa cells, and luteinizing hormone (LH) stimulates the thecal cells, where androstenedione and testosterone are produced. These androgens diffuse into the granulosa cells, where

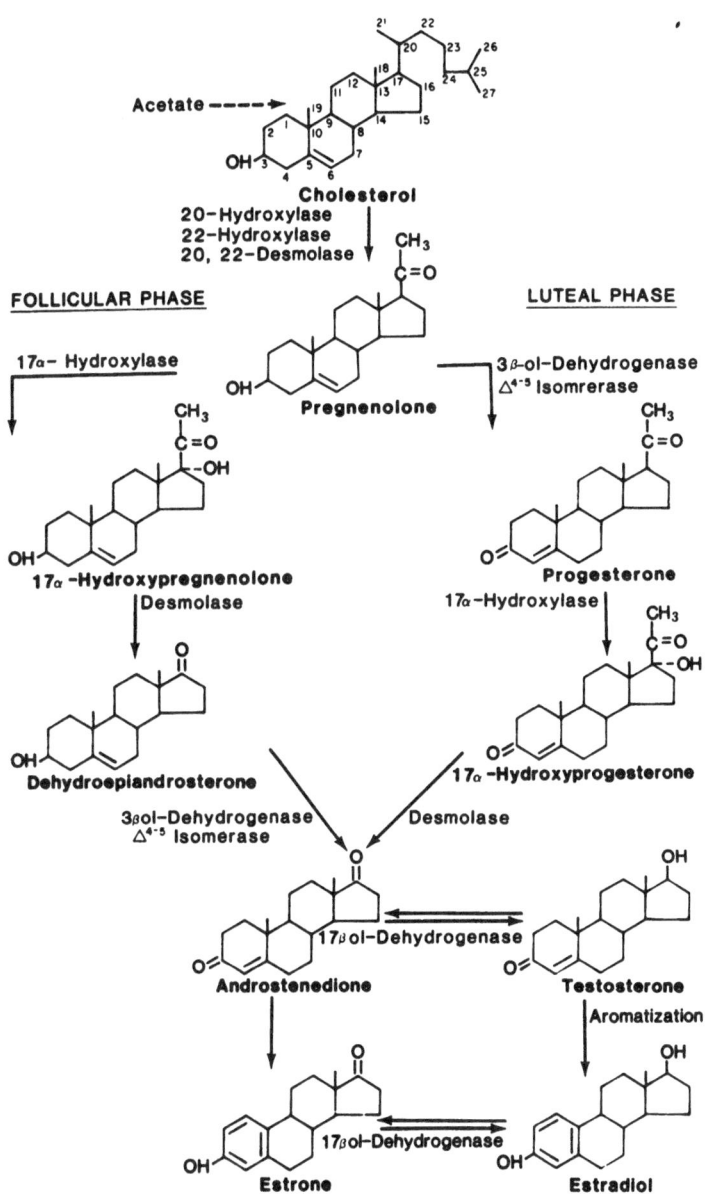

Figure 7-2. Biosynthetic pathway of ovarian steroidogenesis.

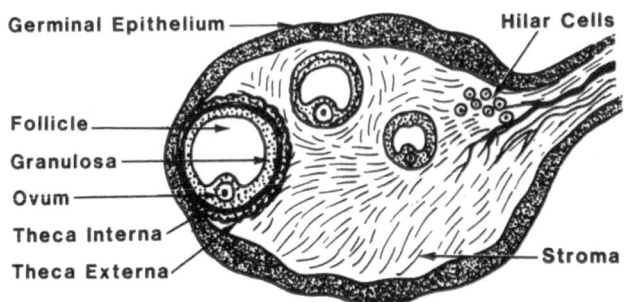

Figure 7-3. Schematic representation of ovarian morphology.

aromatization converts them to estrone and estradiol-17β. Rapid growth of the follicle before ovulation results in marked increases in circulating levels of estrogen. Rising estradiol-17β levels trigger the ovulatory surge of LH and FSH by a positive feedback mechanism. This surge in gonadotropin secretion from the adenohypophysis comes in response to the release of gonadotropin-releasing hormone (GnRH) from the hypothalamus. Secretion of GnRH is apparently dependent on adequate

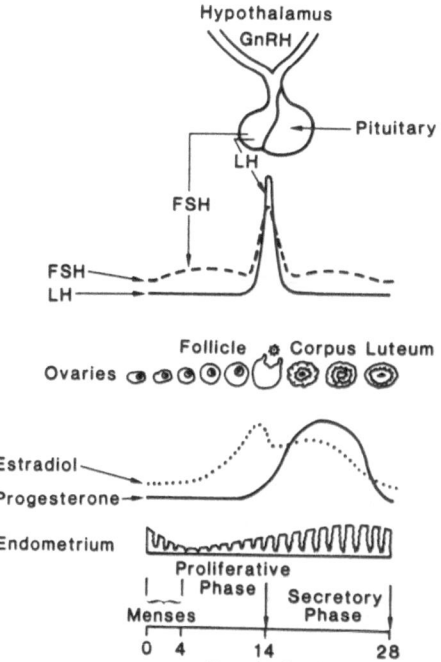

Figure 7-4. Hormonal regulation of menstrual function. FSH, follicle-stimulating hormone; GnRH, gonadotropin-releasing hormone; LH, luteinizing hormone.

estradiol-17β exposure. This involves not only that an adequate level (200 pg/ml) of estrodiol-17β be reached, but that this elevated level of hormone be maintained for a critical period (about 50 hr) as well. Elevated levels of gonadotropins are maintained for approximately 24 hr after which they decline in response to the inhibitory effects of increasing levels of progesterone and estradiol-17β secreted by the corpus luteum (see Figure 7-4).

The maturation of the corpus luteum that occurs postovulation is characterized by hypertrophy and vacuolization of the granulosa cells along with the accumulation of a yellow pigment, lutein (luteinization). Vascularization of the granulosa cells is also achieved. Maximal development of the corpus luteum occurs about 7 days after the LH peak, followed by a 7-day period of regression and declining steroid production. Degeneration of the corpus luteum is inevitable unless a new luteotropic stimulus appears. Chorionic gonadotropin produced by the placenta maintains steroidogenesis in the corpus luteum until the ninth or tenth week of gestation, at which time placental steroidogenesis is sufficient for maintaining pregnancy.

In postmenopausal women, estrogen production is primarily related to the synthesis of androstenedione in the adrenal cortex and its peripheral conversion to estrone. Aromatization of testosterone to estrone in tissues such as liver, muscle, and fat is chiefly responsible for estrogen production in males.

Much of plasma estradiol-17β is metabolized by the liver to estrone and estriol (see Figure 7-5). In addition, these estrogens are subject to

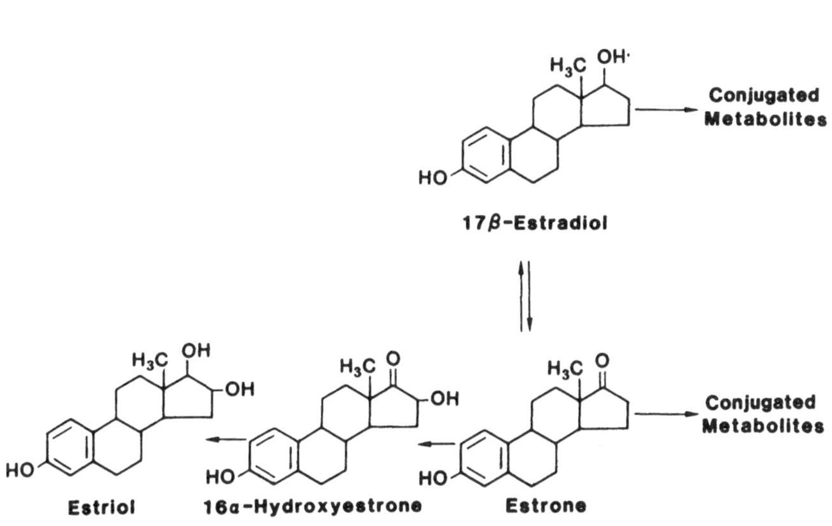

Figure 7-5.   Metabolism of estradiol-17β.

conjugation into glucuronides (C-3 and C-16) as well as sulfates (C-3). Hepatic metabolism of the estrogens markedly reduces their potency and increases their water solubility and renal excretion. Conjugated estrogens circulating in the biliary system are subsequently split by enzymes in the gastrointestinal tract. Most of the free estrogen is reabsorbed, with only a small percentage excreted in the feces.

Most of the synthetic estrogenic steroids are metabolized in a manner similar to that of the natural estrogens. Stilbene derivatives such as DES also undergo oxidation reactions to form short-lived semiquinone and quinone moieties (see Figure 7-6). These entities may be involved in mediating the toxic influences attributed to these nonsteroidal estrogens, particularly the teratogenic and carcinogenic effects.

7.1.5. Mechanism of Action

Estrogen-dependent tissues, such as the uterus, vagina, oviduct, and mammary gland, as well as estrogen-sensitive tissues, including the hypothalamus and anterior pituitary gland, retain radiolabeled estradiol-17β longer than is found in muscle or other estrogen-insensitive tissues. In addition, tritiated estradiol-17β becomes localized in the nuclei of estrogen-responsive tissues. Both the retention and the intranuclear localization of estradiol-17β that occur in estrogen target tissues are the result of an interaction between the steroid and specific molecular entities, referred to as estrogen receptors (see Figure 7-7).

In the absence of estrogen, these receptors appear to be predominantly localized in the cytoplasmic compartment, as evaluated by ligand binding assays. However, two experimental techniques—one a histochemical approach utilizing monoclonal antiboides against estrogen receptors and the other involving enucleation of estrogen-sensitive cells—indicate that estrogen receptors are primarily associated with or within nuclei even in the absence of endogenous estrogen. Nevertheless, when estrogen receptors are characterized (*in vitro*) by sucrose density gradient analysis, the cytoplasmic receptors migrate in the 8S region of hypotonic gradients (molecular weight, 360,000). In the presence of a high-salt

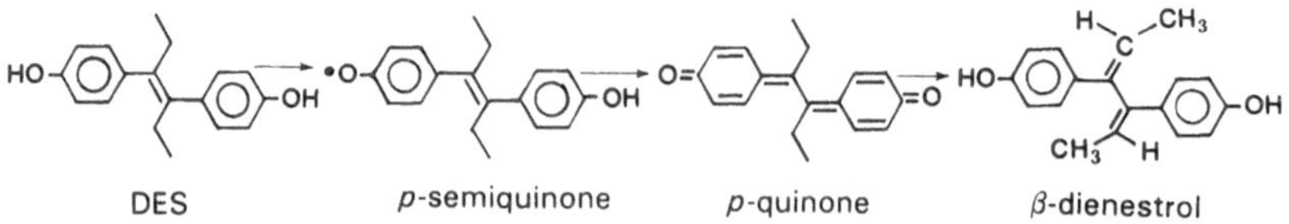

DES   *p*-semiquinone   *p*-quinone β-dienestrol

Figure 7-6. Oxidative metabolism of diethylstilbestrol (DES).

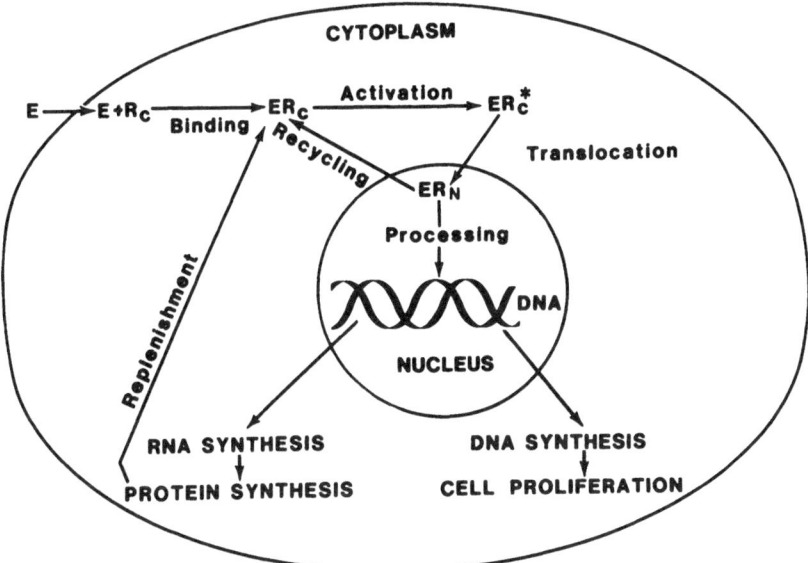

Figure 7-7. Schematic representation of the mechanism of estrogen action. E, estradiol-17β or analogue; R_c, cytoplasmic estrogen receptor; R_n, nuclear estrogen receptor.

solution, the molecular conformation of the cytoplasmic receptor is 4S, a smaller molecule with an estimated molecular weight of 80,000. The significance of salt-induced shifts in the molecular form of the cytoplasmic estrogen receptor is not clear. It seems that the 4S form of the protein is the native receptor and that the 8S molecular conformation represents an aggregated species. A shift from predominantly 8S receptor in low-salt solution to a 4S species in a hypertonic environment apparently represents a dissociation phenomenon.

Cytoplasmic estrogen receptors characteristically exhibit high affinity for estradiol-17β, with an equilibrium dissociation constant of 0.1 nM. The number of these sites in target tissues is generally low, approximating 10,000–20,000 sites per cell. Association of estradiol-17β with the 4S receptor results in a temperature-dependent activation of the cytoplasmic binding site (see Figure 7-7). At low temperature (0–4°C), binding of estradiol-17β to the receptor readily occurs, but this association does not result in activation or transformation of the hormone–receptor complex. At physiological temperature, binding of estrogen to the receptor induces activation of the steroid receptor. Activation of the cytoplasmic estrogen–receptor complex involves a shift in the molecular size or conformation of the receptor, as evidenced by the migration of the hormone–receptor complex in the 5S region of sucrose density gradients rather than in the 4S region. The increase in the apparent molecular size of the activated estrogen receptor suggests that this process involves a dimerization reaction, i.e., the addition of a molecular species of 50,000 M_r to the receptor complex. Alternatively, estrogen binding could induce a conformational change in the shape of the molecule such that sucrose gradient analysis reveals an apparent increase in the molecular weight of the receptor from 80,000 to 130,000.

Activation of the cytoplasmic estrogen receptor is required for subsequent translocation or retention of the complex by target cell nuclei (see Figure 7-7). On the basis of studies using purified antibodies against the estrogen receptor, it is evident that the cytoplasmic receptor is identical, at least relative to immunological criteria, to the nuclear estrogen receptor. Within the nucleus, estrogen receptors appear to interact with specific acceptor sites associated with select regions of DNA. However, it should be noted that the presence of nuclear acceptor sites for estrogen–receptor complexes remains largely conceptual.

It seems probable that there exist at least two nuclear binding sites for estrogen–receptor complexes. A relatively large number of nuclear binding sites with lower affinity for the estrogen–receptor complexes may guide the nuclear receptors to appropriate regions of DNA, where these complexes associate and are retained for prolonged periods (up to 24 hr) at a few higher-affinity acceptor sites. Estrogen receptors are found in association with the nuclear matrix of target cells, which may represent an important site for the regulation of gene expression. It appears that in order for nuclear estrogen receptors to exert full estrogenic activity, they must undergo a poorly understood processing reaction in the nuclear compartment, leading to association of the receptors with the genome.

The interaction between estrogen–receptor complexes and the high-affinity acceptor sites on DNA results in enhanced synthesis of RNA and proteins and in enhanced cellular proliferation. Estradiol-17β initially produces a rise in RNA polymerase II activity that leads to enhanced production of mRNA and proteins. Subsequently, RNA polymerase I activity is stimulated, leading to increased levels of rRNA. Prolonged retention of nuclear estrogen–receptor complexes results in a second rise in RNA polymerase II activity and the initiation of DNA synthesis by 18–24 hr after estrogen treatment in those cell types in which estrogen causes hyperplasia.

Full biological responses to estrogen appear to require both that an adequate number of estrogen receptors enter the nuclei and that these sites remain fully occupied in the nuclei for a critical period of time. This understanding is helpful in explaining the relative potency of estrogenic compounds. Estrone and estriol are recognized as weak estrogens. The fact that these hormones apparently fail to elicit full estrogenic responses in target cells relates to their rapid rate of dissociation from nuclear receptor sites. The increased tendancy to dissociate is a reflection of the lower affinity of these weaker estrogens for the estrogen receptor as compared with 17β-estradiol, DES, or ethinyl estradiol. Continuous administration of estriol or estrone results in full estrogenic responses as a result of complete and prolonged occupancy of nuclear estrogen receptors. Thus, in the physiological state estriol and estrone produce significant estrogenic activity.

The ultimate fate of nuclear estrogen receptors is not well understood. Initially, a larger number of estrogen receptors enter the nuclei under the influence of estradiol-17β than are required to produce full biological responses to estrogen. Although as many as 10,000–20,000 receptors for estrogen may enter the nucleus after administration of supraphysiological doses of estrogen, only 20% of these nuclear estrogen receptors are retained by target cells for a prolonged period (24 hr). In order for nuclear estrogen receptors to exert full estrogenic activity, they must undergo nuclear processing. Since there is often an excess number of nuclear estrogen–receptor complexes, many receptors escape nuclear processing and appear to be recycled to the cytoplasm for subsequent utilization. The mechanism by which recycling of nuclear receptors is accomplished is ill-defined, but it is known to occur independently of protein synthesis. In addition to recycling of nuclear estrogen receptors, estradiol-17β stimulates the replenishment of its receptors in the cytoplasm. Estrogen receptor replenishment results from the *de novo* synthesis of these proteins, as evidenced by the sensitivity of this process to inhibitors of RNA and protein synthesis (Figure 7-7).

7.1.6. Physiological Actions

The biological actions of the estrogens can be separated for convenience into effects on target cell growth and metabolic actions. Many of the effects of estrogen are outlined in Table 7-1. The estrogens are essential for the development of the secondary sexual characteristics in females and for the control of reproduction. These represent the principal physiological roles for the estrogenic steroids.

Estrogens induce the pubertal changes in the uterus, vagina, fallopian tubes, and the breasts and later maintain the integrity of these estrogen-responsive tissues. In this regard, the estrogens stimulate epithelial cell growth and in the breast specifically regulate development

Table 7-1.   Biological Actions of Estrogens

Development of the vagina, cervix, uterus, and fallopian tubes
Development of the uterine endometrium and myometrium
Growth of the ducts and stroma of the breast
Hypothalamic maturation
Distribution of body fat to hips and breast
Metabolic effects in liver and bone

---

of the ductal epithelial cells and breast stroma. The maturation of the hypothalamus to respond cyclically to changes in peripheral estradiol and progesterone levels is related to estrogen influences. Subsequently, estrogens support the physiological processes that ultimately result in production of an ovum and preparation of the uterine endometrium to support implantation. The estrogens also stimulate linear bone growth at puberty and eventually limit this growth by inducing epiphyseal plate closure.

The estrogenic steroids exert a number of metabolic actions in skin, bone, and liver. The normal structure of skin and blood vessels in women is at least partially dependent on estrogens. Bone resorption under the influence of parathyroid hormone is antagonized by estrogens, but these steroids do not stimulate bone formation after puberty. Estrogens increase the coagulability of blood, which is probably related to increases in clotting factors II, VII, IX, and X, to increased plasminogen levels and to reduced levels of antithrombin III. Sodium retention and its attendant accumulation of fluid are promoted by estrogens. These effects are the result of increased plasma renin activity and renin substrate and an elevated rate of aldosterone secretion.

7.1.7.   Therapeutic Uses

One of the principal therapeutic uses of estrogens is in combination with progestins to inhibit ovulation. The contraceptive use of estrogen is discussed in Chapter 8. Estrogens are also used extensively for replacement therapy in estrogen-deficient patients. Estrogen deficiency is usually related to failure of ovarian development, to castration, or to menopause. The major therapeutic uses of the estrogenic drugs are outlined in Table 7-2.

The development of secondary sexual characteristics in patients with failure of ovarian development requires initiation of estrogen therapy. This treatment is usually begun about the age of expected puberty—13 or 14 years. Therapy is initiated with small doses (0.01 mg) of ethinyl estradiol for 3 weeks out of every month. A doubling of dose may be indicated after 3 or 4 months of therapy. Higher doses increase the risk of side effects but may be indicated if no response is achieved. After an initial treatment period of 9 months, progesterone administration is usually added during the last 10 days of the estrogen therapy cycle. This will provide regular and visible menstrual bleeding. Progesterone administration may also protect against adverse side effects attributed to chronic and unopposed estrogen therapy.

Approximately 20–25% of postmenopausal women seek medical attention for menopausal symptoms, which include vasomotor instability (hot flushes and sweating), genitourinary atrophy (atrophic vaginitis and urinary incontinence), and osteoporosis. Generally, small doses of conjugated estrogens (0.625–1.25 mg/day) are adequate to manage the symptoms of menopause (90% effectiveness). Prolonged and unopposed estrogen therapy is not advised, since endometrial hyperplasia may result. Estrogens are usually administered in cyclical fashion to menopausal patients. Either estrogens alone are administered daily for 21 days with a 1-week cessation of therapy or estrogens are administered for 25 days of each month, with an orally active progestin included in the treatment regimen for the last 10 days of estrogen therapy (see Chapter 8).

Although estrogens do not stimulate bone formation, these steroids do antagonize parathyroid hormone-mediated bone resorption, leading to a reduction in the rate of bone loss in postmenopausal women. Unfortunately, there is currently no means of predicting which menopausal women are at high risk of developing severe osteoporosis. To be maximally effective in limiting bone resorption, estrogen therapy must be initiated soon after the onset of menopause before significant bone loss occurs; therapy must be continued indefinitely. Conjugated estrogens at a dosage of 0.625 mg/day are of demonstrated effectiveness in limiting the development of osteoporosis.

Abnormal uterine bleeding may be of organic origin (endometrial

Table 7-2. Therapeutic Uses of Estrogenic Drugs

Contraception
Replacement therapy in hypogonadism and menopause
Osteoporosis
Dysfunctional uterine bleeding
Suppression of postpartum lactation
Breast cancer (estrogen dependent)
Prostate cancer (androgen dependent)

cancer, coagulation defects, endometriosis, polyps, myomas, pregnancy complications) or may be dysfunctional, that is, caused by a disturbance in the balance between estrogen and progesterone stimulation. Often dysfunctional uterine bleeding is associated with anovulatory cycles in adolescence and the premenopausal years. This type of menstrual cycle produces an estrogen-dominated, fragile, hyperplastic endometrium. Periodic profuse bleeding episodes or irregular bleeding result from constant low-level estrogen stimulation. Dysfunctional uterine bleeding may also be caused by an atrophic endometrium produced by progesterone dominance. If the endometrium is hyperplastic, therapy with progesterone is beneficial. The atrophic endometrium responds to administration of an estrogen alone or to a combination of estrogen and progesterone.

Combinations of estrogen and progestins are also used to treat acne and hirsutism in females and for the diagnosis and treatment of amenorrhea. The effectiveness of this treatment is related to the suppression of androgen production through feedback inhibition of gonadotropin secretion and subsequently the suppression of ovarian function (see Chapter 8).

In postpartum patients, estrogens are effective in suppressing lactation. Estrogen therapy must be initiated shortly after parturition and continued for approximately 7 days. This approach is effective in approximately 80% of patients. An important factor in the success of estrogen therapy in the suppression of lactation is avoidance of the suckling stimulus, which elicits prolactin secretion. The mechanism by which estrogen antagonizes postpartum lactation is unclear, but it is probably related to the direct effects of estrogen on breast alveolar cells to decrease their sensitivity to prolactin. It should be noted that suppression of postpartum lactation is more effectively achieved by the administration of bromocriptine (Parlodel), a dopaminergic receptor agonist that is a highly potent inhibitor of prolactin secretion. Since postpartum lactation is dependent on prolactin, bromocriptine therapy (2.5 mg/day) initiated immediately after parturition and maintained for 14 days is very effective in terminating lactation.

Whereas estrogen in low doses will promote the growth of estrogen-dependent neoplastic breast cells, high doses of estrogen actually inhibit the growth of these cells by an undefined mechanism. Estrogen therapy utilizing DES or ethinyl estradiol is effective in approximately 35% of all postmenopausal breast cancer patients. Selection of appropriate patients for estrogen therapy has improved through the utilization of estrogen-receptor analysis. Approximately 70–80% of breast cancers in postmenopausal patients contain cells in which significant levels of estrogen receptors are localized. Two-thirds of estrogen receptor-positive patients benefit objectively from estrogen therapy (high doses of estrogen or endocrine ablative surgery), while the response rate among estrogen receptor-negative patients is 5–10%. Simultaneous presence of progesterone receptor, a biological marker of the functional integrity of the estrogen-receptor pathway in breast cancer cells, improves the probability of response to endocrine therapy to 80%. Fewer than 10% of patients who are negative for both estrogen and progesterone receptors respond to endocrine ablative surgery or to estrogen therapy. It should be noted that endocrine therapy for breast cancer is palliative in nature and that most cases require subsequent cytotoxic chemotherapy. Since the development of estrogen antagonists (antiestrogens), high-dose estrogen therapy for hormone-dependent breast cancer has become less popular. The use of antiestrogens in the management of breast cancer avoids the risks of estrogen-induced tumor flare, hypercalcemia, and cardiovascular accidents. The pharmacology of the antiestrogenic drugs is discussed in Section 7.1.8.

Estrogens are also utilized in the palliative therapy of prostatic adenocarcinoma. Approximately 70–80% of prostatic cancers initially exhibit androgen dependence. In supraphysiological doses, estrogens, like DES, chlorotrianisene, and ethinyl estradiol, suppress gonadotropin secretion in males, thereby inhibiting testicular androgen biosynthesis (see Chapter 6). The absence of testosterone results in regression of the androgen-dependent malignant cells of the prostate gland. The actions of estrogens to restrict the growth of prostatic cancer cells are not related to the direct effects of these hormones on prostatic tissue. The ability of select prostatic cancer patients who will exhibit responses of long duration after estrogen therapy has been improved through the utilization of dihydrotestosterone (DHT) receptor analysis. Patients whose prostatic cancer cells contain high levels of nuclear DHT receptors generally respond better to estrogen therapy and exhibit longer survival (see Chapter 6).

7.1.8. Preparations

The estrogenic drugs available for clinical use are listed in Table 7-3. There are three general groups of estrogens: (1) the natural steroidal estrogens, consisting of estradiol-17β, the esters of estradiol-17β (e.g., estradiol benzoate), estrone, and the conjugated estrogens (estrone sulfate, equilin); (2) the synthetic steroidal estrogens, comprising ethinyl

Table 7-3. Natural and Synthetic Estrogenic Drugs

Drug	Trade name
Natural Steroidal Estrogens	
Estradiol-17β	Estrace, Progynon
Estradiol benzoate	Generic
Estradiol cypionate	Depo-Estradiol Cypionate
Estradiol valerate	Delestrogen
Estrone	Follestrol, Theelin
Estrone piperazine sulfate	Ogen
Esterfied estrogens	Evex, Menest
Conjugated estrogens	Premarin
Synthetic Steroidal Estrogens	
Ethinyl estradiol	Estiny, Feminone
Mestranol	Enovio, Ovulen
Quinestrol	Estrovis
Synthetic Nonsteroidal Estrogens	
Chlorotrianisene	TACE
Diethylstilbestrol	
Benzestrol	
Dienestrol	
Hexestrol	
Methallenestril	
Promethestrol dipropionate	

estradiol, mestranol, and quinestrol; and (3) the synthetic nonsteroidal estrogens exemplified by DES. The molecular structures of the various estrogens are compared in Figure 7-1.

Estradiol-17β is not orally active due to its rapid hepatic inactivation after limited absorption from the intestinal tract. A micronized form of estradiol-17β is available for replacement therapy. Micronization causes a reduction in particle size, thereby increasing surface area, dissolution rate, and subsequent oral absorption. The required daily dosage (1–2 mg) of micronized estradiol-17β is 5–10 times the amount of estradiol-17β produced daily by the premenopausal ovary. Esters of estradiol-17β are administered intramuscularly in aqueous suspension or in oil in order to produce a gradual onset of action; thus, the duration of action is prolonged as well as variable. Estrogens may also be applied topically as well as by transdermal patches (e.g., Estraderm).

Estrone is generally less potent than estradiol-17β and is available as an aqueous suspension or as an oil solution for intramuscular injection. Vaginal suppositories are also available for direct delivery of estrogen in the management of genitourinary atrophy. Conjugated estrogens are sodium salts of the esters of estrone and equilin. The preparations contain 50–65% estrone sodium sulfate and 20–35% equilin sodium sulfate. These drugs can be administered orally, parenterally, or topically. Oral administration is employed for purposes of replacement therapy, while intravenous administration of conjugated estrogens is reserved for the emergency management of dysfunctional uterine bleeding. Esterified estrogens are also sodium salts of sulfate esters of estrogenic substances, principally estrone. Preparations of esterified estrogens contain 75–85% estrone sodium sulfate and 6.5–15% equilin sodium sulfate.

Ethinyl estradiol is the most potent estrogenic drug available. It is structurally related to estradiol-17β. The addition of an acetylene group at the 17α-position of estradiol-17β enhances biological activity due to decreased susceptability to hepatic metabolism. As a result, ethinyl estradiol is highly effective when administered orally. Mestranol represents the 3-methyl ether of ethinyl estradiol and is biologically inert until demethylation occurs *in vivo*.

DES, a derivative of stilbene, is a highly potent, nonsteroidal estrogen. DES and its related analogues, e.g., hexestrol and dienestrol, are slowly inactivated in the liver and are orally active. Chlorotrianisene is a proestrogen with a long duration of action. It must be metabolically converted into a biologically active estrogen. Its long duration of action makes chlorotrianisene unsuitable for treatment of menstrual disorders or for replacement therapy when cyclical therapy is desired. It is used principally in the palliative treatment of prostatic cancer.

Several factors influence the efficacy of estrogenic drugs, as outlined in Table 7-4. Dose, route of administration, absorption efficiency, metabolic clearance, affinity for estrogen receptor, and sensitivity of target tissues contribute significantly to the effectiveness of estrogenic drugs. Clearly, the rate of hepatic metabolism of estrogens is crucial to their degree of effectiveness. Whereas estradiol-17β is orally inactive due to rapid hepatic degradation, ethinyl estradiol as a result of alkylation at the 17α-position is afforded protection from hepatic enzymes and is highly efficacious upon oral administration. While estradiol-17β is not

Table 7-4. Factors Influencing the Efficacy of Estrogenic Drugs

Dose
Route of administration
Absorption efficiency
Metabolic clearance
Affinity for receptor
Tissue sensitivity

well absorbed orally, conjugated estrogens are readily absorbed (70–90%). The sulfate groups are subsequently cleaved enzymatically, and biologically active estrogens are produced. When administered parenterally, both estradiol-17β and estrone exhibit estrogenic activity, yet estradiol-17β is more potent. This difference stems from the fact that estradiol-17β has a considerably higher affinity for the estrogen receptor than does estrone or estriol. The higher affinity of the interaction between estradiol-17β and its receptor results in a decreased tendency for the hormone to dissociate from its receptor. More prolonged occupancy of the estrogen receptor is associated with full biological action if receptor recycling from the nucleus occurs. DES, ethinyl estradiol, and estradiol-17β exhibit similar affinities for the estrogen receptor and are highly potent estrogens.

The relative potencies of estrogenic drugs as determined by bioassay in the rat are presented in Table 7-5. A rank of potency would appear to be ethinyl estradiol > estradiol 17β > mestranol > estrone > estriol. However, the degree of difference in potency differs depending on the specific estrogen-dependent system being studied. When a comparison of equieffective doses of estrogenic drugs is made in humans, a similar relationship is seen as is revealed in Table 7-6. Ethinyl estradiol and mestranol are clearly more potent than the conjugated estrogens, DES or estradiol-17β.

Estrogenic drugs are used frequently in replacement therapy for hypogonadism or in menopause. These drugs can be administered orally, parenterally, or topically. The dose and route of administration depend largely on the drug's molecular structure. Table 7-7 lists estrogenic drugs with respect to dosage for replacement therapy, the dosing interval, and route of administration.

Table 7-5. Relative Potency of Estrogenic Drugs as Determined by Bioassay in the Rat

Drug	Relative response (%)	
	Gonadotropin suppression	Ovulation blockage
Estradiol-17β	100	100
Estrone	30	150
Estriol	10	15
Ethinyl estradiol	300	170
Mestranol	100	85

Table 7-6.   Comparison of Equieffective
Doses of Estrogenic Drugs in Humans

Drug	Required dose[a] (mg)
Estradiol-17β	5.0
Diethylstilbestrol (DES)	5.0
Conjugated estrogens	3.75
Mestranol	0.08
Ethinyl estradiol	0.05

[a] Measured response: (1) suppression of ovulation, (2) vaginal cornification (maximal), (3) endometrial proliferation (maximal), (4) cervical mucus fern (maximal).

Several of these drugs are also employed in the palliative management of hormone-dependent neoplasms of the breast and prostate gland. The estrogenic drugs usually utilized for the treatment of malignant disease are DES, chlorotrianisene, ethinyl estradiol, conjugated estrogens and estrone. The usual dosages and dosing intervals for the use of these drugs in breast and prostate cancer are presented in Table 7-8. The doses of these drugs in the management of malignant disease are significantly higher than doses employed in replacement therapy and should be considered supraphysiological.

Table 7-7.   Estrogenic Drugs Used in Replacement Therapy

Drug	Dose for replacement therapy (mg)	Dose interval	Route of administration
Estradiol-17β	25	3–4 months	SC (implant)
Estradiol-17β (micronized)	1–2	5 days/week	Oral
Estradiol benzoate	0.5–1.5	2–3 days/week	IM
Estradiol cypionate	1–5	Weekly	IM
Estradiol valerate	10–40	1–4 weeks	IM
Estrone	0.1–2	Weekly	IM
Estrone piperazine sulfate	0.35–1.5	Daily	Oral
Conjugated estrogens	0.3–1.25	Daily	Oral
Esterified estrogens	0.3–1.25	Daily	Oral
Ethinyl estradiol	0.02–0.05	Daily	Oral
Diethylstilbestrol	0.2–0.5	Daily	Oral
Hexestrol	0.2–0.1	Daily	Oral

Table 7-8. Estrogenic Drugs Used in the Palliative Therapy of Breast and Prostate Cancer

Drug	Site of malignancy	Dose (mg)	Dose interval	Route of administration
Estone	Prostate	2–4	2–3 days/week	IM
Conjugated estrogens	Breast	10	t.i.d.	Oral
	Prostate	1.25–2.5	t.i.d.	Oral
Ethinyl estradiol	Breast	1	Daily	Oral
	Prostate	0.15–2.0	Daily	Oral
Chlorotrianisene	Prostate	12–25	Daily	Oral
Diethylstilbestrol (DES)	Breast	15	Daily	Oral
	Prostate	1–3	Daily	Oral

7.1.9. Adverse Effects

The chief adverse actions of estrogens used in replacement therapy are nausea, endometrial hyperplasia, and breast tenderness. Males receiving high dosages of estrogens for palliative therapy of prostate cancer will demonstrate indications of feminization, as evidenced by the development of gynecomastia. Adverse effects of the estrogenic drugs are detailed in Table 7-9. In the present context the emphasis is on the untoward effects of estrogen used in replacement therapy; adverse effects of estrogens when combined with progestins for oral contraceptive purposes are discussed in Chapter 8.

Nausea may occur during the initial phase of estrogen therapy. Continued treatment (1–2 weeks) usually results in the disappearance of this untoward effect. If estrogens are taken with food, the probability of GI distress is minimized. Approximately 6–10% of patients taking ethinyl estradiol can be expected to develop nausea. Natural estrogens are less likely to produce nausea and vomiting. Large doses of estrogen used in the endocrine therapy of breast cancer invariably produce nausea, but this problem usually disappears after the second week of therapy.

The development of endometrial hyperplasia after chronic unopposed estrogen therapy must be considered a significant risk and is indicated by abnormal uterine bleeding. Endometrial hyperplasia develops in approximately 12% of patients receiving unopposed estrogen therapy. It should be recognized that the occurence of endometrial hyperplasia places a patient at significantly higher risk for subsequently developing adenocarcinoma of the endometrium. The potential for producing excessive stimulation of the endometrium is clearly related to both the dose of estrogen and the duration of treatment. Higher doses and longer periods of administration of highly potent estrogens are more likely to produce abnormal proliferation of endometrial cells.

Breast tenderness may also plague as many as 12% of patients receiving estrogen replacement therapy. Fullness of the breasts results from the direct stimulatory effects of estrogens on the ductal epithelium as well as to estrogen-induced edema secondary to sodium and water retention. Breast tenderness is an early clinical indication of excessive estrogen dosage. Aggravation of cystic breast disease may also occur after estrogen use and is reversible upon termination of estrogen administration. Cystic mastitis is a reflection of direct stimulatory effects of estrogen on growth of the ductal epithelial cells.

Administration of estrogenic drugs may increase systolic (5–6 mm Hg) and diastolic (1–2 mm Hg) blood pressure. However, hypertension is generally not associated with the use of estrogenic drugs in replacement therapy. The hypertensive actions of estrogens are apparently related to the ability of these steroids to increase plasma renin activity, renin substrate, and the secretion of aldosterone. These effects lead to increased sodium reabsorption and water retention, producing edema.

The effects of estrogen administered in replacement therapy on serum lipids are variable. Total cholesterol is usually reduced slightly, while triglycerides are increased. Concentrations of high-density lipoproteins are elevated by estrogens. The risk of gallbladder disease is significantly increased in patients taking estrogens and is apparently linked to increased levels of cholesterol in the bile.

Estrogens have been associated with reduced glucose tolerance, thromboembolic disease, and increased risk of myocardial infarction.

Table 7-9. Adverse Effects Associated with Estrogenic Drugs

Nausea, vomiting, and diarrhea
Breast tenderness
Aggravation of cystic breast disease
Endometrial hyperplasia
Salt and water retention
Hypertension
Gallbladder disease
Cholestatic jaundice
Thromboembolic disease
Feminization (males)
Teratogenesis
Breast and endometrial malignancy (?)

Generally, these risks are not significant when estrogens are used in dosages for replacement therapy.

High doses of estrogen administered to breast cancer patients in whom bone metastases have been found may produce hypercalcemia, which is reversible after cessation of treatment. In prostatic cancer patients receiving large doses of estrogens, gynecomastia develops as a result of the direct actions of these steroids in stimulating epithelial cell growth in the ducts of the male breast. Galactorrhea is not usually an associated characteristic of feminization in these patients.

Concern remains regarding the role of exogenous estrogens in the etiology of breast and/or endometrial cancer. The evidence has not substantiated a role for estrogen replacement therapy in the development of breast cancer. However, studies have demonstrated increasing support for the risk of estrogen therapy in stimulating adenocarcinoma of the endometrium. This relationship is more evident in those patients receiving estrogens without progesterone opposition.

DES has been definitely linked to the development of clear cell adenocarcinoma of the vagina in the daughters of women who received this estrogen during the first trimester of pregnancy. A variety of other structural abnormalities, including vaginal adenosis, cervical erosion, and transverse fibrous ridges in the vagina and on the cervix have been attributed to *in utero* exposure to DES. Defects in the development of the reproductive system of male offspring from DES-treated mothers have been identified and include epididymal cysts, hypoplastic testes, cryptorchidism, and decreased sperm production. Whether these carcinogenic and teratogenic actions are exclusively related to DES or to all estrogenic drugs is not clear. Recent studies revealing the pathways of oxidative metabolism of DES (see Figure 7-6) suggest that the production of metabolites capable of adversely affecting DNA may be restricted to estrogenic drugs with a stilbene structure (Figure 7-1).

The adverse effects ascribed to estrogenic drugs suggest some relative and absolute contraindications for the uses of these agents in replacement therapy (see Table 7-10). Relative contraindications for estrogen use include a family history of breast or uterine malignancy, severe varicose veins, a history of liver disease, and hypertension. The presence of estrogen-dependent breast or uterine cancer, undiagnosed uterine bleeding, a history of severe thromboembolic disease, and acute liver disease are absolute contraindications for administration of estrogenic drugs in replacement therapy.

Despite the fact that estrogenic drugs exhibit some potentially harmful effects, these agents can be used with relative safety in the management of estrogen deficiency. The current guidelines for prudent use of

Table 7-10. Contraindications for Estrogenic Drugs in
Replacement Therapy

Relative contraindication
    Family history of breast or uterine malignancy
    Uterine leiomyomata
    Varicose veins (severe)
    History of liver disease
    Hypertension
Absolute contraindication
    Estrogen-dependent breast or uterine cancer
    Abnormal genital bleeding (undiagnosed)
    History of thromboembolic disease (severe)
    Liver disease (acute)

estrogens in replacement therapy are outlined in Table 7-11. Following the establishment of an indication for estrogen therapy, it is advisable to select the lowest effective dose of estrogen and the shortest duration of therapy required for the management of symptoms. In chronic estrogen replacement therapy, cyclical administration of estrogen combined with progestin challenge or opposition therapy aids in avoiding estrogenic hyperstimulation and perhaps provides protection from the development of breast and uterine malignancy. Regardless, annual histological evaluation of the endometrium and breast mammography should be conducted in order to detect malignant transformation of these tissues in postmenopausal patients.

7.2. ANTIESTROGENS

There are currently two clinically useful estrogen antagonists: clomiphene citrate (Clomid) and tamoxifen citrate (Nolvadex). The molec-

Table 7-11. Guidelines for the Clinical Use of Estrogenic
Drugs in Replacement Therapy

Lowest effective dose
Shortest duration of therapy required
Cyclical therapy (estrogen for 21–25 days/month)
Progestin challenge therapy (days 16–25 of estrogen therapy)
Histological endometrial evaluation (annual)
Breast mammography (annual)

ular configurations of clomiphene and tamoxifen (see Figure 7-8) are
very similar to those of DES and chlorotrianisene (Figure 7-1). The estrogen antagonists are triphenylethylene derivatives in which the ether
side-chain moiety is essential for antiestrogenic activity.

Like the nonsteroidal estrogenic drugs, the antiestrogens are orally
active and undergo hepatic metabolism. Tamoxifen has recently received
extensive pharmacokinetic study. It is metabolized in the liver to more
polar mono- and dihydroxylated derivatives (see Figure 7-9). The mo-
nohydroxylated derivative exhibits higher antiestrogenic potency than
the parent compound, while the dihydroxylated metabolite is a weaker
antiestrogen. Excretion of both clomiphene and tamoxifen occurs primarily in the feces (60–80%) and to a lesser extent in the urine (20–40%).

Although tamoxifen and clomiphene are characterized as antiestrogens, they are actually partial estrogen agonists. These drugs initially
bind and activate cytoplasmic estrogen receptors in target cells (see Figure 7-7). Furthermore, the drug–receptor complexes are translocated to
the nucleus, where they stimulate the early actions of estrogens. However, the antiestrogen–receptor complexes fail to promote full estrogenic
activity, which involves stimulation of tissue growth and requires prolonged association of the receptor complexes with DNA. In spite of the
failure to induce full estrogenic activity, the antiestrogens do appear to
prevent recycling of the nuclear estrogen receptors to the cytoplasm.
Thus, the antiestrogens deplete target tissues of their cytoplasmic estrogen receptors and produce a state of estrogen insensitivity or estrogen
antagonism.

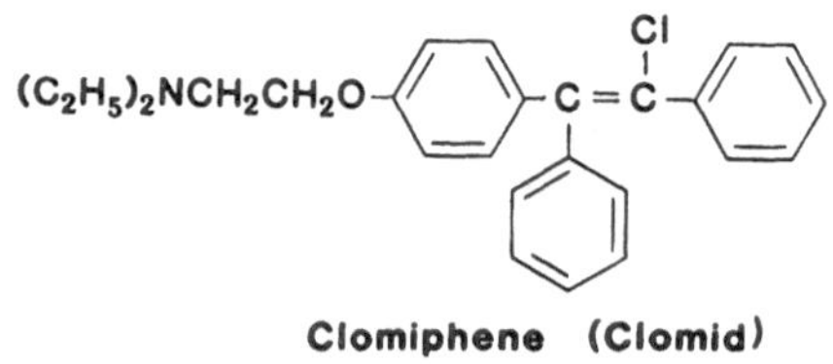

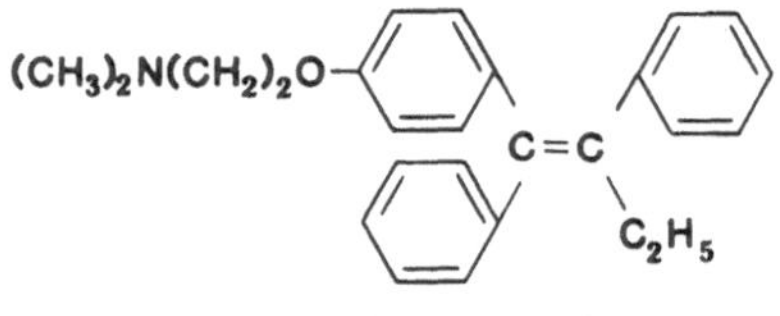

Figure 7-8. Molecular structure of the antiestrogenic drugs.

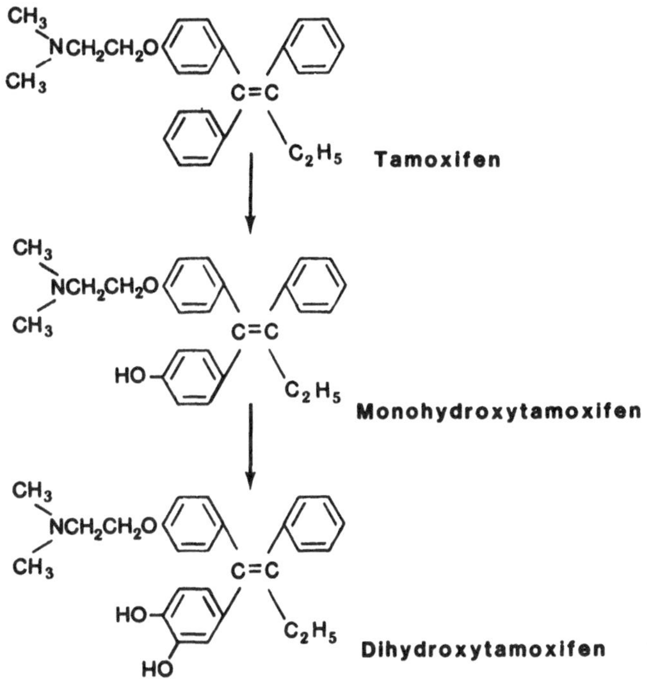

Figure 7-9. Oxidative metabolism of tamoxifen.

The current therapeutic uses of the antiestrogenic drugs are as follows: clomiphene citrate is useful in the induction of ovulation, while tamoxifen is restricted to the palliative management of estrogen-dependent breast cancer.

7.2.1. Clomiphene

Clomiphene therapy in appropriately selected patients stimulates gonadotropin secretion by exerting an antiestrogenic action in the hypothalamus. Within several days after initiation of therapy, gonadotropin levels rise, remain elevated during therapy, and begin to fall approximately 2 days after cessation of treatment. Rising estrogen levels from ovarian follicles stimulated to grow by the initial release of gonadotropins trigger the preovulatory surge of LH. This is a result of positive feedback similar to that occurring in the normal ovulatory cycle (see Figure 7-4). Ovulation usually occurs 13–15 days after initiation of clomiphene treatment. It should be recognized that the presence of ovaries capable of responding to endogenous gonadotropin secretion is a vital prerequisite for the success of clomiphene therapy. Ovarian follicular activity is usually established by the induction of menstrual bleeding after progesterone administration.

Clomiphene therapy is indicated in the induction of ovulation in the infertile anovulatory patient. Anovulation resulting from hypothalamic dysfunction, polycystic ovaries, oral contraceptive-induced amenorrhea, and excessive adrenal androgen production is usually responsive to clomiphene. Patients with polycystic ovarian disease are particularly sensitive to the actions of clomiphene. Patients who exhibit limited pituitary gonadotropin reserve or estrogen deficiency will usually not benefit from clomiphene administration.

The initial dosage of clomiphene is 50 mg taken orally beginning on the fifth day of the cycle and is administered for 5 days. Failure to induce ovulation after two or three cycles at this dosage is followed by increased dosages in 50-mg increments. Increasing the daily dosage above 100 mg/day is rarely more effective; however, dosages of 250 mg/day for 5 days have been used without apparent increase in side effects. Alternatively, increasing the duration of dosing to 7 or 10 days, rather than the dose level, often induces ovulation. By contrast, individuals with polycystic ovarian disease are more sensitive to clomiphene and may respond after 2–3 days therapy. Before initiation of subsequent cycles of clomiphene therapy, patients should be evaluated for pregnancy or ovarian enlargement. Failure to induce ovulation with clomiphene alone may be followed with combination therapy utilizing clomiphene and human chorionic gonadotropin (HCG) to augment the midcycle LH surge. Similarly, GnRH may be combined with clomiphene to enhance the preovulatory LH surge.

Whereas approximately 70–80% of patients receiving clomiphene ovulate, the pregnancy rate approximates only 40%. An explanation for this discrepancy is not currently available. It is possible that the antiestrogen interferes with the uterine environment (e.g., nature of cervical mucus), preventing proper implantation. In addition, ovulation is usually established based on a rise in basal body temperature. It is conceivable that clomiphene induces a thermogenic response through hypothalamic actions independent of an actual ovulatory event. Multiple births occur in 6–10% of pregnancies resulting from ovulation induction by clomiphene. Three-fourths of the multiple births involve twins. A higher frequency of multiple gestation occurs in patients with polycystic ovaries. Clomiphene therapy for ovulation induction is not associated with increased risk of congenital malformations.

The most serious adverse effect attributed to clomiphene therapy is ovarian enlargement or hyperstimulation, with the possibility in severe ascites and pleural effusion. The incidence of ovarian hyperstimulation is related to the duration of treatment, ranging from 2% after 3 days of therapy to 7–8% for 7 days of therapy. Not surprisingly, patients with cystic ovarian disease are more likely to develop ovarian enlargement. The probability of producing ovarian hyperstimulation with clomiphene therapy is lessened by closely monitoring plasma levels of estradiol-17β to establish the degree of follicular development. A period of 1–4 weeks is required for the spontaneous resolution of clomiphene-induced hyperstimulation of the ovaries. Less serious and less common consequences of clomiphene therapy include nausea, vomiting, abdominal discomfort, visual disturbances, headache, abnormal uterine bleeding, dizziness, fatigue, depression, skin rash, hair loss, increased urinary frequency, and dry vaginal mucosa (see Table 7-12). Hot flashes also occur in 5–10% of patients and are related to the antiestrogenic effect of clomiphene. Administration of clomiphene early in pregnancy may be teratogenic.

7.2.2. Tamoxifen

Approximately one-third of patients with metastatic breast cancer will benefit from antiestrogen therapy. Administration of tamoxifen is indicated in the management of breast cancer that has been established as estrogen-dependent based on analysis of steroid hormone receptors.

Table 7-12. Adverse Effects Associated with Antiestrogenic Drugs

Nausea and vomiting
Hot flashes
Ovarian hyperstimulation during induction of ovulation
Blurred vision
Hypercalcemia in malignant disease
Thrombocytopenia and leukopenia (tamoxifen)
Skin rash
Hair loss
Headache
Abnormal uterine bleeding
Dizziness
Dry vaginal mucosa
Increased urinary frequency

Breast cancer cells in about 70–80% of patients contain significant levels of estrogen receptors; about one-half of these tumors also contain progesterone receptors. The presence of progesterone receptors is indicative of the functional integrity of the estrogen-receptor pathway. Sixty percent of estrogen receptor-positive patients and 75% of patients who are positive for both steroid receptors benefit from tamoxifen therapy. Responses to tamoxifen usually extend for 7–18 months, but responses of several years have been observed. By contrast, fewer than 10% of the steroid receptor-negative patients exhibit objective responses after antiestrogen treatment.

Antiestrogenic drugs effectively bind to cytoplasmic estrogen receptors, but these drug-receptor complexes exert little intrinsic activity. Therefore, antiestrogens block the access of endogenous estrogens to their receptors and in this fashion impede the growth of estrogen-sensitive breast carcinomas. Estrogen and progesterone are essential hormones involved in the regulation of normal ductal and alveolar breast cell growth, respectively. Consequently, it is not surprising that the hormone sensitivity of the malignant breast is related to the continued dependence of some transformed cells on at least estrogen or progesterone, or both. Since these steroid hormones initiate their actions through receptor-mediated processes, the responsiveness of these tissues to antiestrogen therapy is directly related to the intracellular localization of these essential receptor proteins.

The usual dosage of tamoxifen is 10 mg twice daily by the oral route. The twice-daily dosing interval is based on the plasma half-life of tamoxifen, which is 9–12 hr. Failure of a response to the initial dose of tamoxifen in properly selected patients should be followed by increasing dosage to 40 mg twice daily. In general, 8–12 weeks of therapy is required to establish efficacy. The slow onset of activity for tamoxifen is probably related to the need for 10–16 weeks of continuous therapy before steady-state plasma levels of tamoxifen are achieved. After the termination of tamoxifen treatment, 4–6 weeks are required for plasma drug clearance to occur. Tamoxifen is usually restricted to use in postmenopausal patients, but premenopausal patients have been successfully treated as well. Higher doses of tamoxifen are usually required in premenopausal patients in order to overcome the actions of higher levels of endogenous estrogens. Since tamoxifen may induce teratogenesis, it should not be administered during pregnancy.

Tamoxifen is well tolerated, and withdrawal of treatment due to side effects occurs in fewer than 3% of patients. The most frequent adverse actions are associated with the drug's antiestrogenic actions. These include hot flushes in 10–20% of cases and nausea and vomiting in about 10% of individuals (see Table 7-12). Atrophic vaginitis, skin rash and hypercalcemia in patients with osseous metastases occur infrequently. Transient thrombocytopenia and leukopenia have also been noted. On occasion, tamoxifen induces tumor flare and bone pain in patients, possibly related to the fact that tamoxifen initially produces weak estrogenic activity. These stimulatory effects of tamoxifen are observed during the first few days of therapy and are usually reversed if the antiestrogen treatment is continued.

RECOMMENDED READINGS

Physiology of the Estrogens

Chappel, S. C., The neuroendocrine regulation of luteinizing hormone and follicle-stimulating hormone: A review, Life Sci. 36:97, 1985.

Clark, J. H., and Markaverich, B. M., The agonistic and antagonistic effects of short-acting estrogens: A review, Pharmacol. Ther. 21:429, 1983.

Fritz, M. A., and Speroff, L., The endocrinology of the menstrual cycle: The interaction of folliculogenesis and neuroendocrine mechanisms, Fertil. Steril. 38:509, 1982.

Gorski, J., Welshons, W., and Sakai, D., Remodeling the estrogen receptor model, Mol. Cell Endocrinol. 36:11, 1984.

Greene, G. L., Sobel, N. B., King, W. J., and Jensen, E. V., Immunochemical studies of estrogen receptors, J. Steroid Biochem. 20:51, 1984.

Katzenellenbogen, B. S., Dynamics of steroid hormone action, Annu. Rev. Physiol. 42:17, 1980.

Keenan, E. J., The physiological and pathophysiological significance of steroid hormone receptors, Gynecol. Obstet. 5:343, 1982.

Knobil, E., The neuroendocrine control of the menstrual cycle, Recent Prog. Horm. Res. 36:53, 1980.

Leung, P. C. K., and Armstrong, D. T., Interactions of steroids and gonadotropins in the control of steroidogenesis in the ovarian follicle, Annu. Rev. Physiol. 42:71, 1980.

O'Malley, B. W., Steroid hormone action in eukaryotic cells, J. Clin. Invest. 74:307, 1984.

Pohl, C. R., and Knobil, E., The role of the central nervous system in the control of ovarian function in higher primates, Annu. Rev. Physiol. 44:583, 1982.

Sherman, M. R., Structure of mammalian steroid receptors: Evolving concepts and methodological developments, Annu. Rev. Physiol. 46:83, 1984.

Thorneycroft, I. H., and Boyers, S. P., The human menstrual cycle: Correlation of hormonal patterns and clinical signs and symptoms, Obstet. Gynecol. Annu. 12:199, 1983.

Whitehead, M. I., Townsend, P. T., Pryse-Danes, J., Ryder, T. A., and King, R. J. B., Effects of estrogens and progestins on the biochemistry and morphology of postmenopausal endometrium, N. Engl. J. Med. 305:1599, 1981.

Pharmacology of the Estrogens

Allegra, J. C., Rational approaches to the hormonal treatment of breast cancer, Semin. Oncol. 10:25, 1983.

Dorfman, R. I., Pharmacology of estrogens, Pharmacol. Ther. 9:107, 1980.

Gambrell, R. D., The menopause: Benefits and risks of estrogen-progestogen replacement therapy, *Fertil. Steril.* **37**:457, 1982.

Geola, F. L., Biological effects of various doses of conjugated equine estrogens in postmenopausal women, *J. Clin. Endocrinol. Metab.* **51**:620, 1980.

Herbst, A., The current status of the DES-exposed population, *Obstet. Gynecol. Ann.* **10**:267, 1981.

Heywood, R., and Wadsworth, P. F., The experimental toxicology of estrogens, *Pharmacol. Ther.* **8**:125, 1980.

JAMA Council on Scientific Affairs, Estrogen replacement in the menopause, *JAMA,* **249**:359, 1983.

Judd, H. J., Meldrum, D. R., Deftos, L. J., and Henderson, B. E., Estrogen replacement therapy: Indications and complications, *Ann. Intern. Med.* **98**:195, 1983.

Mandel, F. P., Geola, F. L., Lu, J. K. H., Eggena, P., Mohinder, M. P., Hershman, J. M., and Judd, H. L., Biologic effects of various doses of ethinyl estradiol in postmenopausal women, *Obstet. Gynecol.* **59**:673, 1982.

Hammond, C. B., and Maxson, W. E., Current status of estrogen therapy for the menopause, *Fertil. Steril.* **37**:5, 1982.

McGuire, W. L., Steroid hormone receptors in breast cancer treatment strategy, *Recent. Prog. Horm. Res.* **36**:135, 1980.

McGuire, W. L., and Clark, G. M., The prognostic role of progesterone receptors in human breast cancer, *Semin. Oncol.* **10**:2, 1983.

Pepperell, R. J., Suppression of lactation, *Med. J. Aust.* **144**:37, 1986.

Place, V. A., Powers, M. S., Darley, P. E., Schenkel, L., and Good, W. R., A double-blind comparative study of estraderm and premarin in the amelioration of post-menopausal symptoms, *Am. J. Obstet. Gynecol.* **152**:1092–1099, 1985.

Powers, M. S., Schenkel, L., Darley, P. E., Good, W. R., Balestra, J.C., and Place, V. A., Pharmacokinetics and pharmacodynamics of transdermal dosage forms of 17β-estradiol; Comparison with conventional oral estrogens used for hormone replacement, *Am. J. Obstet. and Gynecol.* **152**:1099–1106, 1985.

Quigley, M., Postmenopausal estrogen replacement therapy: An appraisal of risks and benefits, *Drugs* **22**:153, 1981.

Ryan, K. J., Postmenopausal estrogen use, *Annu. Rev. Med.* **33**:171, 1982.

Segal, S. J., and Koide, S. S., Clinical uses of estrogens, *Pharmacol. Ther.* **11**:451, 1980.

Segaloff, A., Pharmacological receptor determination in endocrine therapy of breast cancer, *Annu. Rev. Pharmacol. Toxicol.* **20**:429, 1980.

Seibert, K., and Lippman, M., Hormone receptors in breast cancer, *Clin. Oncol.* **1**:735, 1982.

Stampfer, M. J., Willett, W. C., Colditz, G. A., Rosner, B., Speizer, F. E., and Hennekens, C. H., A prospective study of post-menopausal estrogen therapy and coronary heart disease, *N. Engl. J. Med.* **313**:1044–1049, 1985.

Weinstein, M. C., Estrogen use in postmenopausal women—Costs, risks and benefits, *N. Engl. J. Med.* **303**:308, 1980.

Wilson, P. W. F., Garrison, R. J., and Castelli, W. P., Post-menopausal estrogen use, cigarette smoking, and cardiovascular morbidity in women over fifty, *N. Engl. J. Med* **313**:1038–1043, 1985.

Pharmacology of the Antiestrogens

Fabian, C. L., Clinical pharmacology of tamoxifen in patients with breast cancer, *Cancer* **48**:876, 1981.

Heel, R. C., Brogden, R. N., Speight, T. M., and Avery, G. S., Tamoxifen: A review of its pharmacological properties and therapeutic use in the treatment of breast cancer, *Drugs* **16**:1, 1978.

Huppert, L. C., Induction of ovulation with clomiphene citrate, *Fertil. Steril.* **31**:1, 1979.

Furr, B. J. A., and Jordan, V. C., The pharmacology and clinical uses of tamoxifen, *Pharmacol. Ther.* **25**:127, 1984.

Jordan, V. C., Biochemical pharmacology of antiestrogen action, *Pharmacol. Rev.* **36**:245, 1984.

Milgrom, E., Monoclonal antibodies to steroid hormone receptors, *Pharmacol. and Ther.* **28**:389–415, 1985.

Patterson, J. S., Clinical aspects and development of antiestrogen therapy: A review of the endocrine effects of tamoxifen in animals and man, *J. Endocrinol.* **89**:67, 1981.

Rochefort, H., Borgna, J., and Evans, E., Cellular and molecular mechanism of action of antiestrogens, *J. Steril. Biochem.* **19**:69, 1983.

Sorbie, P. J., and Perez-Marrero, R., The use of clomiphene citrate in male infertility, *J. Urol.* **131**:425, 1984.

Sutherland, R. L., and Murphy, L. C., Mechanisms of estrogen antagonism by non-steroidal antiestrogens, *Mol. Cell Endocrinol.* **25**:5, 1982.

Thorneycroft, I. H., Current status of ovulation induction with clomiphene citrate, *Fertil. Steril.* **41**:806, 1984.

Walters, M. R., Steroid hormone receptors and the nucleus, *Endocr. Rev.* **6**:512–543, 1985.

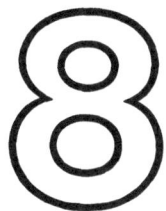

PROGESTINS AND ORAL CONTRACEPTIVES

8.1. PROGESTINS

8.1.1. Introduction

Development and maintenance of the female reproductive system are dependent on the cyclical interaction between estrogens, primarily estradiol-17β, and progesterone. The principal target tissues for these steroid hormones include the uterus, vagina, fallopian tubes, and mammary glands, as well as the anterior pituitary and hypothalamus. Although estrogens are recognized as promoters of cellular proliferation, progestins are known to facilitate cellular differentiation. In addition, progesterone and related drugs exert significant antiestrogenic effects. It is the balance between estrogen and progesterone actions that regulates the state of the female reproductive system. Some of the therapeutically useful derivatives of progesterone share a structural similarity to androgens, and these agents in some instances also produce androgenic or antiandrogenic activity.

8.1.2. History

It was apparent as early as 1897, following the studies by Beard, that ovulation failed to occur during pregnancy. Subsequently, the studies by Haberlandt indicated that hormones derived from the ovary and placenta could be used for regulation of fertility. In 1929 the Corner and Allen bioassay for detecting progestational activity was developed and became instrumental in the isolation of progesterone from the corpus luteum. By 1932, Butenandt had elucidated the structure of progesterone. The observation by Inhoffen in 1938 that alkylation of the 17α-position of the steroid nucleus converted estradiol-17β and testosterone into orally active compounds provided the basis for the development of progestational compounds. Yet the evolution of the orally active synthetic progestins required the availability of significant quantities of progesterone. This was made possible by Marker's recognition in 1943 that the Mexican sweet potato contained high levels of progesterone.

Allen and Ehrenstein revealed in 1944 that 19-norprogesterone possessed oral progestational activity. In 1950 Birch outlined an efficient procedure for synthesizing 19-nortestosterone, which would subsequently become an important precursor for the development of synthetic progestational drugs. Djerassi derived 19-norethisterone in 1951, and norethynodrel was synthesized by Colton in 1952, using 19-nortestosterone as the parent molecule.

Pincus and Chang subsequently demonstrated the antifertility activity of progesterone in females in 1953. By 1957, the initial studies of the clinical use of progestational drugs as orally active contraceptives in females were described by Rice-Wray. During the same year, Enovid, containing norethynodrel, was approved by the Food and Drug Administration for menstrual regulation and was subsequently approved as a contraceptive agent in 1960. Ortho-Novum containing norethisterone was approved as a menstrual regulator in 1957 and was approved for birth control needs in 1962.

Today's principal use of progestational drugs was born during the early 1960s. Currently, at least 28 drug formulations containing a progestin alone or a combination of a synthetic progestin and an estrogenic substance are available for fertility regulation in women. One of six progestins differing in potency and spectrum of action and one of two synthetic estrogens are utilized in these products. It is the difference in hormonal constituents and content that pharmacologically distinguishes the various oral contraceptive agents.

8.1.3. Chemistry

The progestins are classified according to their molecular structure. Progesterone is the endogenous progestational substance produced by the cells of the corpus luteum during normal menstrual cycles and in early pregnancy as well. The placenta serves as an important source of progesterone during later stages of pregnancy.

A number of synthetic progesterone derivatives are available for therapeutic purposes (see Figure 8-1). Direct descendants of progesterone include medroxyprogesterone acetate, megestrol acetate, hydroxyprogesterone capronate, and dydrogesterone. A second group of progestational drugs is derived from 19-nortestosterone, and one of these is usually included in the formulation of oral contraceptive drugs. Included among this group of synthetic progestins are norethindrone,

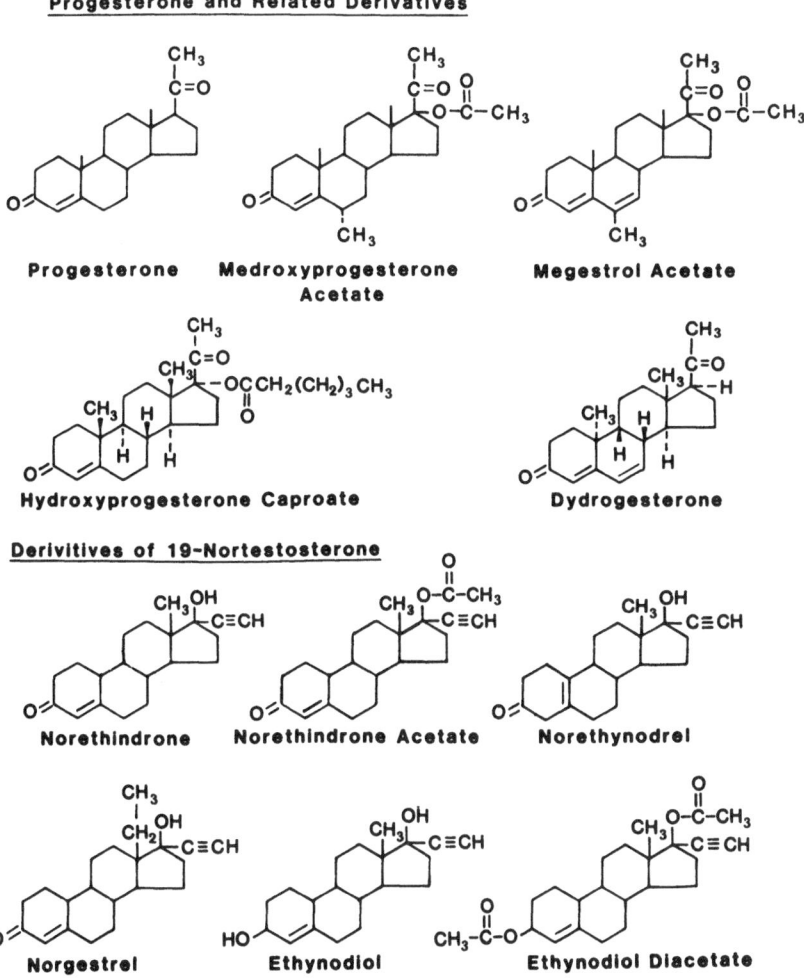

Figure 8-1. Molecular structure of the progestational drugs.

norethindrone acetate, norethynodrel, norgestrel, ethynodiol, and ethy-nodiol diacetate (Figure 8-1).

Progesterone is a 21-carbon steroid, that, in addition to its inherent biological activity and significance, serves as an important substrate of steroidogenesis in all tissues that secrete steroid hormones. One of these metabolites of progesterone is 17α-hydroxyprogesterone, which lacks progestational activity but does represent one of the precursors that lead to the development of orally active progestins. The 6-methyl analogue of this precursor with an acetate group at C-17 is medroxyprogesterone acetate (Figure 8-1). Megestrol acetate is structurally similar to medrox-yprogesterone acetate differing only with respect to the presence of a double bond in the B ring of the steroid nucleus. Further modification at the 17 α-position of progesterone results in the progestational agents, hydroxyprogesterone capronate and dydrogesterone (Figure 8-1).

Ethinyl testosterone-17α (ethisterone) was the first progestin to demonstrate significant oral efficacy. Subsequently, it was established that the 19-nortestosterone derivatives are substantially more effective when administered orally. These compounds lack the angular methyl group at the C-19 position. Although 19-nortestosterone itself is inactive, alkylation at the 17α-position instills progestational efficacy. Norethin-drone is 17α-ethinyl-19-nortestosterone and its isomer, norethynodrel is an effective progestin as well (Figure 8-1). Reduction of the 3-keto group of norethindrone yields the partially reduced derivative of ethinyl es-tradiol, ethynodiol. Both ethynodiol and its 17α-diacetate derivative are potent progestins (Figure 8-1).

8.1.4.   Biosynthesis, Secretion, and Metabolism

Progesterone is synthesized by the cells of the corpus luteum in the ovary and by the placenta. After secretion, the majority (>90%) of pro-gesterone is transported in the blood in association with corticosteroid-binding globulin (CBG). Free progesterone, which is not localized in target cells, is readily metabolized in the liver. The metabolism of pro-gesterone is complex, but a primary metabolite is pregnanediol. Urinary elimination of pregnanediol and related metabolites occurs following conjugation with glucuronic acid. The plasma half-life of progesterone is short and estimated at approximately 5–10 min. It is the rapid hepatic metabolism of progesterone that precludes its administration *via* the oral route. The chief result of the chemical modification of progesterone is a marked reduction in the rate of hepatic clearance for the synthetic progesterone derivatives, resulting in their oral efficacy.

The synthesis of progesterone involves the enzymatic conversion of cholesterol to pregnenolone (see Figure 8-2). Only a small amount of

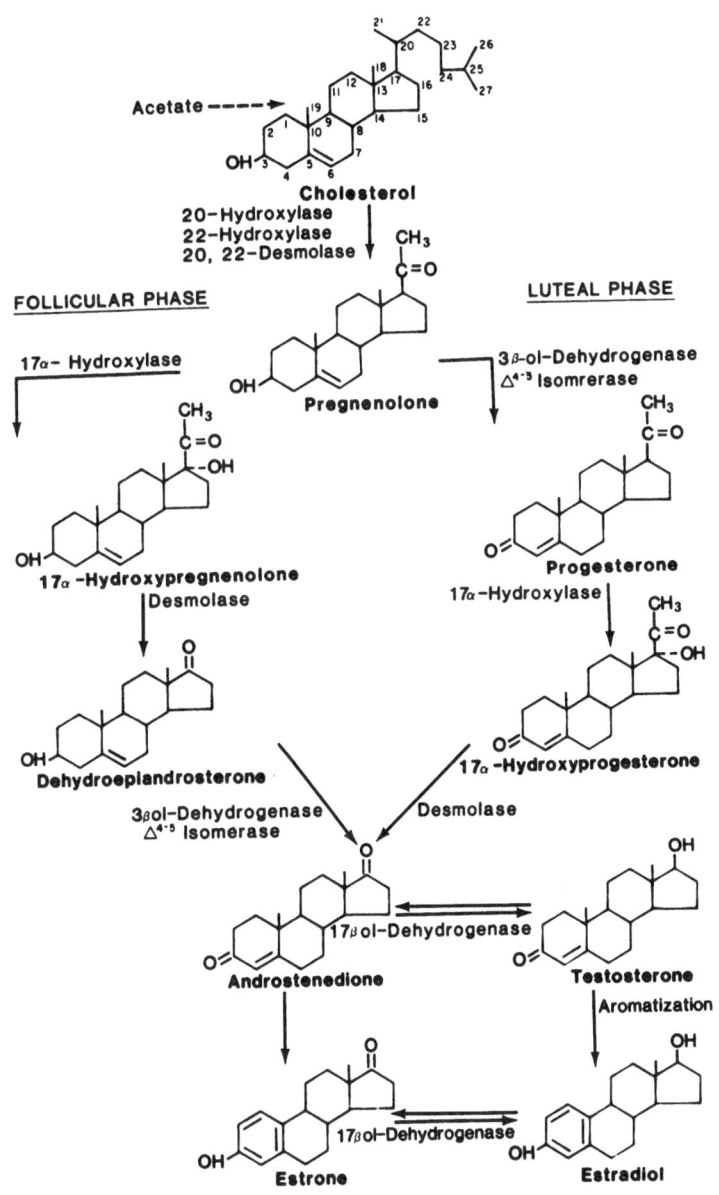

Figure 8-2.   Biosynthetic pathway of ovarian steroidogenesis.

progesterone is produced during the follicular phase of the menstrual cycle. However, after ovulation large quantities of progesterone are synthesized and secreted by the corpus luteum. The enzymatic conversion of pregnenolone to progesterone is mediated by 3β-ol-dehydrogenase Δ^{4-5} isomerase. The pathways of ovarian steroidogenesis are outlined in Figure 8-2.

Preovulatory production of progesterone is estimated at 2–3 mg/day, while synthesis rises to 20–30 mg/day in the luteal phase of the menstrual cycle. The corpus luteum exhibits an active period of growth and steroid production during the 7-day postovulatory peak in luteinizing hormone (LH) levels (see Figure 8-3). If pregnancy fails to occur, the corpus luteum subsequently regresses, and steroid production declines over the next 7-day period. Blood levels of progesterone in adult females (follicular phase), prepubertal females, and in males is less than 1 ng/ml. Postovulation blood levels of progesterone range from 5 to 20 ng/ml. During the menstrual cycle, LH plays a predominant role in the regulation of progesterone synthesis. The effects of LH are mediated by interaction with ovarian receptors that are specific for LH.

During the first 10 weeks of pregnancy, most progesterone is syn-

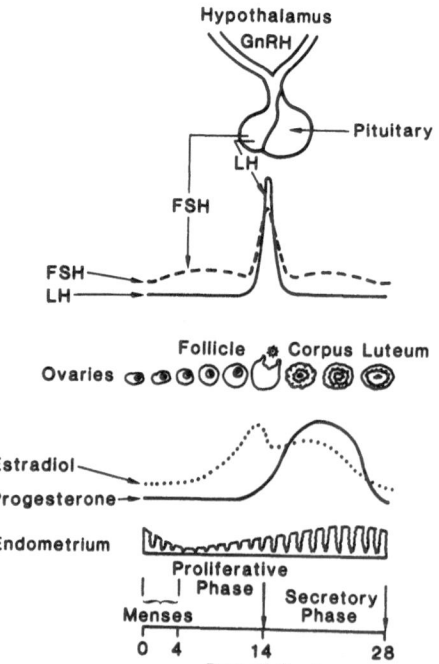

Figure 8-3. Hormonal regulation of menstrual function. FSH, follicle-stimulating hormone; GnRH, gonadotropin-releasing hormone; LH, luteinizing hormone.

thesized and secreted by the corpus luteum. The placenta represents the major source of progesterone by the twelfth week of gestation. The metabolic pathway for the production of progesterone by the placenta is similar to that of the corpus luteum, as depicted in Figure 8-2. At parturition, plasma levels of progesterone range from 10 to 200 ng/ml.

8.1.5. Mechanism of Action

· An understanding of the molecular aspects of the mechanism of progesterone action is well developed but remains incomplete. Progesterone-sensitive target tissues such as the uterus and mammary gland are able to retain progesterone and related synthetic derivatives selectively through specific interactions with protein receptors. These receptors for progesterone appear to be required for mediating the actions of progesterone.

The interaction between progesterone and its receptor is apparently initiated in the cytoplasmic compartment of the cell (see Figure 8-4). In the cytoplasm the progesterone receptor exists in a characteristic molecular conformation, at least as established by *in vitro* receptor characterization studies. In hypotonic sucrose density gradients, the progesterone receptor migrates as a protein with a 7S molecular conformation. During activation of the progesterone receptor complex, the apparent molecular conformation or size of the cytosolic progesterone receptor decreases to that of a 5.5S protein. Molybdate, a phosphatase enzyme inhibitor, stabilizes the cytoplasmic progesterone receptors in their larger molecular conformation. It is evident that purified progesterone receptor is a suitable substrate for phosphorylation and that phosphorylation/dephosphorylation reactions may be involved in the processes of progesterone receptor activation and inactivation. The precise nature of the receptor activation process remains undefined.

Progesterone receptors demonstrate a strict specificity for progesterone and related derivatives as well as a high affinity (K_D = 0.5–1.0 nM) for these compounds. Although the affinity of progesterone for its receptor is lower than that of estradiol-17β for the estrogen receptor, this is not surprising in view of the significantly higher physiological levels of progesterone as compared with circulating estrogens. Therefore, under physiological conditions, significant occupancy of progesterone receptors occurs. The specificity of the interaction between progestins and their receptors is the basis for the selectivity of action associated with these drugs.

The cytoplasmic progesterone receptor is composed of two distinct subunits, distinguished as protein A and B, with molecular weights of

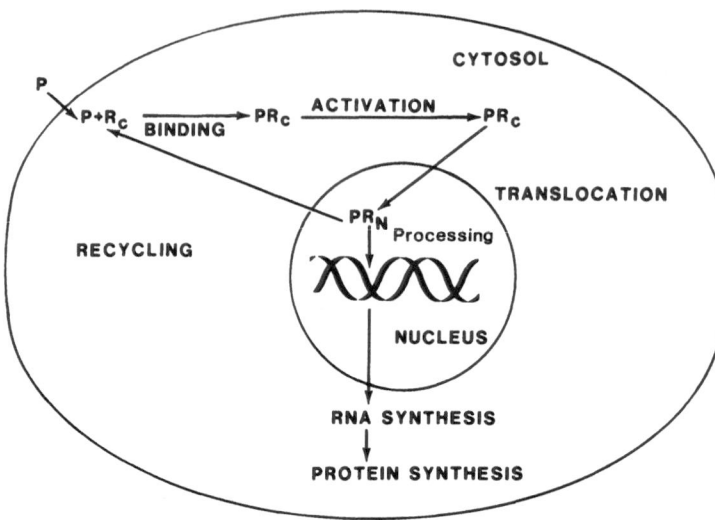

Figure 8-4. Mechanism of progesterone action. P, progesterone; R_C, cytoplasmic progesterone receptor; T_N, nuclear progesterone receptor.

79,000 and 108,000, respectively. After activation of the cytoplasmic receptor, the complex translocates to the nucleus, where the subunits of the receptor bind to separate sites associated with the DNA molecule (see Figure 8-4). Protein A interacts directly with a DNA binding site currently established as an effector site. This region appears to be approximately 150 nucleoside base pairs from the progesterone-activated gene, as revealed by studies of the chicken ovalbumin gene. By contrast, protein B undergoes a high-affinity association with nonhistone chromosomal proteins and is referred to as the specifier unit. The B subunit possesses both a progestin binding site and a phosphorylation site. Both subunits are required for induction of progesterone action. Although unoccupied progesterone receptors can bind DNA, the association of progesterone with its receptor significantly increases the affinity, and presumably the retention, of progesterone receptors for DNA. The nuclear sites to which protein B binds may represent specific areas of DNA, which must be occupied to afford access of protein A subunits to the limited number of effector sites. The region of the genome to which progesterone receptors selectively localize is rich in adenine–thymine base pairs.

Association of occupied progesterone receptors with DNA apparently exposes sites, facilitates association, or increases the retention of RNA polymerase to specific regions of the genome. This leads ultimately to increases in RNA polymerase activity and stimulation of protein synthesis. Progesterone receptors are not generally retained at intranuclear sites for prolonged periods as is observed with estrogen receptors. Progesterone receptors reside in the nucleus for approximately 4–6 hr. The limited nuclear retention of progesterone receptor complexes may explain the fact that progesterone stimulates only synthesis of RNA and proteins without promoting cellular growth. Intranuclear progesterone receptors do apparently undergo a processing reaction shortly after entering the nucleus. The nature of the processing reaction is unknown, as is the ultimate fate of progesterone receptors in the nucleus. It is likely that at least a portion of intranuclear and probably unprocessed receptors for progesterone are recycled to the cytoplasm for subsequent reutilization (see Figure 8-4).

The synthesis of progesterone receptors in estrogen target tissues such as the breast and uterus is largely dependent on estrogen. In this regard, the estrogen dependence of progesterone receptor synthesis is helpful in explaining the need for estrogen priming to induce full progestational sensitivity (see Figure 8-5). Importantly, progesterone antagonizes the synthesis of its own receptors. This effect occurs as a result of progesterone-mediated inhibiton of estrogen receptor functions. Progesterone does not interfere with the nuclear translocation of estrogen

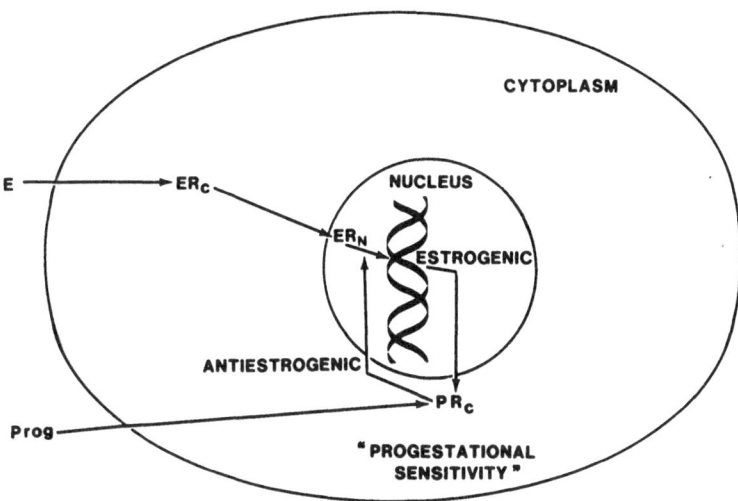

Figure 8-5. Schematic representation of the interaction between estrogen and progestins. E, estrogen; ER, estrogen receptor; P, progestin; PR, progesterone receptor; C, cytoplasmic; N, nuclear.

receptor complexes. Instead, progesterone apparently blocks the estrogen-mediated replenishment of cytoplasmic estrogen receptors (Figure 8-5). Consequently, progesterone-induced inhibition of estrogen receptor synthesis results in the depletion of cytoplasmic estrogen receptors, thereby reducing the number of these receptor complexes entering target cell nuclei. Since progesterone receptor synthesis is dependent on the functional integrity of the estrogen receptor pathway, a decline in the nuclear content of estrogen receptors leads to a depletion of cytoplasmic receptors for progesterone.

The physiological and pharmacological implications of the interaction between estrogens and progestins are evident. Estrogen receptor content of the uterus and breast is highest during the latter portions of the follicular or proliferative phase of the menstrual cycle. During this time, peripheral levels of estradiol-17β are elevated and the uterine endometrium proliferates (see Figure 8-3). Importantly, circulating levels of progesterone are low, resulting in little endogenous antiestrogen activity. Therefore, the antagonistic effects of progesterone on the estrogen receptor content of the uterus and breast are minimal during the first half of the menstrual cycle. Not surprisingly, the levels of progesterone receptor in these tissues rise during the follicular phase of the cycle in response to the rising levels of estradiol-17β and in preparation for the postovulatory increase in progesterone secretion. During the secretory or luteal phase of the cycle, the association of progesterone with its receptors suppresses production of estrogen receptors (antiestrogenic action) and stimulates differentiation of a secretory endometrium (estrogen-dependent progestational action). With time, the antiestrogenic actions of progesterone lead to decreases in progesterone receptor content.

It is evident that there exist significant regulatory influences of estrogen and progesterone on the synthesis of their respective receptors and that the interaction of these hormones is crucial to the control of uterine, breast, and hypothalamic function. The molecular aspects of the interaction between estrogen and progesterone are also pharmacologically significant. The intricate regulation of receptors for estrogen and progesterone explains the requirement for estrogen priming in ensuring progestational responsiveness and also provides the molecular basis for the antiestrogenic actions of progestins, which are exploited clinically.

8.1.6. Physiological Effects

The primary biological actions of progesterone are outlined in Table 8-1. Progesterone is required for cyclically inducing the differentiation

Table 8-1. Biological Actions of Progesterone

Induces secretory differentiation of the uterine endometrium
Decreases contractility of uterine myometrium
Stimulates growth of alveolar epithelium in the breast
Maintains pregnancy
Thermogenic
Stimulates respiration
Estrogen antagonist
Anesthesia (high-dose)

of the estrogen-primed uterine endometrium to the secretory state. Myometrial contractility is subsequently suppressed by progesterone. This effect is related to an increase in intracellular sodium ion concentration and to a decrease in potassium ion content. Not surprisingly, the maintenance of pregnancy requires the presence of adequate progesterone levels. Progesterone is also responsible for stimulating the development of the breast alveolar epithelium. In fact, the proper integration of estrogen and progesterone effects is required for subsequent prolactin-mediated induction of lactation after parturition.

The rise in basal body temperature at the time of ovulation is probably related to the thermogenic actions of progesterone. During the luteal phase of the menstrual cycle and during pregnancy, progesterone stimulates respiration and reduces the arterial partial pressures of CO_2. Anesthetic activity is associated with large doses of certain progestins, including progesterone. High levels of progesterone also stimulate natriuresis by antagonizing aldosterone action in the distal tubule of the kidney. Importantly, large or supraphysiological doses of progesterone inhibit the secretion of LH from the adenohypophysis and consequently inhibit ovulation. This effect provides the rationale for the widespread clinical use of progestational drugs in fertility regulation.

The effects of progestins on plasma lipids are complex. Progestational drugs do appear to elevate plasma triglyceride levels and in some cases may elevate cholesterol levels; however, this effect is inconsistently observed among the various progestins.

8.1.7. Therapeutic Uses

The principal clinical use of progestins is in combination with synthetic estrogens in oral contraceptive preparations. Table 8-2 depicts the various therapeutic uses of progestins. Current approaches to the management of menopausal symptoms include the use of orally active progestins administered cyclically in combination with estrogen replace-

Table 8-2. Therapeutic Uses of the Progestins

Contraception
Menopausal replacement therapy
Amenorrhea
Luteal-phase abnormalities
Premenstrual tension
Dysfunctional uterine bleeding
Endometriosis
Hirsutism
Breast cancer (hormone-dependent)
Endometrial cancer (hormone-dependent)

ment therapy. The progestin challenge is usually reserved for the final 10-day period of a 25-day estrogen replacement regimen. Medroxyprogesterone acetate is usually the drug of choice and is administered at a dosage of 10 mg/day for the 10-day period. This dosing schedule more closely simulates the endogenous dynamics of hormone secretion that occur during the premenopausal state. The objective of this treatment approach is to utilize the antiestrogenic actions of progesterone to minimize or prevent excessive estrogenic stimulation of the uterus and breast that occurs with estrogen-only replacement therapy.

Dysmenorrhea, endometriosis, hirsutism, and dysfunctional uterine bleeding are attributed to excessive estrogenic stimulation, requiring ovarian suppression therapy. Estrogens are clearly contraindicated in these situations, and progestins, particularly the synthetic derivatives of progesterone, have been established as useful. Medroxyprogesterone acetate or norethindrone are usually chosen for management of endometriosis and are administered at dosages of 10–30 mg/day. Currently, danazol, a weakly androgenic agent that lacks estrogenic and progestational activity, is gaining increasing acceptance as a useful hormonal agent for the treatment of endometriosis (see Chapter 6). Dysfunctional uterine bleeding requires assessment for the precise cause of the bleeding, to eliminate the possibility of malignant disease. In the appropriate patient with dysfunctional uterine bleeding, medroxyprogesterone acetate or norethindrone is usually administered at a dosage of 5–20 mg/day beginning on the fifth day of the cycle and terminating on the twenty-fifth day.

Occasionally, progesterone or one of the related synthetic progestins is administered to women who demonstrate difficulty conceiving and who show a slow postovulation rise in basal body temperature. These patients are believed to suffer from ovarian luteal phase defects that can be reversed by progestin supplementation. Progesterone is also employed for diagnostic purposes in establishing whether estrogen stimulation of the uterine endometrium is occurring in amenorrheic women. Intramuscular administration of progesterone, 100–200 mg, or preferably the oral administration of medroxyprogesterone acetate (5–10 mg), for 5–7 days will produce progestin-withdrawal bleeding in amenorrheic women only when the uterine endometrium is estrogen primed. Use of progestin in this manner requires that pregnancy be definitively eliminated as the cause of the amenorrhea, because of the probable teratogenicity to the fetus exposed to progestins during the first few months of gestation.

Progestins are also used in the palliative management of hormone-dependent metastatic cancer of the endometrium and breast. Hormone dependence of these carcinomas is established by steroid receptor analysis. Approximately 80% of progestin receptor-positive endometrial carcinomas respond to megestrol acetate. The dosage of megestrol acetate ranges from 80 to 640 mg/day, and continuous therapy for at least 2 months is required to establish efficacy. Metastatic breast cancer, which has been shown to be hormone dependent based on the presence of estrogen and/or progesterone receptors, is sometimes managed with progestin therapy (megestrol acetate). However, the initial treatment of choice is endocrine ablation (ovariectomy and/or adrenalectomy) or antiestrogen therapy (see Chapter 7) for the palliative management of hormone-responsive breast carcinomas.

8.1.8. Preparations

Clinically useful natural and synthetic progestational drugs are listed in Table 8-3. Progesterone, the natural progestin, is available in an oil vehicle and only for parenteral (intramuscular) administration and is therefore not as convenient for clinical use as are the orally active synthetic progesterone derivatives. Oral administration of progesterone is not feasible in view of the rapid metabolism of progesterone by the liver. Other derivatives of progesterone used in the treatment of menstrual disorders include hydroxyprogesterone capronate and dydroesterone, but like progesterone, these drugs are also administered intramuscularly.

Derivatives of progesterone that are orally active include medroxyprogesterone acetate and megestrol acetate. These drugs are effective in the treatment of menstrual disorders and are also utilized in the palliative management of metastatic hormone-dependent cancers of the endometrium and breast. Norethindrone, norethynodrel and ethynodiol

Table 8-3. Natural and Synthetic Progestational Drugs

Drug	Trade name
Natural	
Progesterone	Lipo-Lutin
Progesterone Derivatives	
Medroxyprogesterone acetate	Provera, Depo-Provera, Curretab, Amen
Megestrol acetate	Megace, Pallace
Hydroxyprogesterone caproate	Delalutin
Dydrogesterone	Duphaston, Gynorest
19-Nortestosterone Derivatives	
Norethindrone	Norlutate
Norethindrone acetate	Norlutate, Aygestin
Norethynodrel	Enovid
Ethynodiol	
Ethynodiol acetate	

diacetate are derivatives of 19-nortestosterone and are used primarily in oral contraceptive formulations.

The various progestins differ in regard to their progestin potency as well as with respect to their antiestrogenic and androgenic activities (see Table 8-4). Relative to progesterone, medroxyprogesterone acetate and megestrol acetate exhibit similar affinity for the progesterone receptor, but these synthetic progesterone derivatives evoke a consider-

Table 8-4. Relative Potency and Related Characteristics of Progestational Drugs

Drug	Relative progesterone receptor affinity	Relative progestational potency	Relative antiestrogenic activity	Androgenic activity
Progesterone	1	1	1	No
Medroxyprogesterone acetate	0.8	35	Yes	No
Megestrol acetate	0.7	25	Yes	No
Norethindrone	0.85	4	7	Yes
Norethindrone acetate	0.06	2	—	—
Norethynodrel	0.05	5	0	No
Norgestrel	0.5	9	74	Yes
Ethynodiol diacetate	0.05	2	Yes	Yes

ably higher degree of progestational potency. Both medroxyprogesterone acetate and megestrol acetate demonstrate antiestrogenic activity, but neither has appreciable androgenic influences. Norethindrone also exhibits high affinity for the progesterone receptor and is a reasonably potent progestin. In addition, norethindrone produces significant estrogenic and androgenic effects (see Table 8-4). Neither norethindrone acetate, norethynodrel, nor ethynodiol diacetate has appreciable affinity for the progesterone receptor. However, these drugs are metabolized *in vivo* to norethindrone (see Figure 8-6); consequently, these drugs produce moderate progestin, antiestrogenic, and androgenic actions. Norgestrel binds to progesterone receptors less strongly than does progesterone but is capable of inducing significant progestational, antiestrogenic, and androgenic actions.

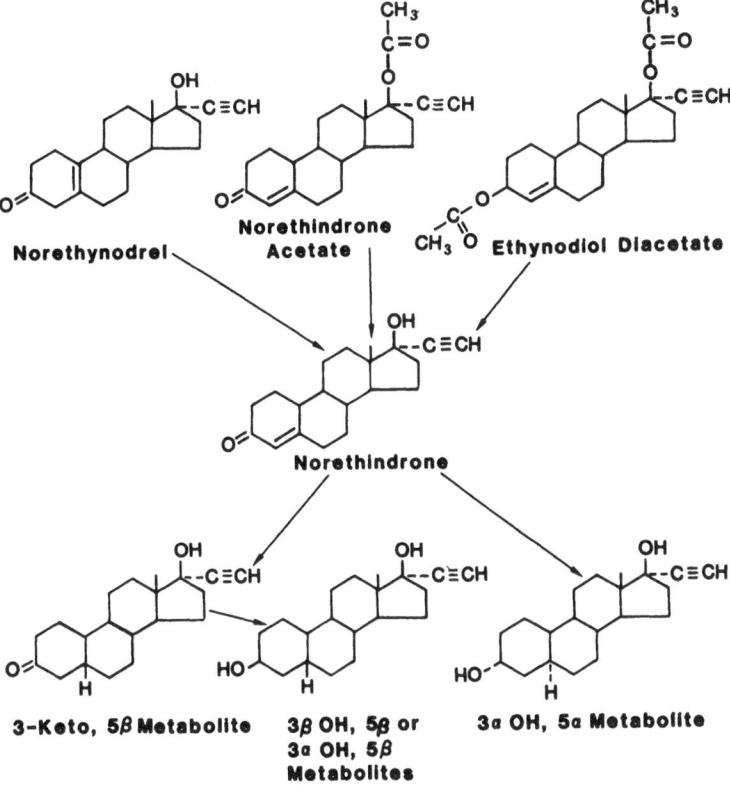

Figure 8-6. Pathways for the metabolism of the 19-norprogestins.

8.1.9. Adverse Effects

The primary untoward effects associated with the use of progestins are related to their androgenic activity (see Table 8-5). Excessive dosages of progestins, especially those that retain relatively strong androgen character, will produce weight gain, acne, and hirsutism. In the management of menstrual disorders, progestin therapy may result in delayed menses, reduced menstrual flow, decreased libido, and uterine cramping. Finally, exposure of the developing fetus to progestins during early pregnancy is associatd with teratogenesis. Progestins are not apparently carcinogenic in adults. In fact, the cyclical administration of progestins during menopausal estrogen replacement therapy reduces the risk of inducing endometrial hyperplasia and carcinoma and probably diminishes the risk of breast cancer in these women as well.

8.2. ORAL CONTRACEPTIVES

8.2.1. Preparations

Three types of oral contraceptives are currently used clinically. The most frequently prescribed preparation is a combination-type agent containing an estrogen and a progestin. Concern over the potential adverse effects attributable to estrogen has led to the development of an alternative approach utilizing continuous progestin administration. Finally, acute treatment with large doses of estrogen is useful for postcoital contraceptive purposes.

The various combination-type oral contraceptives differ principally in the type and quantity of estrogen and progestin present in the formulation (see Table 8-6). Either ethinyl estradiol or mestranol is included

---

Table 8-5. Adverse Effects Associated with Progestational Drugs

Weight gain
Acne
Hirsutism
Decreased libido
Delayed menses
Reduced menstrual flow
Uterine cramps
Teratogenesis

Table 8-6. Combination-Type Oral Contraceptive Agents

Estrogen	Dose (μg)	Progestin	Dose (mg)	Trade name
		I. Monophasic Preparations A. Low Estrogen Dose		
Ethinyl estradiol	35	Norethindrone	0.5	Brevicon
Ethinyl estradiol	35	Norethindrone	0.5	Modicon
Ethinyl estradiol	35	Norethindrone	0.4	Ovcon-35
Ethinyl estradiol	30	Norethindrone	0.3	Lo/Ovral
Ethinyl estradiol	35	Norethindrone	1.0	Norinyl 1/35
Ethinyl estradiol	35	Norethindrone	1.0	Ortho/Novum 1/35
Ethinyl estradiol	30	Norethindrone acetate	1.5	Loestrin 1.5/30
Ethinyl estradiol	20	Norethindrone acetate	1.0	Loestrin 1/20
Ethinyl estradiol	35	Ethynodiol diacetate	1.0	Demulen 1/35
Ethinyl estradiol	30	Levonorgestrel	0.15	Nordette
		B. Intermediate Estrogen Dose		
Ethinyl estradiol	50	Norethindrone	1.0	Ovcon 50
Ethinyl estradiol	50	Norgestrel	0.5	Ovral
Ethinyl estradiol	50	Norethindrone acetate	1.0	Norlestrin 1/50
Ethinyl estradiol	50	Norethindrone acetate	1.0	Zorane 1/50
Mestranol	50	Norethindrone	1.0	Norinyl 1/50
Mestranol	50	Norethindrone	1.0	Ortho Novum 1/50
Ethinyl estradiol	50	Ethynodiol diacetate	1.0	Demulen
Ethinyl estradiol	50	Norethindrone acetate	2.5	Norlestrin 2.5/50
		C. High Estrogen Dose		
Mestranol	150	Norethynodrel	9.85	Enovid 10
Mestranol	75	Norethynodrel	5.0	Enovid 5
Mestranol	100	Norethynodrel	2.5	Enovid E
Mestranol	100	Ethynodiol diacetate	1.0	Ovulen
Mestranol	100	Norethindrone	2.0	Norinyl 2
Mestranol	100	Norethindrone	2.0	Ortho-Novum 2
Mestranol	80	Norethindrone	1.0	Norinyl 1/80
Mestranol	80	Norethindrone	1.0	Ortho-Novum 1/80
Mestranol	60	Norethindrone	10.0	Norinyl 10
Mestranol	60	Norethindrone	10.0	Ortho-Novum 10
		II. Phasic Preparations A. Biphasic		
Ethinyl estradiol	35	Norethindrone	0.5 (days 1–10) 1.0 (days 11–21)	Ortho-Novum 10/11
		B. Triphasic		
Ethinyl estradiol	35	Norethindrone	0.5 (days 1–7) 0.75 (days 8–14) 1.0 (days 15–21)	Ortho-Novum 7/7/7
Ethinyl estradiol	35	Norethindrone	0.5 (days 1–7) 1.0 (days 8–16) 0.5 (days 17–21)	Tri-Norinyl

as the estrogenic component, while one of the 19-nortestosterone derivatives is used as the progestational component. The molecular structure of these hormones is illustrated in Figure 8-7. It is important to recognize that the various preparations differ with respect to estrogen and progestin dosages. In general, the combination-type agents are categorized with respect to their estrogen content (see Table 8-6).

Oral contraceptives containing low, intermediate, and high doses of estrogen are available. Dosages of the highly potent estrogenic drugs, ethinyl estradiol or mestranol of < 50 μg/day are considered low, while dosages of > 100 μg/day represent high dose regimens. As a rule, com-

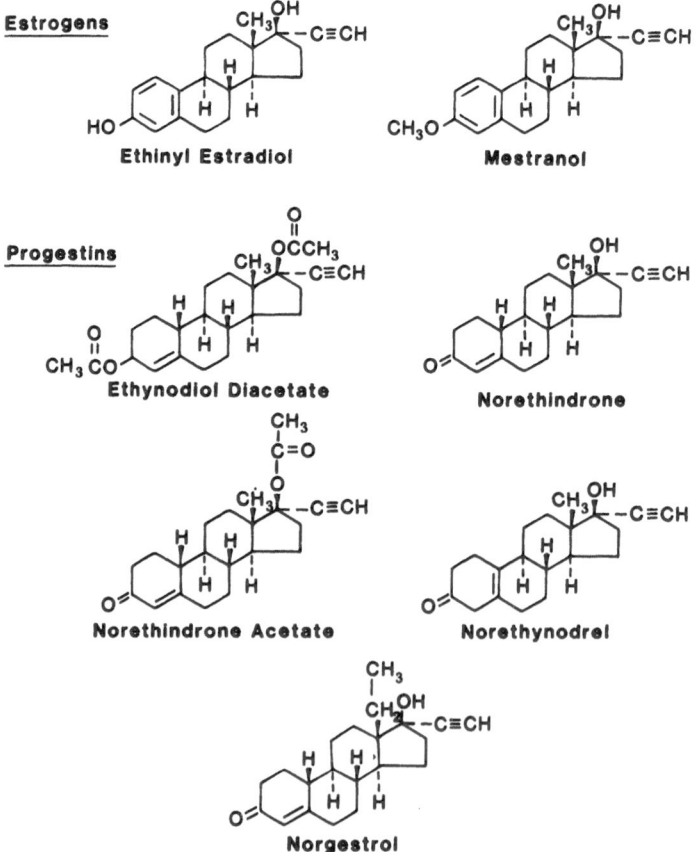

Figure 8-7. Estrogenic and progestational drugs used in oral contraceptives.

bination-type oral contraceptives containing the lowest quantity of estrogen consistent with efficacy and tolerable side effects are preferred. The progestin dosages also vary in most of the available oral contraceptives (see Table 8-6).

Recently a new generation of oral contraceptives has been developed, referred to as phasic contraceptives. These agents are designed to deliver the estrogen and progestin components in a more physiological fashion and to decrease the total dose of steroid administered during a cycle. With the biphasic preparation, the lower progestin : estrogen ratio during the first half of the treatment cycle provides for greater endometrial proliferation. Adequate secretory development results from the higher progestin : estrogen ratio in the second half of the cycle. The intent of the biphasic oral contraceptives is to minimize the incidence of mid- or late-cycle uterine bleeding associated with low-dose oral contraceptives. The triphasic agents utilize a constant low dose of estrogen and vary the progestin doses during the initial, middle, and latter periods of the treatment cycle (see Table 8-6). As with the biphasic preparations, the triphasic dosing regimen is designed to deliver the progestin in a "physiological cycle" and to reduce the total dose of progestin administered during the treatment cycle. It is anticipated that the cardiovascular and metabolic side effects attributable to the progestin will be ameliorated by the triphasic dosing approach. Long-term use of the phasic contraceptives requires continued evaluation.

The combination of different estrogens and progestins in varying dosages results in a group of drugs with a rather broad range of hormonal effects, namely, estrogenic, progestational and androgenic (see Table 8-7). Not surprisingly, the degree of estrogenic activity is related most directly to dosage of estrogen, since ethinyl estradiol and mestranol exhibit similar potency and efficacy in humans. By contrast, the degree of progestational efficacy and androgenic activity is related to the particular progestin and to its dose in the formulation (see Table 8-7). Norethynodrel is the only progestin that does not exhibit significant androgenic activity. The remainder of the 19-nortestosterone derivatives, including norethindrone, norgestrel, and ethynodiol diacetate, produce dose-dependent progestational and androgenic effects.

Currently three oral contraceptive preparations are available that contain a progestin alone (see Table 8-8). Either norethindrone or norgestrel is utilized in these formulations. Furthermore, the dose of progestin employed is lower than that used in conventional combination-type agents. Although the progestin-only contraceptives are less effective than the combination type, this approach may be suitable for patients in whom estrogenic drugs are contraindicated. These agents have

Table 8-7. Relative Estrogenic, Progestational, and Androgenic Potency of Representative Combination-Type Oral Contraceptives

Estrogen	Dose (µg)	Progestin	Dose (mg)	Potency estimates		
				Estrogenic	Progestational	Androgenic
Ethinyl estradiol	35	Norethindrone	0.5	+2	+1	+1
Ethinyl estradiol	30	Norgestrel	0.3	+1	+1	+2
Ethinyl estradiol	20	Norethindrone acetate	1.0	+1	+2	+2
Ethinyl estradiol	30	Norethindrone acetate	1.5	+1	+3	+3
Ethinyl estradiol	50	Ethynodiol diacetate	1.0	+1	+2	+1
Ethinyl estradiol	50	Norgestrel	0.5	+2	+2	+3
Ethinyl estradiol	50	Norethindrone	1.0	+2	+2	+2
Ethinyl estradiol	50	Norethindrone acetate	2.5	+1	+3	+4
Mestranol	80	Norethindrone	1.0	+2	+2	+2
Mestranol	100	Norethindrone	2.0	+2	+3	+3
Mestranol	60	Norethindrone	10.0	+1	+4	+4
Mestranol	150	Norethynodrel	9.85	+4	+3	0

Table 8-8.   Oral Contraceptives Containing Progestin Only

Progestin	Dose (mg)	Trade name
Norethindrone	0.35	Micronor
Norethindrone	0.35	Nor Q.D.
Norgestrel	0.075	Ovrette
Medroxyprogesterone acetate	150 (3 months)	Depo-Provera

not gained widespread acceptance because they fail to produce the structural stability of the endometrium associated with estrogenic stimulation. Consequently, menstrual irregularities ranging from intermittent bleeding to amenorrhea result.

Depot forms of progesterone are also being investigated for purposes of producing long-lasting contraception. Medroxyprogesterone acetate is administered intramuscularly in a depot form at a dosage of 150 mg. Such therapy produces antifertility efficacy for at least 3 months. The efficacy associated with this approach is similar to that observed with the combination-type contraceptives.

Postcoital contraception is produced by administering large doses of estrogen (see Table 8-9). This treatment is most effective when initiated within 24 hr of coitus and must begin within 72 hr. The "morning-after" technique is reserved for emergencies (e.g., rape, incest). Nausea and vomiting are a particular problem with this therapy and are a result of the high estrogen dosages involved. The potential teratogenic effect of estrogen should be considered in the event that therapy fails to intercept implantation.

8.2.2. Mechanism of Action

The combination-type contraceptive agents prevent ovulation by inhibiting gonadotropin secretion. Suppression of LH release results from the inhibitory effects (negative feedback) of the progestational component on the hypothalamus and/or the adenohypophysis (see Figure 8-8). Progestin also produces a thickening of the cervical mucus, rendering it unfavorable to penetration by sperm even in the event of ovulation. The condition of the uterine endometrium may also be altered such that implantation is unlikely; tubal transport of the ovum may be impaired as well. The estrogenic component of the combination-type agent also plays a critical role in conferring antifertility efficacy. Estrogen inhibits follicle-stimulating hormone (FSH) release by a negative feed-

Table 8-9. Postcoital Contraceptive Drugs

Drug	Dosage Regimen
Diethylstilbestrol (DES)	25 mg twice daily for 5 days
Ethinyl estradiol	2.5 mg twice daily for 5 days
Estrone	5 mg three times daily for 5 days
Estrogens (conjugated)	10 mg three times daily for 5 days
Ethinyl estradiol/norgestrel	100 μg ethinyl estradiol and 1 mg dl-norgestrel taken twice at 12-hr intervals

back process leading to ovarian quiescence and suppression of follicular growth and development (see Figure 8-8). Importantly, estrogen stabilizes the endometrium preventing breakthrough bleeding. Finally, estrogen increases progestational sensitivity by increasing the progesterone receptor content of the hypothalamus and other estrogen-sensitive tissues. These hormonal effects combine to produce effective antifertility activity. The theoretical effectiveness, as reflected by the annual pregnancy rate is estimated at 0.1%. However, the actual use effectiveness rate of pregnancy is higher (2–3%). By comparison, the use-effectiveness rate is 3–20% for barrier contraceptive methods and 25–30% for the rhythm method. Pregnancy would be expected to occur in 80–85% of women who utilize no contraceptive method.

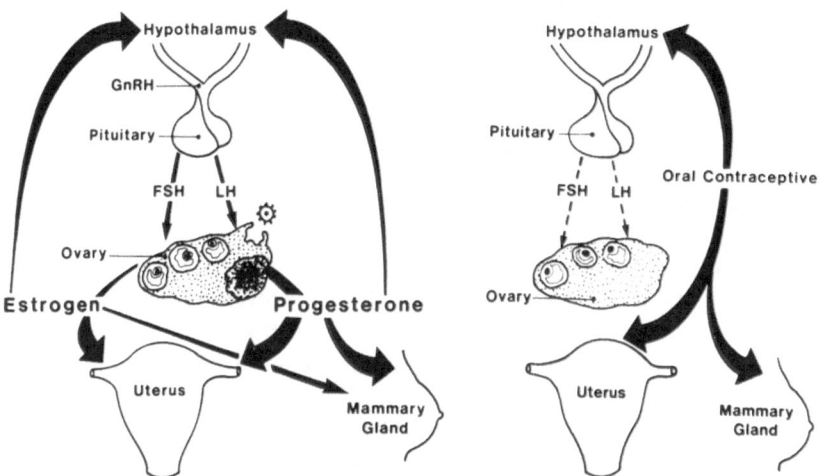

Figure 8-8. Mechanism of action of oral contraceptives.

Oral contraceptives containing only progestin do not reliably inhibit ovulation. The antifertility activity associated with these agents can be attributed to the direct progestin effects on the reproductive tract, including a thickening of the cervical mucus and a decrease in tubal transport of the ovum.

Interception of pregnancy resulting from high-dose estrogen therapy is poorly understood. Estrogenic drugs may disturb the function of the fallopian tubes and thereby interfere with ovum transport. These drugs could also affect the state of the endometrium and consequently block implantation.

8.2.3. Adverse Effects

Many of the side effects associated with the combination-type oral contraceptives are attributed to the estrogenic components. As the dose of estrogen is incresaed, the incidence and severity of untoward effects also increase. The nature of the side effects produced by combination-type contraceptives is often actually a reflection of the balance between estrogenic and progestational effects. Adverse effects attributable to either an excess or a deficiency of estrogen are outlined in Table 8-10. Common and minor problems resulting from excessive estrogenic stimulation include nausea, breast tenderness, edema, and hyperpigmentation (chloasma). Insufficient estrogen dosage results in early uterine bleeding, decreased menstrual flow, or amenorrhea. These latter effects can also result from excessive progestin challenge. Untoward effects produced by either insufficient or excessive progestin dosages are presented in Table 8-11. Noncyclic weight gain, acne, hirsutism, depression, and fatigue are signals of excessive progestin treatment. These effects are closely related to the androgenic potency of the progestin. Excessive uterine bleeding, late uterine bleeding (days 15–21), and delayed withdrawal bleeding may be attributable to either deficient progestin dosage or to excessive estrogenic stimulation.

Normal menstrual cycles generally return within the first 3 months after cessation of oral contraceptive therapy with combination-type agents. However, approximately 1–2% of patients develop postpill amenorrhea. There is some indication that women who experience irregular menstrual cycles before oral contraceptive use are more likely to develop amenorrhea after termination of therapy. Postpill amenorrhea is usually treated with inducers of ovulation, such as clomiphene, or with bromocriptine if hyperprolactinemia is associated with the amenorrhea.

Combination-type oral contraceptives produce significant effects on hepatic function. These drugs increase the incidence of gallbladder dis-

Table 8-10. Side Effects of Oral Contraceptives Related to the Dosage of Estrogen

Estrogen excess	Estrogen deficiency
Nausea and vomiting	Early uterine bleeding (days 1–14)
Dizziness–syncope	Hypomenorrhea
Edema, leg cramps	Small uterus
Irritability	Pelvic relaxation
Bloating	Nervousness
Weight gain (cyclic)	Vasomotor symptoms
Increased female fat distribution	Atrophic vaginitis
Vaginal discharge (clear)	
Uterine growth	
Fibroid growth	
Cystic breast disease	
Breast growth (ducts and stoma)	
Visual changes	
Hyperpigmentation	
Telangiectasia	
Vascular headache	
Hypertension	
Hypermenorrhea	
Dysmenorrhea (also progestin deficiency)	

ease and gallstones as a result of increased cholesterol levels in the bile. Those patients who have developed jaundice during pregnancy and women with a genetic predisposition are at higher risk of developing cholestatic jaundice while using oral contraceptives. These effects of the oral contraceptives are reversible after termination of therapy. Chronic use (>3 years) of oral contraceptives is associated with a higher risk of developing benign hepatic adenomas and focal nodular hyperplasia. This condition can become life-threatening if the adenoma ruptures resulting in hemorrhage.

Carbohydrate metabolism may be altered by oral contraceptives. Utilization of glucose can be decreased, while insulin secretion rises in a compensatory response. At least during the initial year of oral contraceptive use, this effect results from the anti-insulin effects of growth hormone, the secretion of which is stimulated by oral contraceptives. Women who become diabetic during pregnancy or women with a genetic predisposition toward diabetes mellitus are susceptible to the development of glucose intolerance while taking combination-type oral contraceptives. Generally speaking, these drugs are not utilized by diabetics who require medication for the control of blood sugar. The effects of oral contraceptives on carbohydrate metabolism are probably attributable to the progestin component.

Serum lipids are also influenced by oral contraceptive therapy. Notably, triglyceride levels rise by approximately 50%. Low-density lipoprotein (LDL) concentrations rise to a lesser extent, while high-density lipoprotein (HDL) levels may rise or fall. The progestin component is responsible for the elevation of triglycerides and for the decline in LDL. The effects on HDL levels are related to the balance between estrogen and progestins in the combination-type pill. HDL levels are elevated by estrogen and reduced by progestins.

Retrospective and prospective studies have demonstrated that the combination-type oral contraceptives produce significant cardiovascular and hematological effects. The relative risk of developing idiopathic thromboembolic phenomena (deep vein thrombosis and pulmonary embolism) is increased 4–11-fold in oral contraceptive users. The relative risk of developing superficial thrombosis is two to three times higher for women taking combination-type agents. For women with predisposing conditions, particularly a history of thromboembolic disease, the risk increases. Women with blood types A, B, or AB are at a higher risk, further emphasizing the significance of genetic predisposition to oral contraceptive use. The oral contraceptive drugs also stimulate intravas-

Table 8-11. Side Effects of Oral Contraceptives Related to the Dosage of Progestin

Progestin excess	Progestin deficiency
Weight gain (noncyclic)	Late uterine bleeding (days 15–21)
Increased appetite	Hypermenorrhea, dysmenorrhea
Fatigue	(estrogen excess also)
Depression	Delayed withdrawal uterine bleeding
Breast tenderness	Reduced breast size
Breast growth (alveolar)	Weight loss
Dilation of leg veins	
Pelvic congestion	
Decreased duration of menstruation	
Moniliasis	
Oily skin and scalp	
Acne	
Hirsutism	
Rash	
Pruritis	
Chloestatic jaundice	
Amenorrhea (postpill)	

cular clot formation by enhancing platelet number and adhesiveness, elevating blood clotting factors, reducing fibrinolysis, and damaging the vascular endothelium leading to sites of endothelial hyperplasia. Clotting factors VII, VIII, IX, and X and prothrombin are increased by oral contraceptive use, while antithrombin III levels are reduced. The increased risk of deep vein thrombosis is apparently related to the estrogenic component in a dose-dependent manner. Oral contraceptives of the combination-type that contain low estrogen doses are less likely to produce thromboembolic phenomena.

The possibility of fatal or nonfatal stroke is increased among users of oral contraceptives. Risk of thrombolic stroke is increased 10-fold, while that of hemorrhagic stroke is increased two- to threefold. The risk of subarachnoid stroke is also increased. The combination of smoking, hypertension, and the use of oral contraceptives synergistically increases the risk of hemorrhagic stroke.

Oral contraceptive use also increases the risk of circulatory disease such as ischemic heart disease and subarachnoid hemorrhage about fourfold. A group at particular cardiovascular risk are women over 35 years of age who also smoke. The increased risk of myocardial infarction may persist for at least 10 years after discontinuation; however, this increased risk is related to duration of use. Short-term use (0–5 years) is not associated with increased risk of myocardial infarction. Use of combination-type agents for 5–9 years increases the risk about twofold, and a threefold increase in risk is expected among long-term users (>10 years).

It appears that the cardiovascular effects associated with oral contraceptive use are related to the ability of these drugs to amplify the effects of other risk factors, namely, age, smoking, hypertension, diabetes, obesity, and hyperlipidemia. The estrogenic component seems to impart the hematological effect, while the progestin exerts a role in the development of ischemic heart disease.

Women, particularly those over 35 years old who use oral contraceptives are three to six times more likely to develop hypertension than are nonusers. This effect is also related to duration of use. Systolic blood pressure usually rises about 5 mm Hg, while diastolic pressure increases 1–2 mm Hg; however, larger increases in blood pressure may occur. Increased blood pressure probably results from alterations in the renin-angiotensin system involving an increase in angiotensinogen. Decreases in blood pressure are generally observed within the first 6 months after cessation of therapy.

The variety of adverse side effects associated with the use of combination-type oral contraceptives and the potential severity of these untoward effects underscore the need for caution when prescribing these drugs. The relative and absolute contraindications for the use of combination-type contraceptives are presented in Table 8-12. Relative contraindications include age (>35 years), a history of migraine headaches, or gestational diabetes mellitus, varicose veins, hypertension, and the prospect of elective surgery as it relates to the potential for abnormal blood clotting. Absolute contraindications for the use of combination-type contraceptives include thromboembolic disease or a history of such, impaired hepatic function, obstructive jaundice during pregnancy, congenital hyperlipidemia, pregnancy, undiagnosed uterine bleeding, and hormone-dependent cancer of the breast or uterus (see Table 8-12).

Current evidence suggests that oral contraceptives (combination-type) do not increase the risk of developing cancer of the breast, endometrium, or ovaries. In fact, the incidence of benign breast disease is lower in women using oral contraceptives. It is well recognized that fibrocystic breast disease is a significant risk factor in breast cancer. By contrast, patients who have had a previous history of cystic breast disease and who subsequently initiate oral contraceptive therapy may be at substantially increased (11-fold) risk of developing carcinoma of the breast. Combination-type oral contraceptives reduce the risk of endometrial cancer by 50%. Likewise, the incidence of ovarian cancer is lower in women using these drugs. It should be stressed that the precise role

Table 8-12. Contraindications for the Use of Oral Contraceptives

Relative contraindications
  Migraine headache
  Hypertension
  Uterine leiomyomas
  Epilepsy
  Varicose veins
  Gestational diabetes
  Elective surgery
  Women over 35 years of age

Absolute contraindications
  Thromboembolic disease (or past history)
  Impaired liver function
  Breast or uterine cancer (estrogen-dependent)
  Abnormal uterine bleeding (undiagnosed)
  Pregnancy
  Cholestatic jaundice in pregnancy
  Congenital hyperlipidemia

of oral contraceptives in the carcinogenesis of the female reproductive system remains unresolved due to the long latent period exhibited by these carcinomas. It would seem reasonable that the progesterone dominance of the combination-type oral contraceptives could provide a protective (antiestrogenic) milieu and thereby restrict the development of estrogen-dependent breast and uterine carcinomas.

Drugs such as barbiturates and anticonvulsants have been shown to reduce the efficacy of oral contraceptives. This effect is related to the induction of hepatic oxidative metabolism, which reduces the efficacy of the contraceptive agents. This drug interaction could be expected to be of particular significance when low-dose estrogen formulations are being administered. Similarly, some antibiotics including ampicillin and tetracycline reduce the effectiveness of oral contraceptives by decreasing enterohepatic recirculation of the steroid hormones. This is the result of disturbing the bacterial flora of the gut, which are involved in the metabolism of steroid conjugates before recirculation.

RECOMMENDED READINGS

Physiology and Pharmacology of the Progestins

Benagiano, G., Zulli, P., and Diczfalusy, E., Progestogens in therapy, *Serono Symp. Ser.* **3**:1–270, 1983.

Chan, L., and O'Malley, B. W., Mechanism of action of the sex steroid hormones, *N. Engl. J. Med.* **294**:1322, 1976.

Edgren, R. A., Progestagens, in: *Clinical Use of Sex Steroids* (J. R. Givens, ed.), pp. 1–29, Year Book Medical Publishers, Chicago, 1979.

Gambrell, R.D., Menopause: Benefits and risks of estrogen–progestogen replacement therapy, *Fertil. Steril.* **37**:457, 1982.

Gambrell, R. D., Proposal to decrease the risk and improve the prognosis of breast cancer, *Am. J. Obstet. Gynecol.* **150**:119, 1984.

Gambrell, R. D., Bagnell, C. A., and Greenblatt, R. B., Role of estrogens and progesterone in the etiology and prevention of endometrial cancer: Review, *Am. J. Obstet. Gynecol.* **146**:696, 1983.

Gold, R. B., and Wilson, P. D., Depo-Provera: New development in decade-old controversy, *Fam. Plann. Perspect.* **13**:35, 1981.

Grody, W. W., Schrader, W. T., and O'Malley, B. W., Activation, transformation and subunit structure of steroid hormone receptors, *Endocrine Rev.* **3**:141, 1982.

Horowitz, K. B., Wey, L. L., Sedlacek, S. M., and d'Arville, C. N., Progestin action and progesterone receptor structure in human breast cancer: A review, *Recent Prog. Horm. Res.* **41**:249–317, 1985.

Keenan, E. J., The physiological and pathophysiological significance of steroid hormone receptors, *Gynecol. Obstet.* **5**:343, 1982.

Knobil, E., The neuroendocrine control of the menstrual cycle, *Recent Prog. Horm. Res.* **36**:53, 1980.

McCarty, K. S., Jr., Lubahn, D. B., and McCarty, K. S., Sr., Estrogen and progesterone receptors: Physiological and pathological considerations, *Clin. Endocrinol. Metab.* **12**:133, 1983.

McGuire, W. L., and Clark, G. M., Role of progesterone receptors in breast cancer, *J. Sem. Oncol.* **12**:12–16, 1985.

Neumann, F., Progestogens: A short review, *Postgrad. Med. J.* (Suppl. 2) **54**:11, 1978.

O'Malley, B. W., Steroid hormone action in eukaryotic cells, *J. Clin Invest.* **74**:307, 1984.

Renoir, J. M., and Mester, J., Chick oviduct progesterone receptor: Structure, immunology, function, *Mol. Cell Endocrinol.* **37**:1, 1984.

Richards, J. S., Maturation of ovarian follicles: actions and interactions of pituitary and ovarian hormones on follicular cell differentiation, *Physiol. Rev.* **60**:51, 1980.

Rochefort, H., and Chalbos, D., Progestin-specific markers in human cell lines: Biological and pharmacological applications, *Mol. Cell Endocrinol.* **36**:36, 1984.

Whitehead, M. I., Townsend, P. T., Pryse-Davies, J., Ryder, T. A., and King, R. J. B. Effects of estrogens and progestins on biochemistry and morphology of postmenopausal endometrium, *N. Engl. J. Med.* **305**:1599, 1981.

Wilson, J. C., and Brent, R. L., Are female sex hormones teratogenic?, *Am. J. Obstet. Gynecol.* **141**:567, 1981.

Pharmacology of the Oral Contraceptives

Andrews, W. C., Oral contraception: Physiologic and pathologic effects, *Obstet. Gynecol. Ann.* **7**:325:1981.

Back, D. J., Breckenridge, A. M., Crawford, F. E., Mac Iver, M., Orme, M. L. E., and Rowe, P. H., Interindividual variation and drug interactions with hormonal steroid contraceptives, *Drugs* **21**: 46, 1981.

Benagiano, G., and Primiero, F. M., Long acting contraceptives: Present status, *Drugs* **25**:570, 1983.

Bronson, R. A., Oral contraception: Mechanism of action, *Clin. Obstet. Gynecol.* **24**:869, 1981.

Centers for Disease Control, Cancer and Steroid Hormone Study: Oral Contraceptive use and the risk of endometrial cancer, *JAMA* **249**:1600, 1983.

Centers for Disease Control, Cancer and Steroid Hormone Study, Oral contraceptive use and the risk of ovarian cancer, *JAMA* **249**:1596, 1983.

Centers for Disease Control, Cancer and Steroid Hormone Study, Long-term oral contraceptive use and risk of breast cancer, *JAMA* **249**:1591, 1983.

Dalen, J. E., and Hickler, R. B., Oral contraceptives and cardiovascular disease, *Am. Heart J.* **101**:626, 1981.

Della, J. E., and Emery, M. G., Clnical pharmacology and common minor side effects of oral contraceptives, *Clin Obstet. Gynecol.* **24**:879, 1981.

Diczfalusy, E., Gregory Pincus and steroidal contraception: A new departure in the history of mankind, *J. Steroid Biochem.* **11**:3, 1979.

Dixon, G. W., Schlesselman, J. S., Ory, H. W., and Blye, R. P. Ethinylestradiol and conjugated estrogens as postcoital contraceptives, *JAMA* **244**:1336, 1980.

Dorflinger, L. J., Relative potency of progestins used in oral contraceptives, *Contraception* **31**:557–570, 1985.

Droegemaueller, W., and Bressler, R., Effectiveness and risks of contraception, *Annu. Rev. Med.* **31**:329, 1980.

Edgren, R. A. Progestational potency of oral contraceptives: A polemic, *Int. J. Fertil.* **23**:162, 1978.

Edgren, R. A., and Sturtevant, F. M., Potencies of oral contraceptives, *Am. J. Obstet. Gynecol.* **125:**1029, 1976.

Goldzieher, J. W., Estrogens in oral contraceptives: Historical perspectives, *Johns Hopkins Med. J.* **150:**165, 1982.

Greenblatt, R. B., Oral contraceptives: The state of the art, *Clin. Ther.* **8:**6, 1985.

McQueen, E. G., Hormonal steroid contraceptives: A further review of adverse reactions, *Drugs* **16:**322, 1978.

McQueen, E. G., The long term safety of hormonal steroid contraceptives, *Drugs* **16:**460, 1981.

Mishell, D. R., Non-contraceptive health benefits of oral steroid contraceptives, *Am. J. Obstet. Gynecol.* **142:**809, 1982.

Realini, J. P., and Goldzieher, J. W., Oral contraceptives and cardiovascular disease: A critique of the epidemiologic studies, *Am. J. Obstet. Gynecol.* **152:**729, 1985.

Smith, M. A., and Youngkin, E. Q., Current perspectives on combination oral contraceptives, *Clin. Pharm.* **3:**485, 1984.

Speroff, L., The formulation of oral contraceptives: Does the amount of estrogen make any clinical difference?, *Johns Hopkins Med. J.* **150:**170, 1982.

Stadel, B. V., Oral contraceptives and cardiovascular disease, *N. Engl. J. Med.* **305:**612 (pt. 1), 672 (pt. 2), 1981.

Upton, G. V., The phasic approach to oral contraception: The triphasic concept and its application, *Int. J. Fertil.* **28:**121, 1983.

Wilson, E. A., Steroid contraception, in: *Clinical Use of Sex Steroid* (J. R. Givens, ed.), p. 117, Year Book Medical Publishers, Chicago, 1980.

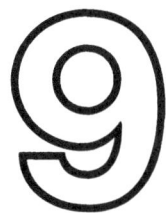

ADRENOCORTICOSTEROID DRUGS

9.1. INTRODUCTION

The adrenocorticosteroids drugs are an important group of therapeutic compounds used for a variety of clinical purposes. It is estimated that annually at least 5 million patients in the United States receive adrenocortical steroids. These agents are used in hormonal replacement therapy as well as for extension of their physiological actions. The adrenocorticosteroids are well recognized for the diversity of their actions underlying their extensive therapeutic use. It is the anti-inflammatory and immunosuppressive activity produced by these steroids that is widely sought for the palliative therapy of many clinical conditions. As would be expected of drugs that influence a multiplicity of tissues, the adrenocortical steroids produce a number of adverse effects. A well-founded appreciation for the pharmacological characteristics of these drugs provides the basis for the rational and safe use of this important group of drugs.

9.2. HISTORY

The muscle wasting disease associated with the destruction of the adrenal glands was initially characterized by Addison in 1855. One year later, Brown-Sequard demonstrated in experimental animals that the adrenal glands are essential for life. It was not until 1932 that Cushing described the classic clinical condition associated with hyperfunction of the adrenal glands.

The period between 1908 and 1930 led to the development of the role of the adrenal gland in carbohydrate metabolism. Bierry and Malloizel demonstrated in 1908 that blood glucose levels were decreased in adrenalectomized dogs, and 2 years later a similar observation was made in patients with Addison's disease. Cori and Cori (1927) systematically studied the adrenal influences on carbohydrate metabolism and noted that hepatic glycogen levels were reduced following adrenalectomy.

The ability of the adrenals to regulate electrolyte balance was established in 1927, when it was noted by Bauman and Kurland that plasma sodium and chloride levels declined, while potassium levels rose, following adrenalectomy. Loeb and associates extended their observations by observing the beneficial effects of dietary sodium on the clinical status of addisonian patients.

Extracts of the adrenal gland became available by 1927, and the findings regarding the effects of these extracts on carbohydrate and electrolyte metabolism were further developed. Long and associates had by 1940 demonstrated that adrenal extracts reversed the changes in carbohydrate metabolism observed in adrenalectomized animals. Kendall had purified glucocorticoids by 1936; with Long he established the effects of these steroid hormones on nitrogen balance. Glucocorticoid-treated animals excreted considerable greater quantities of nitrogen than did adrenalectomized animals. These studies suggested that glucocorticoids raise blood sugar by stimulating the conversion of protein to amino acids and subsequently to glucose *via* increased gluconeogenesis. These investigators also noted the influences of the glucocorticoids on lipid metabolism.

Separation of the glucocorticoid and mineralocorticoid activities was established following the synthesis of deoxycorticosterone during the late 1930s by Steiger and Reichstein. These workers observed that deoxycorticosterone produces only mineralocorticoid activity. Corticosterone was identified in 1937 by Reichstein and by Kendall, and pure formulations exhibiting primarily glucocorticoid activity became available by 1940. Partial synthesis of cortisol was achieved by 1946. The interests of the pharmaceuticals industry subsequently led to the development of many glucocorticoid drugs varying in duration of action and in degree of mineralocorticoid activity.

As early as 1929, Hench had recognized that arthrithic patients sometimes experienced remission when they were pregnant or jaundiced. He reasoned that adrenal hypersecretion during these clinical states was responsible for the remission. The availability of cortisone (1949) led to the use of this steroid in arthritic patients by Hench; dramatic improvements were observed, confirming his early hypothesis. In

1950 Hench, Kendall, and Reichstein were awarded the Nobel Prize for their pioneering studies demonstrating the significance of the adreno-cortical steroids.

It was recognized during the mid-1950s that glucocorticoids regulate the activity of a number of enzymes, and the concept that these steroids produce their effects by modulating enzyme protein synthesis was born. The induction of two key hepatic enzymes involved in gluconeogenesis, namely, tyrosine aminotransferase and tryptophan oxygenase, was studied extensively. By the mid-1960s, it had been established that the molecular basis for glucocorticoid-mediated induction of enzyme synthesis lay in their ability to stimulate transcription of specific mRNAs. The concept that the glucocorticoids regulate the DNA-dependent synthesis of RNA by interacting with specific receptor proteins that exert an intranuclear action developed during the early 1970s. More recently, significant efforts have been focused on the development of a better appreciation for the mechanism of glucocorticoid action through the purification of receptor proteins and from studies of the interaction between corticosteroid receptors and the genome of eukaryotic cells.

9.3. CHEMISTRY

The adrenocorticosteroids are 21-carbon molecules derived from cholesterol. The basic corticosteroid structure is depicted in Figure 9-1. Biological activity is dependent on the presence of a 4,5-double bond and a ketone group at C-3. The presence of a hydroxyl group at C-11 conveys glucocorticoid activity, while its absence results in a steroid (deoxycorticosterone) with predominantly mineralocorticoid activity. The substitution of a hydroxyl group at C-17 yields cortisol or hydrocortisone, which exhibits enhanced glucocorticoid activity. Hydrocortisone is the chief glucocorticoid elicited by the human adrenal cortex. Modifica-

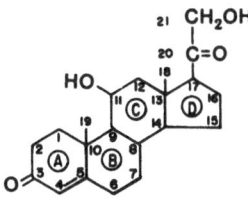

Figure 9-1. Basic molecular structure of the anti-inflammatory adrenal corticosteroids.

Δ^4-Pregnene-11β-21-diol-3, 20-dione

tions of positions involving all four of the rings of the steroid nucleus profoundly change the glucocorticoid and mineralocorticoid potencies, oral availability, and duration of action of the synthetic glucocorticoid derivatives.

9.4. BIOSYNTHESIS, SECRETION, AND METABOLISM

The anatomy of the adrenal gland is depiced in Figure 9-2. Catecholamine synthesis occurs in the inner region or medulla of the adrenal gland. The steroid hormones are synthesized in the outer or cortical region consisting of three distinct zones. Synthesis of the mineralocorticoids occurs in the zona glomerulosa, the outermost region. The zona fasciculata represents the middle portion of the adrenal cortex, where the glucocorticoids are produced. Precursors to the sex steroid hormones are formed in the innermost region, referred to as the zona reticularis. Table 9-1 lists the hormones of the adrenal gland. Epinephrine and lesser quantities of norepinephrine are secreted from the adrenal medulla. The glucocorticoids, cortisol and corticosterone, are synthesized in the adrenal cortex, with cortisol being the principal glucocorticoid in humans. Aldosterone and the less potent deoxycorticosterone represent mineralocorticoids elicited from the adrenal cortex. Dehydroepiandrosterone (DHEA), its sulfate derivative, androstenedione, and small quantities of testosterone represent the primary adrenal androgens. DHEA and an-

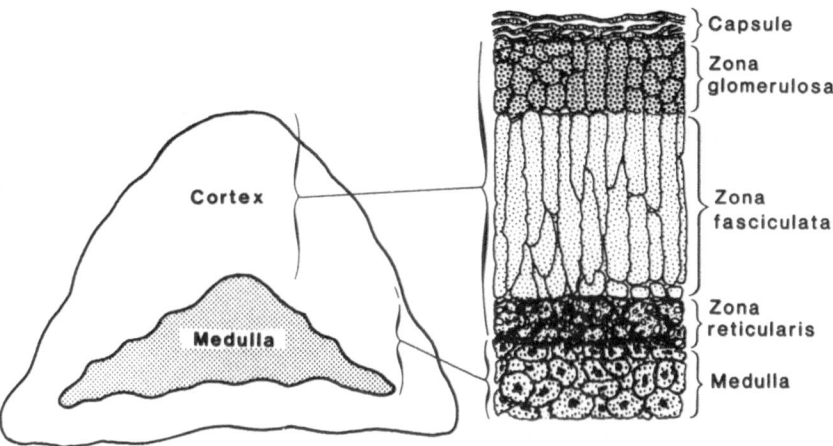

Figure 9-2. Schematic representation of the anatomy of the adrenal gland.

Table 9-1. Hormones of the
Adrenal Glands

Medullary region
Epinephrine
Norepinephrine
Cortical region
Glucocorticoids
Cortisol
Corticosterone
Mineralocorticoids
Aldosterone
Deoxycorticosterone
Sex steroids
Dehydroepiandrosterone (DHEA)
Androstenedione
Testosterone

drostenedione are readily converted by the liver, skin, and adipose tissue to more potent estrogens and androgens such as estrone and testosterone, respectively.

Regulation of the synthesis and secretion of adrenal steroids is portrayed in Figure 9-3. Neural stimuli associated with stress and sensory input converge on the hypothalamus and stimulate the release of corticotropin-releasing hormone (CRH). Stressful stimuli such as trauma, anxiety, severe infections, and hypoglycemia, as well as surgery provoke stimulatory signals arising from the anterior and posterior brain regions. Basal secretion of CRH is modulated in a circadian pattern by neural stimuli emanating from the anterior brain areas. CRH, a peptide, traverses the hypothalamic–adenohypophyseal vasculature and selectively associates with specific, plasma membrane-associated receptors in pituitary corticotrophs (see Chapter 2). The release of adrenocorticotropic hormone (ACTH) from the adenohypophysis promptly follows CRH stimulation. Before its release, ACTH is processed from a larger precursor molecule, pro-opiomelanocortin, which also contains amino acid sequences for lipotropin (LPH), α- and γ-melanocyte-stimulating hormone, (α-MSH and γ-MSH), β-endorphin, and corticotropinlike intermediate lobe peptide (CLIP). Subsequently, ACTH stimulates ACTH receptors in the adrenal cortex, elevating cAMP and leading to the stimulation of glucocorticoid synthesis and secretion.

Systemic glucocorticoids act back upon cells in the hypothalamus and the anterior pituitary gland to limit excessive production of glucocorticoids. Two types of feedback inhibition are involved, differing in their rate of onset. A rapid feedback system acts immediately and is

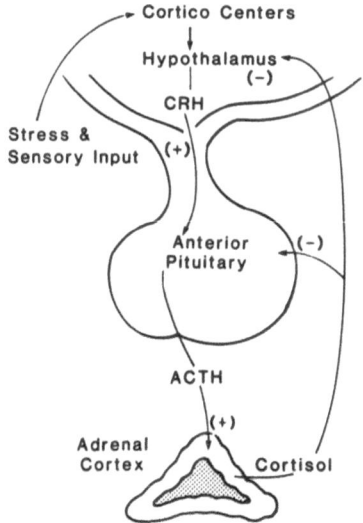

Figure 9-3. Regulation of adrenocortical function.

involved in minute-to-minute physiological control. The delayed system operates more slowly and is involved in the suppression of ACTH produced by exogenous glucocorticoids. The latter type of feedback inhibition can produce significant difficulties to the patient receiving prolonged glucocorticoid therapy. In these cases, the hypothalamus and adenohypophysis can remain suppressed for up to 1 year. Lack of endogenous glucocorticoids (e.g., Addison's disease) results in excessive ACTH secretion due to the absence of glucocorticoid-mediated feedback inhibition. Since ACTH is derived from a larger precursor peptide, proopiomelanocortin, which contains the amino acid sequence for MSH, addisonian patients often exhibit hyperpigmentation, produced by excessive secretion of MSH.

The synthesis of mineralocorticoids occurring in the zona glomerulosa is not regulated by ACTH. Rather, changes in blood volume and blood pressure control the synthesis and the release of aldosterone *via* the renin-angiotensin system (see Figure 9-4). Renal renin secretion increases when blood volume is low and converts angiotensinogen (derived from the liver) to angiotensin I. Conversion of angiotensin I to angio tensin II results in the stimulus for aldosterone secretion. Aldosterone enhances sodium retention and stimulates potassium exchange in the distal renal tubule. Increased sodium retention and concomitant reabsorption of water produce increases in blood volume and blood pressure that signal for a reduction in aldosterone synthesis and release. Approximately 30–150 μg of aldosterone is secreted daily.

The enzymatic steps involved in the synthesis of adrenocortical steroids are outlined in Figure 9-5. Glucocorticoids and mineralocorticoids are derived from cholesterol, as are the other steroid hormones. The conversion of cholesterol to pregnenolone is the rate-limiting step; this reaction is catalyzed by desmolase. Pregnenolone production occurs in mitochondria and is regulated by ACTH through a cAMP-dependent process. Pregnenolone is subsequently transported to the endoplasmic reticulum, where the synthesis of the adrenalcortical steroids proceeds by two pathways. One metabolic route involves the conversion of pregnenolone to progesterone, to corticosterone, and subsequently to aldosterone. The alternative pathway proceeds from 17α-hydroxyprogesterone to 11-deoxycortisol and results in cortisol production. These biosynthetic pathways for the glucocorticoids involve the 17-, 21-, and 11-hydroxylase systems that are localized in the endoplasmic reticulum, except for 11-hydroxylation, which occurs within mitochondria. The synthesis of aldosterone requires hydroxylation at C-18 to produce corticosterone as a precursor. Synthesis of dehydroepiandrosterone and androstenedione result from the further metabolism of 17α-hydroxypregnenolone and 17α-hydroxyprogesterone (Figure 9-5).

Glucocorticoids are synthesized and secreted in a circadian manner. ACTH release and plasma cortisol levels are highest in the early morning

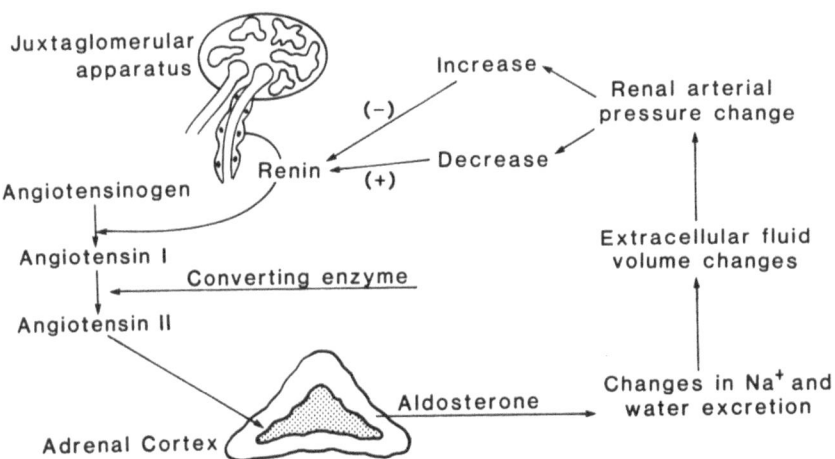

Figure 9-4. Aldosterone and the renin-angiotensin system.

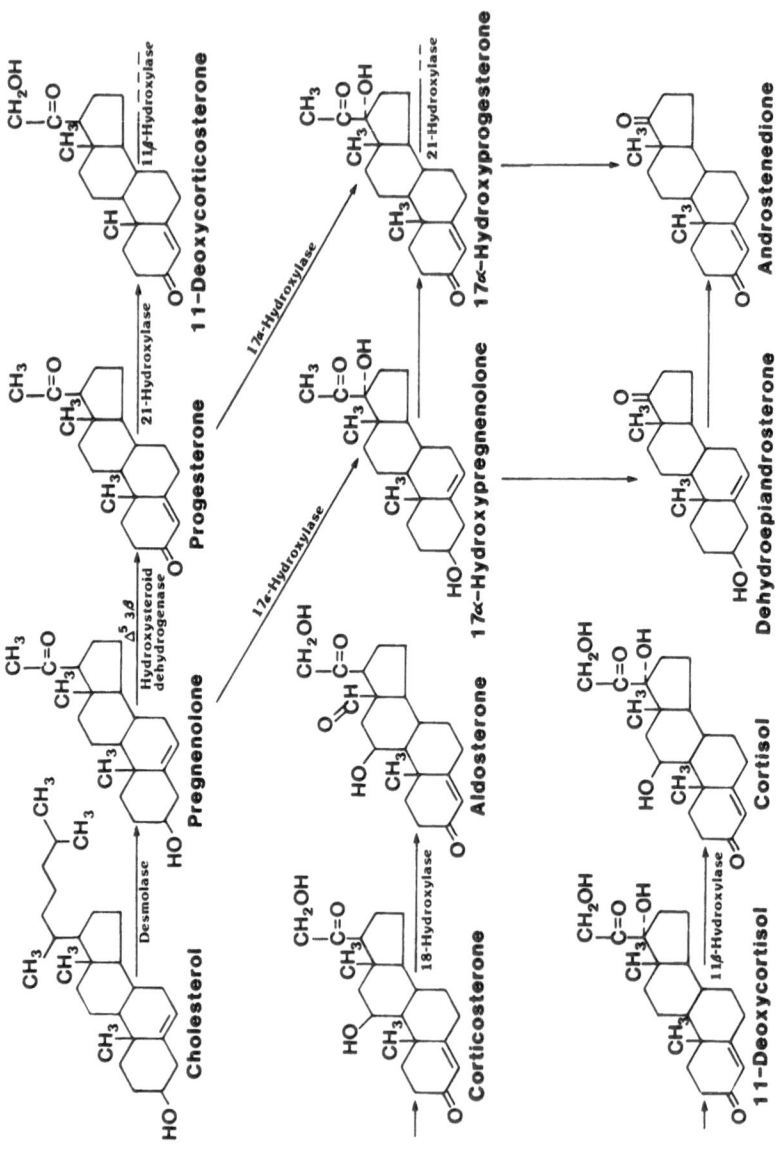

Figure 9-5. Biosynthesis of the adrenocortical steroids.

hours, when conventional light–dark and sleep cycles are followed. In the normal, unstressed adult, approximately 20 mg of cortisol is secreted daily. Plasma cortisol levels range from 1–5 μg/ml at midnight (during sleep) to approximately 15–20 μg/ml between 6 and 8 AM. The circadian pattern of cortisol secretion provides the basis for the alternate-day dosing regimens used to minimize suppression of the hypothalamic/pituitary axis by exogenous corticosteroids. Alternate-day therapy is discussed subsequently (see Section 9.9).

Approximately 90% of plasma cortisol is bound to proteins, namely, corticosteroid-binding globulin (CBG) and to albumin. Seventy-five percent is associated with CBG, and the remaining 15% is bound to albumin. CBG exhibits greater specificity and affinity but a lower capacity for glucocorticoid binding than does albumin. Binding of these steroids to CBG is not required for biologic activity. Corticosteroids are soluble in plasma at effective levels; synthetic glucocorticoids are highly efficacious, yet they do not bind to CBG. Consequently, CBG acts as a reservoir, providing a constant supply of cortisol to target cells. Protein binding of the glucocorticoids also prolongs their plasma half-life by reducing their rate of metabolic clearance. Suppression of ACTH release is also not as marked, since only free glucocorticoids could be expected to enter the hypothalamus and pituitary gland. Pregnancy, chronic estrogen therapy, and thyroxine increase CBG levels as well as total plasma levels of cortisol. The relative amount of free cortisol does not change under these conditions.

Unbound cortisol is rapidly removed from the circulation. The plasma half-life of cortisol is approximately 100 min. Less than 2% of cortisol is excreted unchanged in the urine. The primary site of catabolism is the liver. Metabolism of cortisol either decreases or abolishes its activity. The major steps of cortisol metabolism include (1) reduction of the 4–5 double bond in the A ring of the steroid nucleus, and (2) hydroxylation of the 3-keto group (see Table 9-2). Glucuronide conjugation increases water solubility, reduces protein binding, and increases the elimination

Table 9-2. Hepatic Catabolism of Cortisol and Cortisone

Reaction	Product
Reduction of 4,5-double bond (ring A)	Dihydrocortisol and dihydrocortisone
Reduction of 3-keto group (ring A)	Tetrahydrocortisol and tetrahydrocortisone
Reduction of C-20	Cortol and cortolone
Glucuronidation at 3α-position (ring A)	Reduced conjugates
Oxidative removal of side chain at C-17	17-Ketosteroids
Hydroxylation of C-6	6α-Hydroxycortisol and 6α-hydroxycortisone

rate of glucocorticoid metabolites. Additional, less important steps in the metabolism of cortisol are outlined in Table 9-2.

9.5. MECHANISM OF ACTION

The adrenal steroids interact with specific intracellular receptor proteins in order to produce a significant number of their many actions (see Figure 9-6). Receptors for aldosterone are distinct from those that recognize glucocorticoids. Corticosteroid receptors are initially localized in the cytoplasm and, following activation, are translocated to the nucleus. Two forms of the cytosolic glucocorticoid receptor probably exist. One form cannot readily bind hormone, and a second form is endowed with the capacity to associate with glucocorticoids. Phosphorylation of the receptor protein conveys the capability of binding corticosteroids. Molybdate ion, an inhibitor of phosphatase enzyme, as well as phosphate sources including ATP and pyridoxal phosphate, stabolize glucocorticoid receptors. The precise role of phosphorylation and dephosphorylation of the corticosteroid receptors has not been elucidated.

Glucocorticoid–receptor complexes ultimately act within the nucleus, presumably at specific effector regions of the genome. Association of

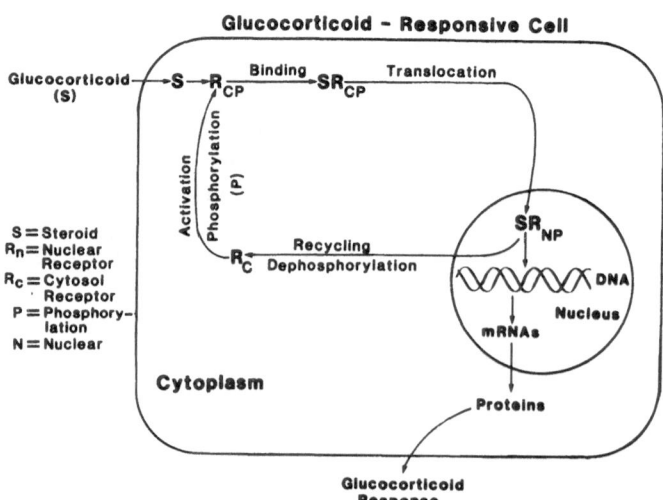

Figure 9-6. Schematic representation of the molecular mechanism of glucocorticoid action. S, steroid; R_n, nuclear receptor; R_c, Cytosol receptor; P, phosphorylation; N, nuclear.

the receptor complexes at these sites stimulates DNA-dependent synthesis of RNA leading to increases in mRNAs. These molecular transcripts code for the synthesis of specific proteins responsible for eliciting glucocorticoid effects. It is likely that expression of only a small portion of the genome is affected by glucocorticoid–receptor complexes. Significant advances in our understanding of the molecular events underlying glucocorticoid action can be expected to result from present hybridization and recombinant DNA studies.

An appreciation for the basic steps of glucocorticoid action is significant in understanding the pharmacology of these drugs. Importantly, since the glucocorticoids effects depend on the transcription of mRNA and translation of the specific gene products, it is not surprising that there is an appreciable time lag (hours) before the onset of glucocorticoid actions. Likewise, there is a significant variation in the duration of steroid effects due to the variable rates of degradation of the critical gene products.

9.6. PHYSIOLOGICAL AND PHARMACOLOGICAL ACTIONS

A characteristic of adrenal steroids is the diversity of their actions (see Table 9-3). The pharmacological actions of these hormones and their derivatives are merely an extension of their physiological effects. Glucocorticoid influences on carbohydrate and lipid metabolism are both anabolic and catabolic in nature.

Anabolic actions include stimulation of gluconeogenesis and increased glycogen storage. The elevated rate of gluconeogenesis is attributable to the induction of specific hepatic enzymes. Hyperglycemia and related actions are the product of the catabolic effects of the glucocorticoids. These hormones stimulate the conversion of proteins in skeletal muscle and connective tissue into amino acids, which are then converted in the liver to glucose. Hepatic enzymes involved in gluconeogenesis and induced by glucocorticoids include glucose 6-phosphatase, fructose 6-diphosphatase, phosphoenopyruvate carboxykinase, tyrosine aminotransferase and tryptophan pyrrolase. The net effect of the glucocorticoids is to oppose the actions of insulin, that is, to promote hyperglycemia and glucosuria. Lipolysis in peripheral adipose tissue is stimulated by glucocorticoids, causing increases in circulating levels of glycerol and free fatty acids. Many of the lipolytic actions of the glucocorticoids may be related to their ability to enhance the actions of epinephrine. Glucocorticoids are not necessarily lipolytic in all adipose tissue. In fact, lipogenesis is enhanced in the abdominal fat stores, ex-

Table 9-3. Physiological and Pharmacological Actions of the Adrenal
Steroids

Anabolic actions
  Stimulate gluconeogenesis
  Stimulate hepatic glycogen storage
  Hyperglycemia
Catabolic actions
  Stimulate conversion of proteins to amino acids
  Stimulate lipolysis
Electrolyte balance
  Antagonize actions of vitamin D and impair calcium absorption
  Stimulate sodium reabsorption and potassium excretion (mineralocorticoids)
Immune system
  Decrease infiltration by lymphocytes
  Decrease lymphocyte and thymocyte populations (antimitotic)
  Suppress cell-mediated hypersensitivity
  Impair phagocytosis
Cardiovascular system
  Decrease permeability of capillary endothelium
  Inotropic (positive) action on myocardium
  Facilitate vasoconstriction
Central nervous system
  Euphoria
  Reduce seizure threshold

---

plaining the redistribution of body fat in patients receiving excessive
glucocorticoid therapy or individuals with Cushing's disease.

The adrenal steroids also produce pronounced effects on ion balance. Glucocorticoids antagonize the actions of vitamin D in the gastrointestinal (GI) tract, thereby lowering the plasma levels of calcium.
The potent mineralocorticoid, aldosterone, stimulates the reabsorption
of sodium and excretion of potassium in the distal tubule of the renal
nephron.

A basis for much of the therapeutic utility of the glucocorticoids is
founded in their ability to suppress the immune system as well as to
produce anti-inflammatory activity. Antagonism of inflammation involves the complex interaction of these hormones with several components of the reticuloendothelial system (RES). Glucocorticoids decrease
the permeability of the capillary endothelium, restricting the movement
of leukocytes from the circulation to sites of inflammation. These steroids
also produce antimitotic activity in certain cell types, particularly the
small lymphocytes and thymocyte populations. Consequently, the number of circulating lymphocytes is reduced as is their ability to enter sites
of inflammation. Lysosomal membranes are stabilized by corticosteroids,

but the steroid concentrations required to produce this effect are considerably higher than needed to produce anti-inflammatory activity.

Glucocorticoids produce suppressive effects at virtually evey step of the immune response. Phagocytosis of antigens is impaired, migration of cells to areas of inflammation is decreased, and, in sufficient doses, cell-mediated hypersensitivity reactions are depressed. Since the T lymphocytes are primarily responsive to glucocorticoids and are not involved in humoral immunity, the production of antibodies is not affected by these steroid hormones. The suppressive effects of the corticosteroids on cell-mediated immunity are important to their use in preventing rejection of transplanted organs. Clearly, these drugs do not interfere with the antigen–antibody reaction, but they do interfere with the inflammatory response produced by this interaction.

The cardiovascular and CNS effects of the glucocorticoids are not well understood. These hormones restore circulatory function in shock resulting from hemorrhage, anaphylaxis, endotoxin, snake venom, or trauma. This effect may be related to the positive intropic actions of the glucocorticoids on the myocardium. The glucocorticoids also appear to provide permissive actions that enhance adrenergic stimulation of vasoconstriction in small vessels. The CNS effects of the glucocorticoids include euphoria and decreases in seizure threshold. It is possible that these effects of the glucocorticoids are related to alterations in carbohydrate metabolism, electrolyte balance, and cerebral blood flow.

9.7. PREPARATIONS

The glucocorticoid and anti-inflammatory drugs can be distinguished according to differences in their duration of action and potency (see Table 9-4). Agents demonstrating a short duration of action include hydrocortisone and cortisone. Synthetic derivatives of cortisol such as prednisone, prednisolone, methylprednisolone, fluprednisolone, triamcinolone, and paramethasone are thought to have intermediate duration of action. Both betamethasone and dexamethasone are synthetic derivatives that produce a long duration of action. Extending the action of these drugs stems largely from chemical modification of the glucocorticoid structure. The rate of hepatic degradation is reduced, oral activity is conferred, and in most cases anti-inflammatory potency is increased and mineralocorticoid activity is reduced but not eliminated.

The molecular structures of the anti-inflammatory glucocorticoid drugs are presented in Figure 9-7. Modification of cortisone and cortisol by addition of a 1,2-double bond results in prednisone and prednisolone,

Table 9-4. The Glucocorticoid and
Anti-inflammatory Steroids[a]

Short duration of action
  Hydrocortisone (Cortex, Hydrocortone)
  Cortisone (Cortone)
Intermediate duration of action
  Prednisone (Deltasone, Meticorten, Ovasone)
  Prednisolone (Delta-Cortef, Sterane)
  Methylprednisolone (Medrol)
  Triamcinolone (Aristocort, Kenacort)
  Paramethasone (Haldrone)
  Fluprednisolone (Alphadrol)
Prolonged duration of action
  Betamethasone (Celestone)
  Dexamethasone (Decadron, Dexone, Hexadrol)

---

[a] Proprietary names in parentheses.

respectively. These compounds are more potent glucocorticoids and anti-inflammatory agents and produce significantly less mineralocorticoid activity than do cortisol or cortisone. Prednisone is converted to the active metabolite, prednisolone, by hepatic metabolism. Addition of a methyl group at the 6α-position of ring B confers slightly greater glucocorticoid activity in methylprednisolone. When cortisol is halogenated with a fluorine atom at C-9, all adrenocortical activity is enhanced, particularly the mineralocorticoid efficacy of 9α-fluorohydrocortisone, fludrocortisone (see Table 9-5). Hydroxylation or methylation at the 16-position of 9α-fluoroprednisolone is employed to produce triamcinolone, dexamethasone, or betamethasone. These compounds are potent glucocorticoid and anti-inflammatory agents. Importantly, these drugs produce very little mineralocorticoid activity (see Table 9-5). It should be emphasized that none of the adrenocorticosteroid drugs is completely lacking in glucocorticoid or mineralocorticoid activity. Choice of drug, dose, dosing regimen, and duration of dosing greatly influence the extent of adrenocorticoid effects.

Chemical modification of cortisol in general increases the affinity of the derivative for the glucocorticoid receptor (see Table 9-6). The affinity of prednisolone and triamcinolone, intermediate-acting glucocorticoids, for the corticosteroid receptor is about twice that of cortisol. Not surprisingly, the biological half-life of these drugs is increased to 12–36 hr, as compared with 8–12 hr for cortisol. Similarly, betamethasone and dexamethasone demonstrate a fivefold higher affinity for the corticosteroid receptor and a long biological or tissue half-life of 36–54 hr.

In accordance with higher affinity for the corticosteroid receptor, the anti-inflammatory potency of the synthetic derivatives is also mark-

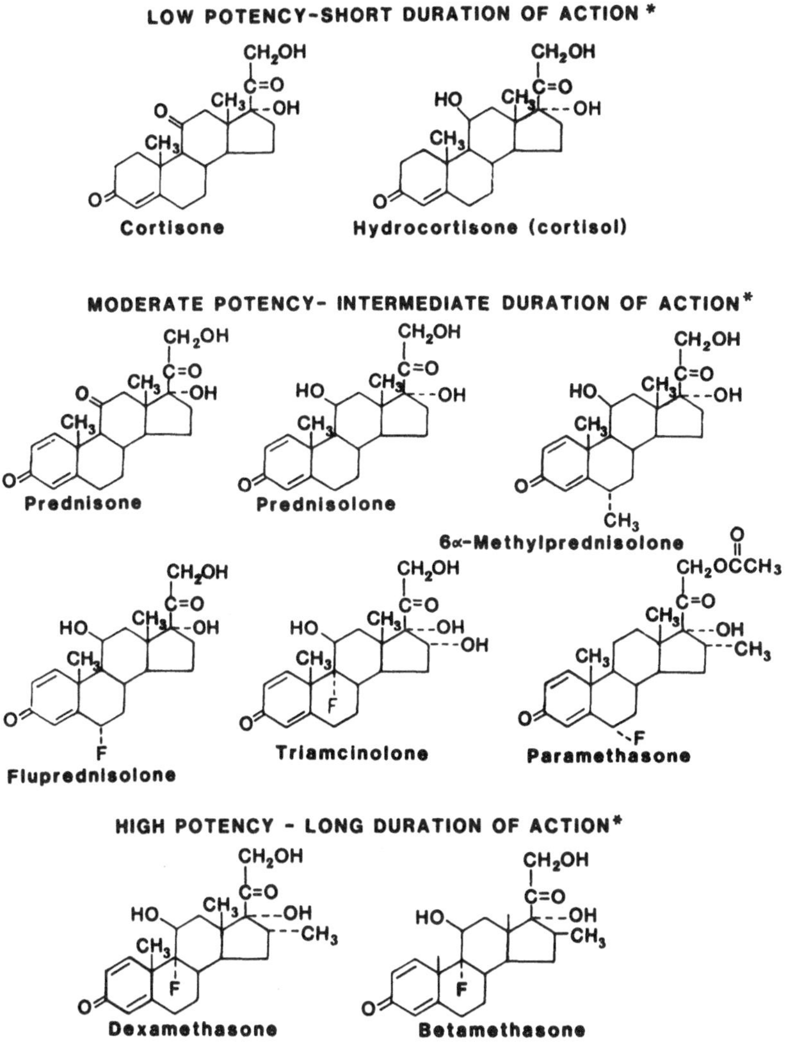

LOW POTENCY-SHORT DURATION OF ACTION *

Cortisone   Hydrocortisone (cortisol)

MODERATE POTENCY- INTERMEDIATE DURATION OF ACTION*

Prednisone   Prednisolone

6α-Methylprednisolone

Fluprednisolone

Triamcinolone   Paramethasone

HIGH POTENCY - LONG DURATION OF ACTION*

Dexamethasone   Betamethasone

*Duration of action also related to dose and/or dose regimens

Figure 9-7. Molecular structure of the glucocorticoid and anti-inflammatory steroid drugs.

edly increased. Betamethasone and dexamethasone are approximately
25–30 times more potent than cortisol, while prednisolone and triamcinolone are three to five times more potent. The increased potency and
prolonged activity of the synthetic steroids are also attributable to their
longer plasma half-lives. Decreases in rates of hepatic catabolism despite

Table 9-5. The Anti-inflammatory and Mineralocorticoid
Potencies of the Adrenocortiosteroid Drugs

Drug	Relative anti-inflammatory potency	Relative mineralocorticoid potency
Cortisol	1	1
Prednisolone	4	0.5
Methylprednisolone	5	0.5
Triamcinolone	5	0.1
Betamethasone	25	0.05
Dexamethasone	30	0.05
Fludrocortisone	10	125

reduced plasma protein (CBG) binding of the synthetic derivatives explains the three- to fourfold increase in their elimination half-lives (see
Table 9-6).

The potency and spectrum of activity of the glucocorticoid drugs
greatly influence their clinical utility. Hydrocortisone and cortisone are
relatively potent glucocorticoid and anti-inflammatory drugs possessing
a significant degree of mineralocorticoid activity. Consequently, these
agents are useful in replacement therapy for adrenocortical insufficiency.
The more potent glucocorticoids, prednisolone and prednisone, lack
sufficient mineralocorticoid activity to be used as the sole adrenocortical
steroid in replacement therapy. Their use for this purpose requires the
concomitant use of a mineralocorticoid such as fludrocortisone (see Table
9-7). Methylprednisolone, triamcinolone, paramethasone, betamethasone and dexamethasone are not generally used for replacement therapy
due to their high degree of glucocorticoid potency and very low mineralocorticoid efficacy. The usual oral dosages of glucocorticoid drugs used

Table 9-6. Pharmacological Characteristics of the Glucocorticoid and
Anti-inflammatory Steroids

Drug	Relative glucocorticoid affinity	Relative anti-inflammatory potency	Biological half-life (hr)	Plasma half-life (min)
Cortisol	1.0	1	8–12	80
Prednisolone	2.1	3–5	12–36	200
Triamcinolone	1.9	3–5	12–36	200
Betamethasone	5.4	25	36–54	300
Dexamethasone	7.1	30	36–54	300

Table 9-7. Recommended Oral Dosages of the Adrenocorticosteroid Drugs

Drug	Glucocorticoid replacement dose (mg/day)	Anti-inflammatory dose (mg/day)
Hydrocortisone	25–50	20–240
Cortisone	35–70	25–300
Prednisolone	5–10[a]	5–60
Prednisone	5–10[a]	5–60
Methylprednisolone	Not recommended	4–48
Triamcinolone	Not recommended	4–48
Paramethasone	Not recommended	2–24
Betamethasone	Not recommended	0.6–7.2
Dexamethasone	Not recommended	0.75–9

[a] Requires administration of a mineralocorticoid during replacement therapy.

in the management of adrenal insufficiency vary due to differences in potency (see Table 9-7). Not surprisingly, the dosages of these drugs that are needed to produce significant anti-inflammatory activity are higher than are those used in replacement therapy.

Drugs that primarily exhibit mineralocorticoid activity as well as antagonists of aldosterone are available for clinical use (see Table 9-8). Deoxycorticosterone and fludrocortisone are the primary mineralocorticoids. The former is a natural steroid and the latter a synthetic derivative (see Figure 9-8). Aldosterone, the highly potent naturally occurring mineralocorticoid, is not available for therapeutic use. Fludrocortisone is advantageous in that it is orally active, while deoxycorticosterone must be administered intramuscularly. These drugs are important in replacement therapy for adrenocortical insufficiency when steroids with salt-retaining activity are indicated. Deoxycortisone is administered in doses of 1–2 mg/day, with the maintenance dose being about 1 mg/day. Deoxycorticosterone pivalate is a long-acting, microcrystalline suspension

Table 9-8. Mineralocorticoid Agonist and Antagonist Drugs[a]

Agonists
    Deoxycorticosterone (Doca Acetate)
    Fludrocortisone (Florinef)
Antagonist
    Spironolactone (Aldactone)

[a] Proprietary names in parentheses.

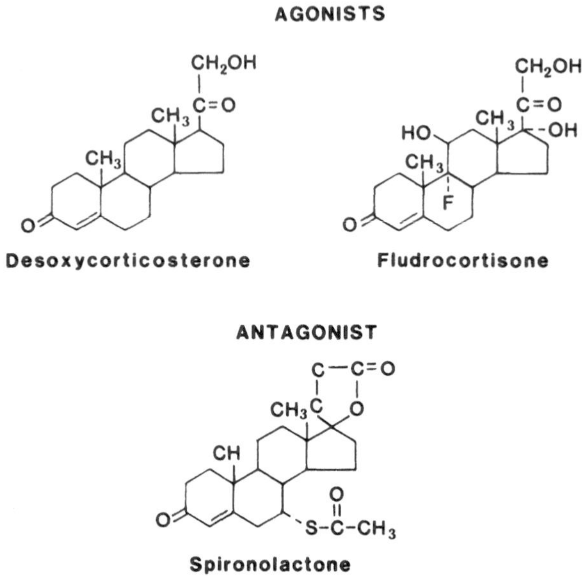

AGONISTS

Desoxycorticosterone   Fludrocortisone

ANTAGONIST

Spironolactone

Figure 9-8. Molecular structures of the mineralocorticoid agonists and antagonist drugs.

(aqueous) that can be administered in doses ranging from 25 to 100 mg every 4 weeks for maintenance therapy. Fludrocortisone, the halogenated derivative of cortisol, is considerably more potent than cortisol in regard to stimulating sodium reabsorption (Table 9-5). It is administered orally in doses of 50–100 µg/day for chronic primary adrenocortical insufficiency and up to 300 µg/day for salt-losing forms of congenital adrenal hyperplasia.

Spironolactone is an aldosterone antagonist with a steroidlike structure used as a diuretic drug in the management of edema (see Figure 9-8). It is usually used in conjunction with a more potent diuretic belonging to either the thiazide or loop diuretic class. The daily dose of spironolactone ranges from 50 to 100 mg. Spironolactone is poorly absorbed from the GI tract, explaining its delayed onset of action. Maximal effects do not occur until the third day of therapy. Upon discontinuation of therapy, the effects of spironolactone diminish gradually over 2 or 3 days. Antagonism of aldosterone action is attributed to the competitive blockade of the mineralocorticoid receptors in the cells of the distal renal tubule. Consequently, sodium and water excretion is enhanced (two- to threefold), and potassium reabsorption increases. In addition to its hyperkalemic action, spironolactone also produces endocrine effects. Doses exceeding 50 mg/day often produce gynecomastia. Decreased libido and impotence may also occur. Spironolactone can also alter menstrual function. The endocrine effects of spironolactone seem to relate to its antiandrogenic activity (see Chapter 6) and probably to its ability to inhibit gonadal steroidogenesis.

Several different formulations of the glucocorticoid drugs are available for therapeutic purposes (see Table 9-9). In general, the base forms of these drugs are orally effective, while the sodium phosphate or succinate derivatives are administered intravenously for emergencies or intramuscularly for maintenance therapy. The acetate, acetonide, hexacetonide, and tebutate ester forms of the glucocorticoid drugs are administered intra-articularly or into soft tissue sites such as tendons or directly onto dermatological lesions (see Table 9-9).

The various routes of administration available for the delivery of glucocorticoid drugs provide advantages in the therapeutic use of these

Table 9-9. Formulations of the Adrenocorticosteroid Drugs and Routes of Administration

Drug	Formulation	Route of administration
Hydrocortisone	Base	Oral
	Acetate	Intra-articular
	Cypionate	Oral
	Sodium phosphate	IV or IM
	Sodium succinate	IV or IM
Cortisone	Acetate	Oral or IM
Prednisolone	Base	Oral
	Acetate	IM or intra-articular
	Sodium phosphate	IV or IM
	Tebutate	Intra-articular
Prednisone	Base	Oral
Methylprednisolone	Base	Oral
	Acetate	IM or intra-articular
	Sodium succinate	IV or IM
Triamcinolone	Base	Oral
	Acetonide	IM, intra-articular
	Diacetate	Oral, IM, or intra-articular
	Hexacetonide	Intra-articular
Paramethasone	Acetate	Oral
Betamethasone	Base	Oral
	Sodium phosphate	IV or IM
	Acetate/sodium phosphate	IM or intra-articular
Dexamethasone	Base	Oral
	Acetate	IM or intra-articular
	Sodium phosphate	IV or IM

agents. The oral route offers convenience for chronic dosing such as replacement therapy and in the palliative management of inflammatory diseases (see Table 9-10). However, not all formulations of these drugs are suitable for oral administration. Emergencies resulting from adrenocortical insufficiency or from allergic reactions require delivery of large doses of the glucocorticoids and a relatively rapid onset of action. Intravenous administration is usually employed in these emergencies. When oral administration is precluded, or when sustained systemic release of the glucocorticoid drugs is desired, the intramuscular injection of these agents is advantageous. Limitations of the systemic actions of the glucocorticoids can be approached by administering these drugs intra-articularly or into soft tissue areas, to control inflammation in joints and tendons, topically for dermatological needs and by inhalation for effects directed at the bronchi. These selected routes of administration provide for direct delivery of significant glucocorticoid dosages in order to enhance efficacy and also limit systemic drug delivery. The incidence and degree of glucocorticoid side effects are also lessened when these routes are selected.

9.8. THERAPEUTIC USES

The ability of adrenocortical steroids to produce glucocorticoid, antiinflammatory, and antiallergic activity as well as suppression of the lymphoid system has resulted in the extensive therapeutic use of this group of drugs (see Table 9-11). Adrenal steroids are used for two principal reasons. First, they are utilized as replacement hormonal therapy in adrenal insufficiency resulting from Addison's disease, adrenalec-

Table 9-10. Significance of the Route of Administration for the Adrenocorticosteroid Drugs

Route of administration	Significance
Oral	Convenient for chronic therapy and dosage is easily regulated
Intravenous	Rapid onset of action in emergency
Intramuscular	Sustained systemic release or if oral administration is precluded
Intra-articular	Localized drug delivery
Topical	Localized drug delivery
Inhalation	Localized drug delivery

Table 9-11. Therapeutic Uses of the Adrenocorticosteroid Drugs

Replacement therapy: adrenocortical insufficiency
Addison's disease
Adrenalectomy
Congenital adrenal hyperplasia
Palliative therapy: anti-inflammatory and immune suppression
Arthritis and tendonitis
Allergy and asthma
Dermatological disorders
Organ transplantation
Hematological disorders
Cerebral edema
Shock
Gastrointestinal disorders
Hypercalcemia
Collagen vascular disorders
Neuromuscular disorders (myasthenia gravis)
Specialized therapy
Fetal respiratory distress syndrome
Idiopathic nephrotic syndome

tomy, or congenital adrenal hyperplasia. Second, advantage is taken of their potent anti-inflammatory and immunosuppressive actions.

Replacement therapy in primary adrenocortical insufficiency is designed to simulate the normal secretory pattern of the glucocorticoids. Therefore, two-thirds of the daily glucocorticoid dose is administered in the early morning and the remaining one-third dosage is administered in the evening. The doses employed for replacement therapy are much lower than those indicated for anti-inflammatory purposes (Table 9-7). Hydrocortisone and cortisone are preferred for replacement therapy in view of their ability to produce both glucocorticoid and weak mineralocorticoid activity. If necessary, a mineralocorticoid like fludrocortisone is administered once daily to control orthostatic hypotension. The use of prednisolone or prednisone in replacement therapy requires the administration of a mineralocorticoid. In cases of secondary and tertiary adrenocortical insufficiency, replacement therapy is generally identical to primary disease; however, mineralocorticoids are not required, since endogenous secretion of aldosterone suffices. Acute adrenal insufficiency (crisis) may result from adrenal or pituitary failure (neurosurgery, head trauma or hemorrhagic shock), from insufficient adrenal replacement therapy, from inadequate corticosteroid therapy in stressed patients (glucocorticoid-dependent), or from the rapid withdrawal of glucocorticoids after chronic, high-dose therapy. Management of acute adrenal crisis necessitates prompt administration of salts, fluids, and glucocorticoids. Intravenous administration of hydrocortisone followed by intramuscular injection of cortisone acetate provide rapid and sustained corticosteroid action required to control acute adrenal insufficiency.

Patients receiving glucocorticoid replacement therapy, including mineralocorticoids, require supplemental doses during periods of stress. The dosage required is generally two to three times the replacement dose but must be adjusted in proportion to the degree of stress. Mild illness such as upper respiratory infections necessitates a doubling of glucocorticoid dosage. However, patients undergoing surgery need a fivefold increase in dosage from the preoperative period through the postoperative interval. If the postsurgical period is uncomplicated, the dosage is reduced gradually over a 2–5-day period and the usual replacement therapeutic regimen reinitiated.

The anti-inflammatory and immunosuppressive effects of the glucocorticoids are utilized often in the management of a number of clinical manifestations. Prednisone is usually employed, although prednisolone appears equally effective. Adrenocortical steroids with minimal mineralocorticoid activity may be more appropriate for the patient with hypertension or congestive heart failure.

The symptoms associated with many allergic states (bronchial asthma, allergic rhinitis, hayfever) are relieved by glucocorticoids. Theophylline and antihistamines remain the primary therapeutic agents in these clinical conditions, with the glucocorticoids reserved for the management of acute episodes. In an emergency related to anaphylaxis and status asthmaticus, the glucocorticoids are used in an adjunctive capacity with epinephrine, cardiorespiratory support, and a theophylline derivative for status asthmaticus. Topical glucocorticoid therapy relieves the symptoms of allergic, inflammatory, and pruritic dermatoses. Psoriasis, alopecia areata, and cheloids may be treated by intralesional instillation of glucocorticoids.

A major therapeutic use of the adrenocortical steroids is in the adjunctive management of rheumatoid arthritis for which they are utilized in addition to nonsteroidal anti-inflammatory drugs. Generally, intra-articular administration is preferred so as to minimize the systemic toxicity of the glucocorticoids. Bursitis and tendonitis are occasionally managed with local injections of depot forms of the glucocorticoids when lesser forms of therapy are ineffective.

Prevention and treatment of graft rejection are common clinical uses of the glucocorticoid drugs. Their efficacy is attributable to immunosuppression. The antimitotic actions of adrenocortical steroids on lymphocytes are important in the management of selected hematological malignancies, including lymphocytic leukemia, lymphomas, and multiple myeloma. The responsiveness of malignant reticuloendothelial cells seems to require the presence of significant levels of glucocorticoid receptors.

Cerebral edema produced by brain tumors, particularly metastatic disease, is quite responsive to glucocorticoid therapy. The edema caused by brain abscesses also responds to glucocorticoids, but edema resulting from closed head injuries is less sensitive to steroid therapy. Dexamethasone is generally used to treat cerebral edema, since large doses must be administered and dexamethasone exhibits little mineralocorticoid activity, which would compromise therapeutic results.

Shock resulting from adrenocortical insufficiency as well as septic shock is responsive to glucocorticoids. These drugs improve tissue perfusion and limit capillary permeability, thereby lessening fluid and protein leakage into the extracellular fluid space. The effectiveness of adrenal steroid therapy in cardiogenic, hypovolemic, or traumatic shock is less evident.

Hypercalcemia caused by increased intestinal absorption of calcium is managed with glucocorticoids. Their efficacy is related to antagonism of vitamin D action. Inflammatory bowel disorders and Crohn's disease are also treated with adrenocortical steroids.

Patients with severe myasthenia gravis, a neuromuscular disorder, may receive glucocorticoids. The effect of the steroids is to suppress the production of immunoglobulins that specifically bind to and ultimately initiate the degradation of the acetylcholine (ACh) receptors at the neuromuscular junction. The immunosuppressive actions of the glucocorticoids are also employed in the management of collagen vascular disorders, including systemic lupus erythematosus (SLE), polymyositis, dermatomyositis, polyarteritis nodosa, polymyalgia rheumatica, and mixed tissue disease.

The death of premature infants may result from respiratory distress syndrome (RDS). Antenatal administration of glucocorticoids reduces the incidence and severity of this syndrome. The adrenocortical steroids enhance the production of lung surfactant by pneumomonocytes (type 2). Effectiveness is maximal if delivery occurs 24–48 hr after administration and is lost after 7 days. Betamethasone and dexamethasone are the drugs of choice and are usually administered intramuscularly twice at 24-hr intervals. This approach is not appropriate for patients with severe preeclampsia or with conditions in which immediate delivery is required for maternal or neonatal survival.

Remission of idiopathic nephrotic syndrome in children is induced by glucocorticoids. Approximately 80–90% of patients respond within 4–8 weeks. Two-thirds of responsive patients do not relapse or otherwise demonstrate only moderate recurrent disease.

9.9. ADVERSE EFFECTS

Many potential adverse effects are associated with the therapeutic uses of the adrenal steroids. These include effects on nearly every organ system (see Table 9-12). The incidence of untoward actions produced by the adrenocortical steroids is related to several significant aspects of their pharmacology. These include dose, frequency, route of administration, duration of therapy, patient age, as well as clinical condition (see Table 9-13).

Cardiovascular and renal toxicity associated with the glucocorticoids

Table 9-12.   Adverse Effects of the Adrenocorticosteroid Drugs

Cardiovascular and Renal
  Sodium retention
  Edema
  Hypertension
  Hypokalemia
Musculoskeletal and skin
  Myopathy
  Osteoporosis
  Growth suppression (children)
  Redistribution of body fat
  Skin thinning
  Prolonged wound healing
Central nervous system
  Psychoses
  Psychic dependence
Ophthalmic system
  Increased intraocular pressure (glaucoma)
Immune system
  Increased susceptibility to infection
  Masking of infection
Gastrointestinal tract
  Peptic ulceration (?)
Endocrine system
  Hypocalcemia
  Hyperglycemia
  Hypothalamic and pituitary suppression

Table 9-13.   Factors Influencing the Incidence
of Adverse Effects Produced by the
Adrenocorticosteroid Drugs

Dose
Dosing interval
Route of administration
Duration of therapy
Patient age
Clinical status of patient

---

includes excessive salt retention, edema, and hypertension, as well as
hypokalemia. These effects are attributable to excessive mineralocorticoid activity.

Adrenal steroids produce a number of undesired effects on the
musculoskeletal system and the skin. Myopathy results from the excessive breakdown of skeletal muscle proteins to their amino acid consi-
tuents. Osteoporosis may be aggravated by the adrenocorticosteroid-
mediated suppression of osteoblast function and from the inhibition of
calcium absorption from the GI tract. In children, the glucocorticoids
will induce premature epiphyseal plate closure and consequently suppress growth. Redistribution of body fat to the abdomen, shoulders,
and face results from excessive and prolonged glucocorticoid therapy.
Thinning of the skin is caused by steroid-induced breakdown of the
collagen fibrils, and wound healing is impaired.

The CNS may also be adversely affected by the glucocorticoids.
Euphoria may be evoked initially. Some of this effect is probably related
to the drug-mediated lessening of symptoms as well as the direct effects
on psyche. Psychic dependence is possible, making withdrawal of therapy problematical.

Topical application of glucocorticoids to the eyes can increase intraocular pressure by decreasing fluid outflow. This occurs most frequently in patients with open-angle glaucoma. Diabetics are also at risk.

The immune system is impaired in patients receiving large doses
of glucocorticoids; accordingly, their susceptability to infection is increased. There is an increased risk of developing fungal, bacterial, and
viral infections. The presence of herpes simplex keratitis represents an
especially hazardous situation. Since the symptoms of infection are masked
by the glucocorticoids, these infections may become severe before they
are diagnosed.

It is uncertain whether the adrenocortical steroids increase the incidence of peptic ulcer. These drugs alter the gastric mucosal barrier,

antagonize repair of the gastrointestinal epithelium, and in some patients may increase secretion of gastric acid. There is evidence indicating that large doses (>1 g/day) of glucocorticoids increase the incidence of peptic ulcers. Likewise, patients with cirrhosis or nephrotic syndrome are also at risk. This effect may be related to the higher levels of unbound corticosteroids in patients exhibiting hypoalbuminemia.

Several untoward effects on the endocrine system are observed in patients receiving adrenocortical steroids. Hypocalcemia may occur due to the antagonistic effects of the glucocorticoids on the actions of vitamin D. These drugs can also aggravate diabetes mellitus and convert latent disease as a result of their hyperglycemic actions. A particularly important effect of the adrenal glucocorticoids is their capacity to suppress hypothalamic and adenohypophyseal function. Like most of the adverse effects attributed to the glucocorticoids, this action is an extension of their physiological action. Suppression of the hypothalamic–pituitary axis is a reflection of the negative feedback influences of these steroids.

Large doses of the glucocorticoids administered for short periods (1–3 days) produce only temporary suppression of the hypothalamus and anterior pituitary gland. Withdrawal of corticosteroid therapy in this situation is accomplished with little difficulty. More prolonged therapy extending for a month or more requires gradual withdrawal of glucocorticoid therapy. Reduction of dosage usually begins by administering a single daily dose in the morning, thereby minimizing suppression of the hypothalamic–pituitary axis. Thus, suppression is minimized, since endogenous adrenal steroids are already elevated each morning. Gradual reduction in dose to replacement dose levels is subsequently initiated. Replacement dosages are then administered on alternate days and are finally discontinued. The recovery of hypothalamic and pituitary function occurs in phases with plasma ACTH levels returning to normal before the development of a normal adrenocortical secretory pattern. Recovery can occur rapidly or require a year or more for completion. Children demonstrate a tendency for quicker recovery. A greater degree of suppression is produced by dexamethasone and betamethasone as compared with the other, less potent, glucocorticoids. The greatest degree of hypothalamic–pituitary suppression occurs after parenteral administration followed in degree by oral administration. Topical application of the glucocorticoids is less likely to induce suppression of the hypothalamus and the pituitary gland.

The suppression of adrenocortical function produced by the glucocorticoids is highly dependent on the duration of exposure rather than on the degree of exposure. Consequently, suppression of the hypothalamic–pituitary axis can be minimized by administering large doses of these steroids on alternate days.

The regimen of alternate-day therapy involves administering a 48-hr dose of an intermediate-acting glucocorticoid (e.g., prednisone, prednisolone, or methylprednisolone) every other morning. This approach more closely simulates the natural circadian rhythm of glucocorticoid secretion. Importantly, less suppression of the hypothalamus and adenohypophysis results, since the level of exogenously administered steroids is highest in conjunction with normally elevated levels of endogenous adrenocortical steroids. Restoration of the hypothalamic and pituitary responsiveness occurs on the days when glucocorticoids are not administered. Alternate-day therapy is advantageous, since it produces less suppression of the hypothalamus and adenohypophysis, reduces the incidence of other adverse effects associated with glucocorticoid therapy, and is convenient. Alternate-day therapy is the preferred treatment approach for maintenance therapy whenever it is feasible and is usually initiated after the clinical condition is controlled by a daily dosing regimen. Asthma, systemic lupus erythematosis (SLE), nephrotic syndrome, and ulcerative colitis are generally well managed by the alternate-day approach. Other severe disease states, including hematological malignancy, rheumatoid arthritis, and giant cell arteritis, are not amenable to alternate-day therapy with glucocorticoids.

9.10. INHIBITORS OF ADRENOCORTICAL STEROID BIOSYNTHESIS

Antagonists of adrenocortical steroid synthesis are useful in assessing adrenal function and in limiting steroid secretion in certain clinical conditions. The molecular structure of the inhibitors of adrenocortical steroid synthesis is shown in Figure 9-9.

Metyrapone inhibits 11β-hydroxylase (11-hydroxylation) and interferes with the synthesis of cortisol and corticosterone, leading to the secretion of 11-deoxycortisol. The decline in systemic cortisol levels results in a lower degree of feedback influence on the hypothalamus and anterior pituitary gland. Consequently, ACTH secretion rises and stimulates further secretion of 11-deoxycortisol. Metyrapone is used clinically to establish the ability of the adenohypophysis to secrete ACTH and is the most commonly used drug in the assessment of adrenal function. Oral doses (750 mg) are administered every 4 hr for 24 hr. Blood levels of 11-deoxycortisol and urinary levels of 17-hydroxycorticosteroids are

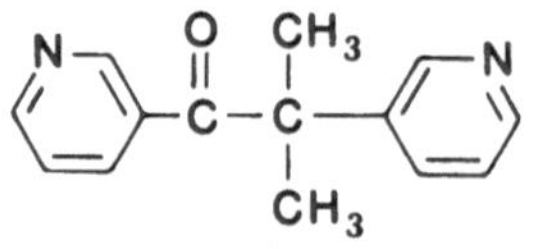

Metyrapone (Metopirone)

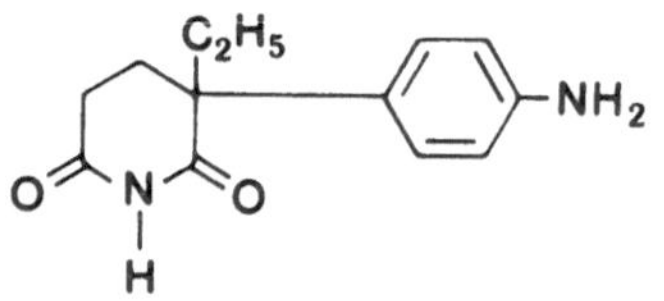

Aminoglutethimide (Cytadren)

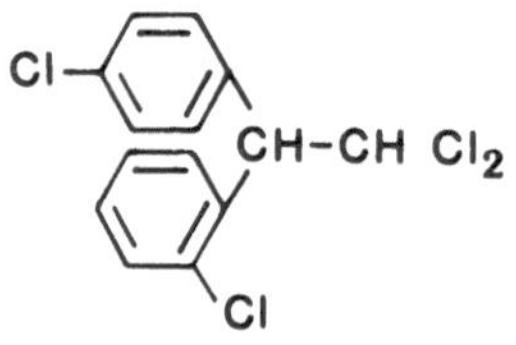

Mitotane (O,P'-DDD)

Figure 9-9. Inhibitors of adrenocortical steroid biosynthesis.

monitored. Gastrointestinal distress and transient dizziness may be produced by metyrapone.

Patients whose adrenal insufficiency is caused by pituitary failure will not respond to metyrapone. In addition, patients being considered for withdrawal from glucocorticoid therapy may not respond to metyrapone but will respond to either ACTH or to insulin-induced hypoglycemia. Metyrapone is useful in distinguishing Cushing's disease from autonomously secreting carcinomas of the adrenal gland. Metyrapone will elicit release of ACTH and increase the urinary excretion of corticosteroids in patients with adrenocortical hyperplasia. If pituitary release of ACTH is suppressed by an autonomous adrenal tumor, metyrapone fails to stimulate secretion of ACTH and excretion of corticosteroids.

Aminoglutethimide inhibits the conversion of cholesterol to pregnenolone and consequently impairs the synthesis of all adrenal steroids. It also antagonizes aromatase activity, thereby suppressing the peripheral conversion of androstenedione to estrone and estradiol-17β. In effect, aminoglutethimide produces a "medical adrenalectomy." Therefore, aminoglutethimide is useful in the palliative management of hormone-dependent cancer of the breast. Its efficacy is attributable to inhibition of adrenal androgen synthesis and to suppression of the peripheral production of estrogen. Glucocorticoids are administered concomitantly in order to prevent enhanced ACTH release, which would surmount the adrenal inhibitory effects of aminoglutethimide. The side effects produced by aminoglutethimide are considerably greater than those associated with tamoxifen, the antiestrogen and drug of choice for the palliative management of hormone-dependent breast cancer (see Chapter 7). Patients who respond initially to tamoxifen and who subsequently experience recurrent disease often benefit from aminoglutethimide therapy.

Aminoglutethimide is orally active and is eliminated by renal excretion (50%) and by hepatic metabolism (50%). The initial elimination half-life for aminoglutethimide is 13 hr but, after 1–2 weeks of therapy, the half-life of elimination declines to 7 hr. This pharmacokinetic alteration is probably related to the induction of hepatic drug metabolism.

Initial oral dose in the management of breast cancer is 250 mg twice daily for the first 2 weeks of therapy in order to minimize side effects. Subsequently, 250 mg of aminoglutethimide is administered four times each day. Approximately 40% of patients experience lethargy, and 10% demonstrate ataxia during the first few weeks of therapy. Tolerance to these effects usually develops as a result of the induction of hepatic drug metabolizing enzymes. Skin rash and GI distress are also common side effects. Orthostatic hypotension occurs in about 10% of patients, and supplements of mineralocorticoids may be required.

Recently, another adrenocortical inhibitory agent has been approved by the FDA for use in the treatment of Cushing's syndrome. Trilostane (Modrastane) is an enzymatic inhibitor of adrenal steroidogenesis. However, this new agent does not appear to offer any particular advantage over existing adrenocortical inhibitors.

RECOMMENDED READINGS

Physiology of the Adrenocorticosteroids

Baxter, J. D., Glucocorticoid hormone action, *Pharmacol. Ther.* **2**:605, 1976.

Cupps, T. R., and Fauci, A. S., Corticosteroid-mediated immunoregulation in man, *Immunol. Rev.* **65**:133, 1982.

Dannenberg, A. M., The anti-inflammatory effects of glucocorticosteroids, *Inflammation* **3**:329, 1979.

Edelman, I. S., and Marver, D., Mediating events in the action of aldosterone, *J. Steroid Biochem.* **12**:219, 1980.

Homo-Delarche, F., Glucocorticoid receptors and steroid sensitivity in normal and neoplastic human lymphoid tissues, A review, *Cancer Res.* **44**:431, 1984.

Kontula, K., Glucocorticoid receptors and their role in human disease, *Ann. Clin. Res.* **12**:233, 1980.

Leung, K., and Munck, A. Peripheral actions of glucocorticoids, *Annu. Rev. Physiol.* **37**:245, 1975.

Marver, D., Aldosterone action in target epithelia, *Vitamin Hormone* **38**:57, 1980.

Mulrow, P. J., and Forman, B. H., The tissue effects of mineralocorticoids, *Am. J. Med.* **53**:561, 1972.

Munck, A., Guyre, P. M., and Holbrook, N. J., Physiological functions of glucocorticoids in stress and their relation to pharmacological actions, *Endocrinol. Rev.* **5**:25, 1984.

Parillo, J. E., and Pauci, A. S., Mechanisms of glucocorticoid action on immune process, *Annu. Rev. Pharmacol. Toxicol.* **19**:179, 1979.

Pearl, W. S., Renin-angiotensin system, *N. Engl. J. Med.* **292**:302, 1975.

Ringold, G. M., Steroid hormone regulation of gene expression, *Ann. Rev. Pharmacol. Toxicol.* **25**:529–566, 1985.

Ringold, G. M., Dobson, D. E., Grove, J. R., Hall, C. V., Lee, F., and Vannice, J. L., Glucocorticoid regulation of gene expression: Mouse mammary tumor virus, a model system, *Recent Prog. Horm. Res.* **39**:387, 1983.

Rousseau, G. G., Control of gene expression by glucocorticoid hormones, *Biochem. J.* **224**:1, 1984.

Rousseau, G. G., Structure and regulation of the glucocorticoid hormone receptor, *Mol. Cell Endocrinol.* **38**:1, 1984.

Schmidt, T. J., and Litwack, G., Activation of the glucocorticoid-receptor complex, *Physiol. Rev.* **62**:1131, 1982.

Yasuda, N., Greer, M. A., and Aizaiwa, T., Corticotropin-releasing factor, *Endocrinol. Rev.* **3**:123, 1981.

Pharmacology of the Adrenocorticosteroids

Axelrod, L., Glucocorticoid therapy, *Medicine* **55**:39, 1976.

Burry, H. D., Use and abuse of corticosteroids in rheumatic diseases, *Drugs* **19**:447, 1980.

Byyny, R. L., Withdrawal from glucocorticoid therapy, *N. Engl. J. Med.* **295**:30, 1976.

Carpenter, P. C., Cushing's syndrome: Update of diagnosis and management, *Mayo Clin. Proc.* **61**:49, 1986.

Chamberlain, P., and Meyer, W. J., Management of pituitary-adrenal suppression secondary to corticosteroid therapy, *Pediatrics* **67**:245, 1981.

Collins, T. R., and Byyny, R. L., Clinical use of glucocorticoids, *Compr. Ther.* **6**:63, 1980.

Conn, H. O., and Blitzer, B. L., Non-association of adrenocorticosteroid therapy and peptic ulcer, *N. Engl. J. Med.* **294**:473, 1976.

Dixon, R. B., and Christy, N. P., On various forms of corticosteroid withdrawal syndrome, *Am. J. Med.* **68**:224, 1980.

Fass, B., Glucocorticoid therapy for nonendocrine disorders: Withdrawal and coverage, *Ped. Clin. N. Am.* **26**:251, 1979.

Fauci, A. S., Alternate-day corticosteroid therapy, *Am. J. Med.* **64**:729, 1978.

Fauci, A. S., Dale, D. C., and Balow, J. E., Glucocorticosteroid therapy: Mechanisms of action and clinical considerations, *Ann. Int. Med.* **84**:304, 1976.

Flick, M. R., and Murray, J. F., High-dose corticosteroid therapy in the adult respiratory distress syndrome, *J.A.M.A.* **251**:1054, 1984.

Garger, E. K., Realistic guidelines of corticosteroid therapy in rheumatic disease, *Semin. Arthritis Rheum.* **11**:231, 1981.

Gwinup, B., and Johnson, B., Clinical testing of the hypothalamic-pituitary-adrencortical system in states of hypo- and hyper-cortisolism, *Metabolism* **24**:777, 1975.

Lagerquist, L. G., and Tyler, F. H., Diagnosis and treatment of disorders of the adrenal cortex, *Pharmacol. Ther.* **1**:259, 1976.

Loeb, J. N., Corticosteroids and growth, *N. Engl. J. Med.* **295**:547, 1976.

Meikle, A. W., and Tyler, F. J., Potency and duration of action of glucocorticoids: Effects of hydrocortisone, prednisone and dexamethasone on human pituitary-adrenal function, *Am. J. Med.* **63**:200, 1977.

Melby, J. D., Clinical pharmacology of systemic corticosteroids, *Annu. Rev. Phamacol. Toxicol.* **17**:511, 1977.

Miller, J. A., and Munro, D. D., Topical corticosteroids: Clinical pharmacology and therapeutic use, *Drugs* **19**:119, 1980.

Munck, A., Guyre, P. M., Holbrook, N. J., Physiological functions of glucocorticoids in stress and their relation to pharmacological action, *Endocr. Rev.* **5**:25–45, 1984.

Pickup, M. E., Clinical pharmacokinetics of prednisone and prednisolone, *Clin. Pharmacokinetic.* **4**:111, 1979.

Quinn, S., and Snader, T. C., Corticosteroid therapy for septic shock: Review and analysis, *Drug Intel. Clin. Pharm.* **14**:247, 1980.

Rose, J. Q., Yurchak, A. M., and Jusko, W. J., Dose-dependent pharmacokinetics of prednisone and prednisolone in man, *J. Pharmacokinet. Biopharm.* **9**:389, 1981.

Santen, R. J., Worgul, T. J., Lipton, A., Harvey, H., Boucher, A., Samoylik, E., and Wells, S. A., Aminoglutethimide as treatment of postmenopausal women with advanced breast carcinoma, *Ann. Int. Med.* **96**:94, 1982.

Shapiro, G. G., Corticosteroids in the treatment of allergic disease—Principles and practice, *Ped. Clin. N. Am.* **30**:955, 1983.

Sprung, C. L., Paragiota, V. C., Marcial, E. H., Pierce, M., Gelbard, M. A., Long, W. M., Duncan, R. C., Tendler, M. D., and Karpf, M., The effects of high-dose corticosteroids in patients with septic shock, *N. Engl. J. Med.* **311**:1137, 1984.

Todd, J. K., Ressman, M., Caston, S. A., Todd, B. H., and Wiesenthal, A. M., Corticosteroid therapy for patients with toxic shock syndrome, *J.A.M.A.* **252**:3399, 1984.

Weintraub, M., and Bakst, A., Trilostane: A new inhibitor of adrenal cortical hormone synthesis, *Hosp. Form.* **20**:1051–1054, 1985.

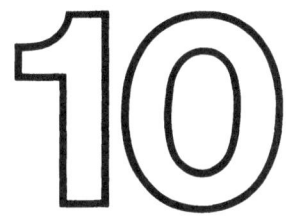

INSULIN AND ORAL HYPOGLYCEMIC AGENTS

10.1. INSULIN

10.1.1. History of Diabetes Mellitus

About 100 years have elapsed since the classic experiments of von Mering and Minkowski demonstrated that pancreatomized dogs exhibited signs and symptoms resembling those seen in diabetes mellitus. The pioneering efforts of Banting and Best revealed that pancreatic extracts could sustain the life of patients suffering from severe diabetes, thereby providing the link between insulin deficiency and the disease. Insulin was subsequently crystallized by Abel and was eventually chemically synthesized in the laboratory. Recently, synthetic insulin derived from recombinant DNA technologies has been approved for clinical trials. Therapy employing animal insulin has been used in the clinical management of diabetes mellitus for many years. Despite the experience with hormone replacement therapies, it is now recognized that diabetes mellitus is a very complex metabolic disorder, and the simple concept that its pathogenesis is due solely to insulin deficiency is no longer tenable. Indeed, contributing to the reduced production of insulin are contributing factors such as excess glucagon, which aggravate both hyperglycemia and ketosis. Insulin resistance, as demonstrated in insulin-dependent diabetes mellitus (IDDM) (i.e., type I), is yet another complicating factor and may be due to both a decrease in insulin receptors and a postreceptor defect.

Certain rare forms of diabetes mellitus appear to be due to molecular abnormalities involving insulin itself or the insulin receptor. A small number of patients with IDDM also seem to demonstrate certain HLA

229

genotypes. Epidemiological studies utilizing gene-typing techniques have identified at least five allelic combinations of HLA and Bf genes associated with marked susceptibility to IDDM. On the basis of such findings, it has been suggested that pancreatic insult by viruses or perhaps other factors may cause the immune system to initiate damaging changes to the islet cells.

The etiology of IDDM or type I diabetes mellitus, which affects about 500,000 patients in the United States is not completely understood, but there is growing evidence that it might be an autoimmune disease. Interestingly, preliminary clinical trials have reported some improvement in the therapeutic management of IDDM using immunosuppressive drugs such as cyclosporin. Such experimental therapies are of no value in non-insulin-dependent diabetes mellitus (NIDDM), or type II diabetes mellitus (see Table 10-8).

10.1.2. Chemistry of Insulin

The molecular configuration of insulin and proinsulin reveals its relationship to connecting peptide (C-peptide) (see Figure 10-1a). Of course there are species differences with respect to amino acid residues (see Figure 10-1b and Table 10-1). There are a few more differences in the A chain than in the B chain of the insulin molecule. Pancreatic human insulin has the same amino acid composition found in the *Escherichia coli* bacterial systems genetically engineered to produce human rDNA insulin.

The molecular structure and amino acid sequence of insulin indicate that it is a simple protein (Figure 10-1). Proinsulin is a precursor form of insulin and is a single polypeptide chain consisting of about 80 amino acids, depending on the species. The C-peptide contains about 30 amino acid residues, but species variations are known to occur. C-peptide, a portion of the insulin precursor molecule, is secreted by the β cells along with insulin. Measurement of C-peptide levels has been used in assessing residual β-cell function in diabetes mellitus and in diagnosing islet cell tumors.

Insulin is a small globular molecule. The insulin molecule consists of two polypeptide chains (an A chain and a B chain) connected by disulfide bonds. It consists of 51 amino acids. The oxidation of disulfide linkages in the insulin molecule causes a reduction in biological activity. This hormone can exist in different states of polymerization, depending on temperature, pH, concentration of zinc, and other factors. In its monomeric form, insulin has a molecular weight of 5734. The amino acid sequence and composition of animal insulins (e.g., bovine, ovine,

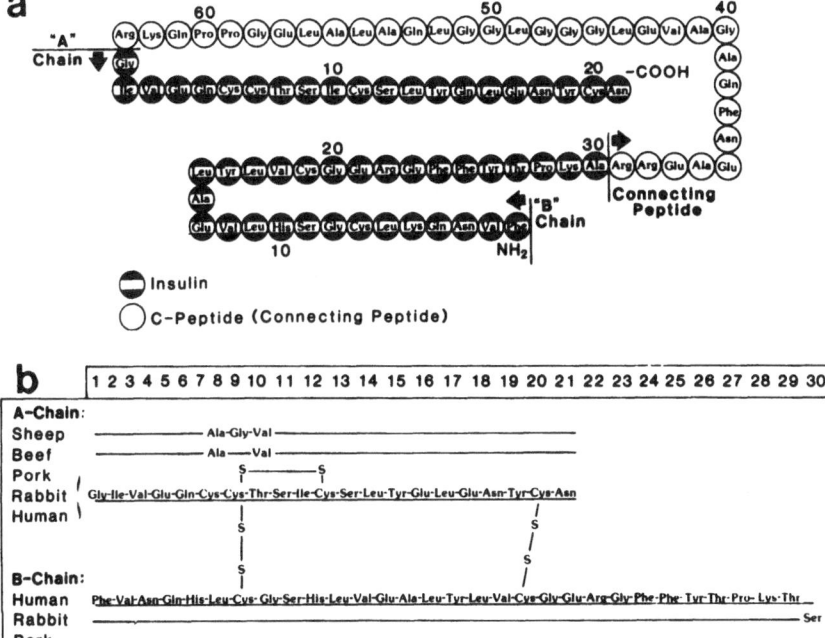

Figure 10-1.   (a) The primary structure of porcine proinsulin. (b) Amino acid sequence differences of human, rabbit, pork, beef, and sheep insulins as modeled after Kahn and Rosenthal. Differences in the A chain are at residues 8, 9, and 10, whereas the only difference in the B chain is the B-30 residue at the carboxy terminus.

Table 10-1.   Some Differences in Amino Acid Composition among Various Mammalian Insulins

Specie	Positions			
	A chain			B chain
	8	9	10	30
Beef	Alanine	Serine	Valine	Alanine
Sheep	Alanine	Glycine	Valine	Alanine
Pork	Threonine	Serine	Isoleucine	Alanine
Human	Threonine	Serine	Isoleucine	Threonine
Dog	Threonine	Serine	Isoleucine	Alanine
Sperm whale	Threonine	Serine	Isoleucine	Alanine
Rabbit	Threonine	Serine	Isoleucine	Serine
Horse	Threonine	Glycine	Isoleucine	Alanine

porcine) differs from human insulin, but fortunately their biological actions are similar (see Table 10-1). While immunological differences between animal and human insulin are minimal, insulin resistance can be troublesome in the therapeutic management of certain diabetic patients (see Adverse Effects).

Insulin actually belongs to a family of biologically active polypeptides. This family includes insulin-like Growth Factor I (IGFI) (also known as somatomedin C), insulin-like growth factor II (IGFII), relaxin, and nerve growth factor. Each of these peptides has its own receptor, although there is some degree of cross-reactivity. IGFI and IGFII can bind to the insulin receptor, but with a rather low affinity. The IGFI receptor even possesses a subunit very similar to that of the insulin receptor. Insulin itself can bind to the IGFI receptor, but again with low affinity.

10.1.3. Secretion and Metabolism

Glucose affects pancreatic β-cell metabolism by acting as a physiological metabolite capable of enhancing both insulin secretion and biosynthesis. The A and B chains of insulin are not synthesized separately, but are assembled on the ribosomes in the form of a larger, single-chained polypeptide called *proinsulin*, or big insulin (Figure 10-1). Some species have may more than one proinsulin. Proinsulin is immunologically similar to insulin. Proinsulin has relatively little biological activity. Proinsulin is proteolytically cleaved to insulin in the rough endoplasmic reticulum (RER) of the β cell. While these are species variation in C-peptide, their hypoglycemic actions are insignificant. The Golgi apparatus seems to be involved in the sacculation of insulin-containing granules. After a physiological stimulus, insulin-containing granules situated nearest to the β-cell plasma membrane fuse with the membrane (exocytosis) and subsequently empty their stored content of hormone into the extracellular space. The C-peptide is retained within the secretory granules along with insulin and is subsequently released with the hormone. A microtubular system of the β cell seems to play an important role in the migration of insulin-containing granules through the cytosol.

The insulin stored within the granules of the β cell can be rapidly mobilized and secreted into the blood. Although glucose itself seems to be the most important physiological stimulus, several pharmacological agents and other hormones can stimulate the release of insulin. Arginine and leucine as well as certain other hexoses and pentoses are effective stimuli for the secretion of insulin. In addition, glucagon, ACTH, growth hormone, secretin, and pancreozymin can enhance insulin secretion.

Several electrolytes, including potassium, sodium, and calcium, can affect the secretion of insulin.

Insulin secretion is a continuous process but, after the ingestion of carbohydrates, blood levels of the hormone can rise severalfold. Only very small amounts of insulin reach peripheral tissues because the liver readily metabolizes substantial amounts of the hormone. The secretion rate of insulin in normal human subjects is about 1–2 mg/24 hr, and of this amount hepatic insulinases inactivate about 50% of the hormone. Insulinases cause a reductive cleavage and hydrolysis of the molecule, leading to a loss in its biological actions.

Insulin that has not been allowed to exert its many and diverse metabolic actions by interacting with its receptor is readily degraded by enzymatic action. Of course, the activity of insulin is rapidly lost by proteolytic enzymes.

10.1.4. General Biochemical Events and Actions

The biochemical actions of insulin are initiated by specific, high-affinity interactions with receptors located on the outer surface of the plasma membrane. The insulin–receptor interaction is reversible, and apparently insulin is not chemically altered when in contact with its receptor. These receptors can be saturated, and the binding sites for the hormone can be destroyed by proteolytic enzymes. Once the insulin–receptor complex is formed, insulin can initiate many biochemical actions. Such actions are undoubtedly triggered by the interaction of insulin with cell-surface protein receptors. The kinetics of the insulin–receptor interaction have received considerable attention but the mechanism of action is not yet understood.

While most attention seems to focus on the membrane initiated action of insulin, at least two intracellular organelles, namely, the Golgi apparatus and the nucleus, might be sites of the action of insulin.

An early event in the mechanism of action of insulin is probably triggered by the oxidation of specific sulfhydryl groups located in the plasma membrane.

Sulfhydryl groups may be involved in transport processes involving glucose and amino acids. However, any final explanation of the molecular interactions must consider such diverse cellular events as (1) a rapid activation of membrane glucose and amino acid transport systems, (2) activation of pyruvate dehydrogenase and glycogen synthetase, (3) enhanced protein synthesis, (4) inhibition of lipolysis, and (5) hepatic gluconeogenesis. Table 10-2 lists some of the metabolic effects of insulin.

Table 10-2.   General Summary of Insulin's Actions on
Certain Metabolic Processes

Metabolic process[a]	Insulin state[b]	
	Excess	Deficient
Glycogenolysis	Decreases	Increases
Gluconeogenesis	Decreases	Increases
Glycogen synthesis	Increases	Decreases
Ketogenesis	Decreases	Increases
Lipogenesis	Increases	Decreases
Lipolysis	Decreases	Increases
Protein synthesis	Increases	Decreases

[a] Metabolic process or response is organ/cell specific.
[b] Increases or decreases reflect the change in the rate of the metabolic process.

It is unlikely that intracelluar levels of either cAMP or cGMP exclusively mediate all the biochemical effects produced by insulin. Cellular calcium appears to play an important role in the mechanism of action of insulin.

Insulin stimulates the synthesis of all proteins in muscle. Ribosomes obtained from the heart and skeletal muscles of diabetic animals do not synthesize proteins nearly as well as those ribosomes obtained from normal animals. Furthermore, insulin stimulates the assembly of polysomes and the synthesis of protein by ribosomes in a manner that does not require RNA synthesis.

Glucose transport into the muscles is accelerated by insulin; an action that is so rapid that it is doubtful that the synthesis of new transport (i.e., carrier) molecules is required. The hormone appears to exert its effects on glycogen synthesis and glucose transport without entering the cell.

Insulin exerts a general anabolic action upon hepatic metabolism. This hormone stimulates hepatic RNA synthesis and activates hepatic glycogen synthetase by a mechanism that may involve a decrease in cellular cAMP. Insulin can inhibit gluconeogenesis and increase glycogenesis by regulating the level of cAMP.

The action of insulin on adipose tissue is due, in part, to an enhancement of both glucose transport and its cellular conversion to fatty acids and glycerol within the fat cells. Furthermore, insulin will retard lipolysis by inhibiting the hormone-sensitive lipases situated in adipose cells. Pyruvate dehydrogenase activity in adipose tissue and other tissues is enhanced by insulin.

Both insulin and glucagon affect lipoprotein metabolism, as do certain ovarian hormones. A highly atherogenic abnormality in serum lipoprotein levels is present in patients with diabetes mellitus.

10.1.5. Insulin Receptors

Hormones operate by means of a cell receptor, and the hormone exerts its effect(s) only when its target cell(s) acknowledges it and binds the hormone to a specific receptor (see Figure 10-2). Insulin interacts with its target tissues initially by way of a highly specific, high-affinity receptor located at the cell surface. The insulin receptor(s) has been purified. It is an intrinsic membrane protein but can be solubilized in a state whereby it retains its insulin-binding properties. The insulin receptor is now known to be a glycoprotein consisting of three polypep-

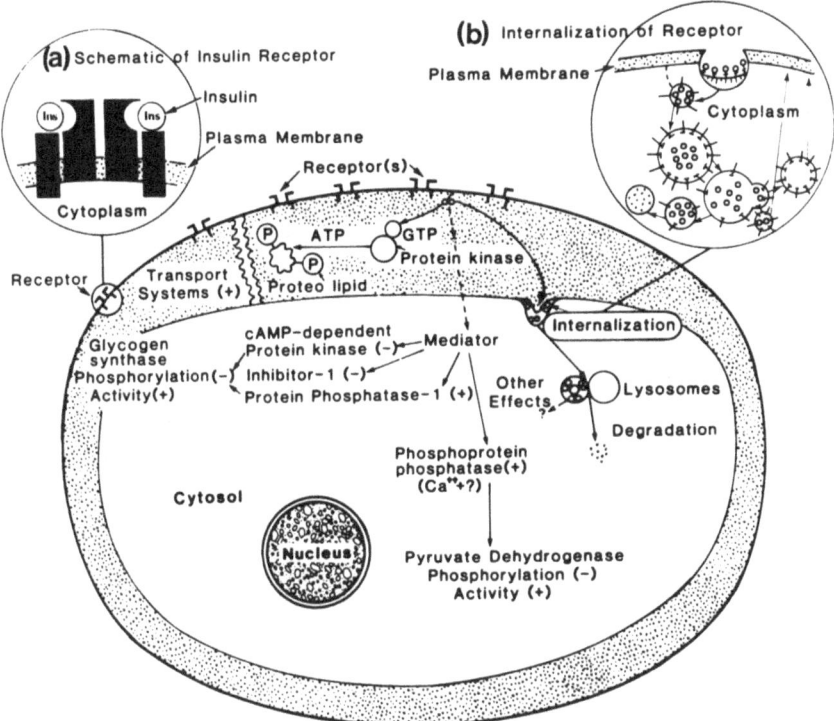

Insulin interacts with a plasma cell membrane receptor and initiates a cascade of metabolic actions within the cell.

Figure 10-2. Insulin: receptors(s), internalization, and cellular events.

tides. These three polypeptides have molecular weights of 135,000, 90,000, and 45,000 and are named α, β, and β_1, respectively. A schematic model of the proposed subunit structure of the insulin receptor has been suggested by Jacobs and Cuatrecasas (see Figure 10-2a). Such a model is schematized as having a complex carbohydrate chain. Disulfide bonds are proposed for linking the various subunits of the insulin receptor.

The molecular weight of the native insulin receptor is approximately 350,000. Each receptor is believed to be able to bind two molecules of insulin. This high-molecular-weight insulin receptor is a disulfide-linked heterotetramer containing two copies of the α and copies of the β. Through denaturization and reducing agent treatment, these subunits (i.e., 3 or 4) can be isolated. The insulin receptor exists in two states where in the predominant state includes all four subunits covalently coupled by disulfide bonds. The physiological significance of two such insulin receptors remains unknown. The β_1 component of the receptor is a proteolytic fragment of β, whether this molecular clipping represents any important physiological event also remains unknown. It has been suggested that β_1 may represent physiological processing of the insulin receptor and, as such, may be involved in its cellular internalization events (see Figure 10-2b).

While the β_1 component of the insulin receptor might be involved in the process of internalization, the α subunit is important for binding. However, β and β_1 may contribute to the binding of insulin.

The principal role of the insulin receptor involved the transmission of biochemical events from the outside of the cell to the interior of the cell. Possibly, the insulin receptor is a transmembrane protein. Because membrane glycoproteins are situated on the exterior surface of the plasma membrane, the α, β, and β_1 subunits must be exteriorized. In addition, the β subunit may be exposed to the internal surface of the membrane, suggesting that this component of the receptor spans the membrane and is also exposed to the cell's interior.

The number of insulin receptors expressed per cell varies considerably. The mature erythrocyte may contain several hundred, while the adipocyte may contain several hundred thousand insulin receptors. The insulin receptor half-life is brief, believed to be measured in hours. Thus, the receptor has a rapid turnover, with its concentration being regulated by insulin itself. However, other hormones (e.g., cortisol, HGH) and factors (e.g., diet) can affect insulin-receptor concentrations.

10.1.6. Receptor-Mediated Internalization

After binding to its receptor(s) located on the surface of the cell, insulin along with its receptor is internalized (see Figure 10-2b). Occupied insulin receptors rapidly redistribute, leading to the formation of clusters on the cell surface. These clusters of insulin receptor form in coated pits that are invaginated regions on the cell membrane. In some cells, these coated pits may be seen to pinch off rapidly or to bud to form thin-walled vesicles containing internalized insulin. The internalized insulin is juxtaposed to the plasma membrane, where is subsequently migrates to the Golgi region of the cell.

Once insulin has been internalized, it is vulnerable to degradation, but the degree of this degradation depends on the particular cell. Some cells such as the hepatocyte may degrade most of the internalized insulin, whereas other cells exert little action on the hormone. Unlike the degradation fate of insulin itself, the insulin receptor either remains on the surface of the cell or somehow escapes degradation. Possibly, the receptor is recycled back to the cell membrane. Small amounts of the internalized receptor appear to be sequestered in an intracellular pool or proteolytically degraded most likely by lysosomes.

The transmembrane signaling caused by insulin leads to a host of cellular actions. A number of enzymatic and metabolic actions are initiated, but the hormone's action on enzymes is indirect and mediated through intervening step(s) that are yet to be disclosed, e.g., second messenger(s). Interestingly, the β subunit of the insulin receptor can be phosphorylated. Tyrosine phosphorylation has been suggested as an early initiating event in insulin-induced cellular proliferative responses. However, it is not established whether the insulin receptor is a protein kinase or acting as a substrate for an extrinsic protein kinase. A search for intracellular mediators for insulin's action continues. The interaction of insulin with its receptor does generate a mediator(s) that activates pyruvate dehydrogenase. Possibly, insulin–receptor interaction activates a protease that cleaves the mediator from a precursor situated with the plasma membrane.

10.1.7. Factors Affecting Insulin and Insulin Resistance

Several physiological factors (e.g., glucose levels, secretion), pathological states, and drugs can affect insulin secretion, modifying the therapeutic management of the patient with diabetes mellitus (see Table 10-3). Increases in the plasma levels of the adrenocortical hormones, epinephrine, thyroxine, and certain anterior pituitary hormones can alter the body's requirements for insulin. Epinephrine causes hepatic glycogenolysis and a transient hyperglycemia. So-called steroid diabetes frequently caused by the overzealous use of anti-inflammatory steroids can produce hyperglycemia, leading to increased insulin requirement. Thyrotoxicosis is accompanied by an increased blood glucose level, hence

Table 10-3.   Some Conditions Altering Insulin
Requirements

Decreased
  Liver dysfunction
  Hypothyroidism
  Renal dysfunction
  Nausea and vomiting
Increased
  Hyperpyrexia (fever)
  Hyperthyroidism
  Severe infections
  Ketoacidosis (diabetic)
  Trauma/surgery/stress
  Increased food intake/weight gain
  Reduction or cessation of physical exercise
  Pregnancy
  Withdrawal of oral hypoglycemic agents
  Deep X-ray therapy/ultraviolet-ray burns

---

an increase in the body's requirement for insulin. Physiological or psychological stress can also increase the patient's insulin requirements. Several physiological factors can reduce the insulin requirements or lead to hypoglycemia (see Table 10-4).

Autoantibodies against the insulin receptor have been detected in the serum of patients with acanthosis nigricans type B who exhibit severe insulin resistance. Such antibodies can inhibit the binding of insulin to its receptor. These antibodies are characterized chemically as polyclonal immunoglobulin, primarily of the IgG class. It is possible that insulin–receptor autoantibodies develop as a result of perturbation of the immune system aggravated by intermittent sepsis.

Various metabolic or pathological states have been associated with insulin resistance (refer to Table 10-7; see also Table 10-3). Several of these conditions are attributable to altered nonpancreatic hormonal secretory activity such as found in Cushing's disease (corticosteroids), acromegaly (growth hormone), and thyrotoxicosis (thyroxine). Estrogen excesses, such as those seen in pregnancy, hormone-producing tumors, or administration of drugs possessing estrogenic activity are often associated with insulin resistance. While current evidence fails to demonstrate any insulin receptor defect in resistant states, it is possible that the activities of several enzymes are modified in certain of these pathological states. Of the available insulin preparations, highly purified porcine insulin posseses the least antigenic activity.

Efforts have been made to classify insulin resistance on the basis of pathophysiology. Such a classification of insulin resistance includes (1) abnormal insulin molecule, (2) circulating antagonists of insulin action, and (3) target cell defects in the pathways for insulin action. A structurally abnormal insulin has been described, but it is apparently very rare. Such an abnormal insulin molecule has been reported in a non-insulin-dependent diabetic with fasting hyperglycemia and hyperinsulinemia, but with surprisingly normal sensitivity to exogenous insulin.

Nearly all patients treated with exogenous insulin, including human insulin, develop insulin-binding IgG antibodies within a few months. Fortunately, such antibodies are rarely troublesome and such forms of resistance do not significantly interfere with the hormone replacement therapy. Switching to less immunogenic insulin preparations or occasionally the use of adrenocorticol steroids to affect the insulin-induced altered immunity are effective therapies. Apparently these antibodies limit the access of insulin to its receptor. No receptor abnormalities have been associated with this type of insulin resistance.

Table 10-4. Causes of Hypoglycemia

Decreased glucose production predominant
  Drugs
    Ethanol
    Oral hypoglycemic drugs
    Salicylates
    Insulin
  Hormonal deficits
    Glucocorticoids
    Growth hormone
    Thyroid hormones
    Catecholamines
    Glucagon
  Extensive hepatic destruction
    Chronic renal failure
    Ketotic hypoglycemia of childhood
    Congenital enzyme defects
    Neonatal hypoglycemic
Increased glucose utilization predominant
  Extrapancreatic tumors
    Pregnancy
    Severe exercise
    Renal glycosuria
Decreased glucose production and increased glucose utilization
  Hyperinsulinism (e.g., tumor)
  Extrapancreatic tumors that secrete hypoglycemic substances

Hormonal antagonists as witnessed in the instance of cortisol, growth hormone, glucagon, and catecholamines produce insulin resistance. These hormones cause insulin antagonism through a variety of mechanisms, including interference with the peripheral uptake of glucose (e.g., cortisol), enhanced hepatic glycogenolysis (e.g., glucagon), influencing β-cell secretion (e.g., catecholamines), and impairment of insulin-sensitive processes within target cells and on the expression of insulin receptors.

It is recognized that some nondiabetic obese patients exhibit elevated levels of insulin, but the clincial significance of this type of insulin resistance has not been well characterized despite suggestions of a postreceptor defect. A similar postreceptor defect has been postulated for insulin resistance in the nonobese type II diabetic, but this hypothesis awaits confirmation.

Some pathological states are also related to more moderate forms of tissue resistance to insulin. Insulin-receptor antibodies have been reported in some patients who have symptomatic diabetes yet who have concomitant medical histories of other possible autoimmune diseases, often referred to as the type B syndrome of insulin resistance with insulin-receptor autoantibodies. In addition, a type A syndrome of insulin resistance has been described that might involve a genetically determined disorder of insulin receptors. Finally, two other rare syndromes entail tissue resistance to insulin: (1) leprechaunism, and (2) lipoatrophic diabetes. In this latter syndrome, the etiology may be congenital or acquired, or a combination of both factors.

10.1.8. Uses and Preparations

Table 10-5 lists some clinical situations wherein the use of insulin is indicated. Insulin is the only effective means of controlling the insulin-dependent-type I form (e.g., juvenile form) of the disease. Furthermore, some severe forms of non-insulin dependent-type II (e.g., maturity-onset) diabetes mellitus that cannot be controlled by the combination of diet, exercise, and oral hypoglycemic agents require insulin therapy. Some adults with severe carbohydrate intolerance require insulin from the onset of therapy. Oftentimes, brief periods of insulin therapy may be indicated for the adult diabetic patient during periods of stress, infection, and occasionally during the second and third trimester of pregnancy.

Because insulin is a polypeptide hormone, it must be administered either subcutaneously or intramuscularly in order to escape gastric proteolytic enzymes. Orally administered insulin is chemically inactivated by gastric peptidases. Recently, the U.S. FDA has approved the clinical

Table 10-5. Indications for the Use of Insulin

Insulin-dependent diabetes mellitus (type I) (IDDM)
Ketoacidosis
Hyperosmolar nonketotic coma
Selected forms (e.g., labile) of type II diabetes mellitus
Acute hyperglycemia complicated by
  Infection
  Steroid therapy
  Pregnancy
  Surgery/trauma

testing of Nazlin, a nasally administered insulin. In some emergency conditions, such as diabetic coma or severe diabetic acidosis, regular crystalline insulin may be injected intravenously.

The pharmacokinetic profiles of various insulin preparations are shown in Table 10-6. Insulins can be categorized according to their duration of action. So-called fast-acting preparations (e.g., regular crystalline or Semilente) begin to exert their hypoglycemic effects as early as 30 min after administration. Intermediate-acting preparations have a more delayed onset of action but act for a longer period of time (e.g., NPH or Lente). Protamine zinc and Ultralente are often referred to as long-acting insulin preparations. Most of these preparations can be obtained in different dosages, ranging from 20, 40, 80, and 100 U/ml. The number of daily injections will vary depending not only on the preparations employed, but on the severity of the disease as well. There is little or no therapeutic justification for the combined use of oral hypoglycemic drugs and insulin.

Insulin injection (regular insulin, crystalline zinc insulin) is indicated in diabetic hyperglycemia and is administered subcutaneously about 30 min before meals up to three or four times per day. Insulin injection is also indicated in diabetic ketoacidosis and may be injected in intravenously (bolus) plus subcutaneous injections. Additional units (subcutaneous) may be needed. In diabetic ketoacidosis, insulin injection can be administered intravenously plus intramuscularly. The rate of insulin administration should be decreased in a manner whereby plasma glucose levels eventually reach about 250 mg%.

Globin zinc insulin (globin zinc) is customarily administered subcutaneously about 30–60 min before breakfast. Unlike insulin injection (i.e., regular insulin), globin zinc insulin should not be mixed with other types of insulin preparations because of its acidity.

Insulin zinc suspension (Lente insulin) is given subcutaneously, usually 30–60 min before breakfast, but sometimes an additional dose

Table 10-6. Pharmacokinetic Profile of Animal Insulin Preparations

Type of insulin	Preparation[a,b] + (units/ml)	Relative effectiveness (hr)					
		Subcutaneous response			Intravenous response		
		Onset	Peak	Duration	Onset	Peak	Duration
Insulin injection (regular insulin, crystalline zinc insulin)	U 40, mixed U 80, mixed U 100, mixed, beef, pork	$\frac{1}{2}$–1	3–5	12–16	$\frac{1}{4}$–$\frac{1}{2}$	$\frac{1}{2}$–1	1–2
	U 500,[c] pork	Prolonged: to 24 hr			Not for i.v. use		
Prompt insulin zinc suspension (Semilente)	U 40, mixed, beef U 80, mixed, beef U 100, mixed, beef	$\frac{1}{2}$–1	5–7	18–24	Not for i.v. use		
Isophane insulin suspension (NPH insulin)	U 40, mixed U 80, mixed U 100, mixed, beef, pork	1–1$\frac{1}{2}$	8–12	18–24	Not for i.v. use		
Insulin zinc suspension (Lente insulin)	U 40, mixed, beef U 80, mixed, beef U 100, mixed, beef, pork	2–4	8–12	24	Not for i.v. use		
Globin zinc insulin (globin insulin)	U 40, mixed U 80, mixed U 100, mixed	2	8–16	24	Not for i.v. use		
Protamine zinc insulin (PZI insulin)	U 40, mixed U 80, mixed U 100, mixed, beef, pork	4–6	14–20	36	Not for i.v. use		
Extended insulin zinc suspension (Ultralente)	U 40, mixed, beef U 80, mixed, beef	4–6	16–18	36	Not for i.v. use		

[a] Mixed = mixture of beef and pork insulins.
[b] Proinsulin content may vary from 1 ppm to 50,000 ppm.
[c] The U 500 preparation is available only for the treatment of selected insulin-resistant diabetic patients.

is required, depending on the severity of the disease. Insulin zinc suspension in 40-, 80-, or 100-U/ml strengths is available as a mixture of beef and pork insulins, and also as beef-only insulin.

Extended insulin zinc suspension (Ultralente) is administered subcutaneously, usually 30–60 min before breakfast. Ultralente is compatible with other types of insulins.

Prompt insulin zinc suspension (Semilente insulin) is administered subcutaneously. An additional dose about $\frac{1}{2}$ hr before a meal or bedtime may be required, depending on the severity of the disease. Prompt insulin zinc suspension is available in 40-, 80-, and 100-U/ml strengths. Semilente can be mixed with other types of insulin.

Protamine zinc insulin suspension (PZI insulin) is injected subcutaneously and is available in strengths of 40, 80, and 100 U/ml as a mixture of beef and pork insulin.

Truly human insulin is secreted only by the human pancreas. Natural human insulin is in reality endogenous, pancreatic, or islet cell cultured. Other human insulins are only "human" in the context of possessing the amino acid sequence and tertiary structure of natural human insulin. Such insulins are fully synthetic, i.e., derived from amino acids, but the nomenclature "totally synthetic insulin" is usually reserved for total chemical synthesis in the laboratory. So-called semisynthetic human insulin is principally a natural product obtained from natural genes translated in the pig pancreas *in situ*. Novolin R is a short-acting human insulin product, while Novolin L is an intermediate-acting Lente human insulin product. Novolin N (NPH human insulin isophane suspension) is a semisynthetic formulation.

rDNA human insulin (Humulin) has recently become available for therapeutic use. There are probably no significant therapeutic advantages to the use of rDNA human insulin over that of highly purified animal insulins. However, rDNA human insulin might be used in the 5% of the diabetic population who are particularly allergic to animal insulins. In addition, rDNA human insulin reportedly affords a better removal of blood ketones in the diabetic. rDNA human insulin is available in a sterile aqueous solution (Humulin S) and in a sterile suspension of isophane human insulin (Humulin I). Human insulin suspension of isophane should not be administered intravenously. Each preparation

Table 10-7. Various Metabolic and Pathological States Associated with Insulin Resistance and/or Changed Insulin Requirements

Acromegaly	Diabetes mellitus
Cushing's syndrome	Oral contraceptives
Obesity	Myotonic dystrophy
Phenochromocytoma	Starvation
Pancreatic α-cell tumors	Streptozotocin-induced diabetes
Pregnancy	Uremia

of human insulin is available in 40- and 80-U/ml strengths. These preparations are somewhat shorter acting than originally anticipated. The absorption time after an intramuscular injection of rDNA human insulin is slightly longer than for porcine insulin; their metabolic clearance rates by the kidney are similar.

Humulin R is regular insulin, while Humulin N is comparable to NPH insulin. The duration of action of Humulin R is about 6–8 hr; Humulin N has a duration of action of less than 24 hr.

Presumably several possible therapeutic benefits are derived from human insulin. Among those benefits touted for human insulin are (1) its consistent absorption profile, (2) increased potency, (3) patient acceptance, and (4) unlimited source.

Clearly, the semisynthetic human insulins will, for the time being, cost more than animal insulins. The therapeutic advantages of human insulin products seem dubious despite the presumed reduced incidence of antigenicity.

A rather recent innovation in the method of administration of insulin has been the so-called insulin pump. Such improved technologies in drug delivery systems has led to the development of at least six different types of insulin pumps. Many more types of insulin pumps are currently under engineering development. Basically, there are two types of pump systems: the open loop and the closed loop.

The open-loop system uses a microcomputer to regulate the flow of insulin from a syringe attached to a catheter connected to a needle inserted subcutaneously into the diabetic patient. The microcomputer is programmed to adjust the rate of flow of insulin with the therapeutic objective of controlling blood glucose levels between 70 and 100 mg/d. The site of injection is usually changed every 2–3 days. The open-loop system requires that patients self-test their blood glucose levels and make the necessary adjustments in the programming of the microprocessor.

The second type of pump system is the closed-loop system. The closed-loop system automatically reads blood glucose levels and adjusts the rate of insulin delivery. Unfortunately, the closed-loop system is not conducive to use in the ambulatory diabetic patient but might be used in a hospital setting, where the diabetic patient is anticipating surgery. Currently, the physical size of the closed-loop delivery system is comparable to that of a small TV set.

The volume of most of these insulin pumps varies from about 3 to 6 ml, with some pumps requiring a diluting vehicle (e.g., saline). Most forms of insulin can be used in these pumps, and it is not uncommon to mix regular insulin and NPH (or Ultralente) together.

10.1.9. Adverse Effects

The dosage and administration of insulin can vary widely and must be tailored to meet a particular patient's requirements for the hormone. Perhaps the most commonly seen side effects of insulin therapy are hypoglycemia, hypokalemia, and varying degrees of allergic reactions. Mild allergic reactions are not uncommon and result from the injection of foreign proteins (*viz.* insulin of animal origin) into the diabetic patient. Hypoglycemia can lead to such CNS symptoms as tremors, nervousness, stimulation of autonomic nervous system functions, and even convulsions or unconsciousness. Changes in electrocardiogram due to insulin treatment is related to hypokalemia.

Other complications can arise from insulin therapy. Some peculiar and annoying side effects of insulin therapy are lipodystrophy, insulin lipoma, and localized infections at the site of the hormone's injection. The incidence of lipodystrophy is not very great; when it does occur, the condition seems to abate by more frequent changes in the site of injection and by the use of an intramuscular rather than a subcutaneous route of injection.

10.2. ORAL HYPOGLYCEMIC AGENTS

Oral hypoglycemic agents are most likely to be effective in those patients with only milder forms of non-insulin-dependent diabetes mellitus (NIDDM) (Type II) wherein their capacity to secrete endogenous insulin is only partially impaired. Ordinarily, such diabetics are at least 30–40 years of age. Furthermore, such patients have probably never experienced ketoacidosis and usually have clinically recognized symptoms of diabetes for less than 10 years. The aforementioned characteristics exemplify the form of the disease once referred to as maturity-onset diabetes currently known as type II, or NIDDM. Type II diabetes has a more gradual onset and is characteristic of a gradual exhaustion of β cells. There may be some residual β cells in the type II diabetic, whereas in the type I diabetic patient (e.g., juvenile) there may be a complete absence of β cells. Type I is usually seen before the age of 30. Typical characteristics of juvenile (type I) and maturity-onset (type II) diabetes are depicted in Table 10-8.

Some milder forms of diabetes mellitus that do not respond to dietary management alone can be treated with oral hypoglycemic agents. Insulin remains the drug of choice in severe cases of diabetes and in

Table 10-8. Characteristics of IDDM and NIDDM[a]

Characteristic	IDDM (Juvenile form)	NIDDM (Maturity-onset)
Onset (age)	Under 30 years	Approximately 40 years
Type of onset	Abrupt	Gradual
Nutritional status at onset	Usually undernourished	Usually obese
Clinical symptoms	Polydipsia, polyphagia, and polyuria	Often none
Ketosis	Frequent, unless diet, insulin, and exercise are properly coordinated	Infrequent (except in the presence of infection or stress)
Endogenous insulin	Negligible	Present, but relatively ineffective because of obesity
Related lipid abnormalities	Hypercholesterolemia frequent, particularly when control is suboptimal; all lipid fractions elevated in ketoacidosis	Cholesterol and triglycerides often elevated; carbohydrate-induced hypertriglyceridemia common
Insulin therapy	Required	Required in only 20–30% of patients
Hypoglycemic drugs	Should not be used	Efficacious
Diet	Mandatory along with insulin for blood glucose control	Diet alone frequently sufficient to control blood glucose

[a] IDDM, insulin-dependent diabetes mellitus (type I); NIDDM, non-insulin-dependent diabetes mellitus.

juvenile diabetes. Although insulin has the disadvantage of having to be injected, it still is without question the most uniformly effective preparation in the treatment of diabetes mellitus. The success of oral hypoglycemic drug therapy is usually based on restoration or normal blood glucose levels and the absence of glycosuria.

Despite the fact that the sulfonylurea chemical class of oral hypoglycemia agents was introduced into clinical medicine during the 1950s, the blood glucose-lowering properties of certain antibacterial drugs of the sulfonamide group were recognized as early as 1930. Carbutamide, an arylsulfonylurea compound, was discovered to be a very effective agent in lowering glucose levels in normal individuals and in certain mild forms of diabetes.

There are two major chemical classes of oral hypoglycemic drugs, i.e., the sulfonylurea drugs and the biguanide derivatives. The biguanides (*viz.* phenethylbiguanide or phenformin) have been withdrawn from the market in the United States because they have caused an increased incidence of fetal hyperlactic acidosis.

10.2.1. Sulfonylureas

During the past two decades, literally thousands of sulfonamide-related agents have been synthesized and bioassayed for their hypoglycemic properties. Less than a dozen of these agents have been identified as being clinically useful, and only about one-half of these are used to any extent in the United States. Two oral hypoglycemic sulfonylurea, long available in Europe, have recently been approved for the treatment of type II diabetes mellitus. These agents are purported to be the second generation of oral sulfonylurea hypoglycemic agents. These agents, specifically glyburide and glipizide, offer no advantage over previously available oral hypoglycemic drugs.

The chemistry of representative sulfonylurea drugs is depicted in Figure 10-3. There are structural similarities to the sulfonamide antibacterial agents. The degree and the rate of metabolism also vary with the particular sulfonylurea. The pharmacological profile of the sulfonylurea drugs is depicted in Table 10-9. Approximately 75% of tolbutamide is oxidized in the liver to an inactive metabolite—carboxytolbutamide. Acetohexamide is rapidly reduced to several derivatives, the main metabolite being hydroxyhexamide (see Figure 10-4). Tolazamide has a slower rate of absorption than is displayed by the other sulfonylureas, and it is metabolized to at least three compounds, all of which have less hypoglycemic potency than that of the parent drug. Chlorpropamide has a relatively long biological half-life due to its affinity for serum proteins, hence slow excretory rate. It may be seen that the hepatic and renal drug-metabolizing enzyme system exerts somewhat different metabolic fates on the various sulfonylurea. Expectedly, these metabolizing sites affect not only the duration of action of the agent, but its hypoglycemic actions as well.

The primary mechanism of action of the sulfonylureas involves a direct stimulation of insulin release from the β cells of the islets of Langerhans (see Figure 10-5). In the presence of viable β cells, i.e., insulin-secreting β cells, the sulfonylurea drugs enhance the release of endogenous insulin, thereby leading to hypoglycemia. This release appears to be mediated by a decrease in the cell membrane potassium-ion permeability. ATP-sensitive K^+ channels or a protein closely associated with it may be the receptor through which sulfonylureas act to stimulate insulin secretion. The sulfonylureas, particularly at high doses, may also exert nonpancreatic actions by causing a reducing outflow of hepatic

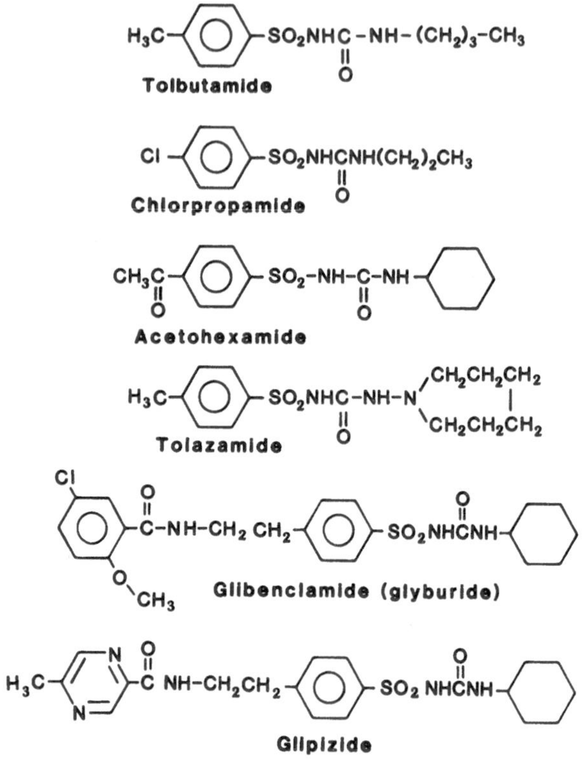

Figure 10-3. Chemical structures of common sulfonylurea oral hypoglycemic agents.

Table 10-9. Pharmacokinetics of Selected Sulfonylurea Agents

Drug	Approximate half-life (hr)	Metabolic fate	Metabolite(s)	Relative activity
Acetohexamide	6	Reduced	Active	+ +
Chlorpropamide	36	Relatively unchanged	Few	+ + + +
Tolazamide	6	Oxidized	Less active	+ + + +
Tolbutamide	6	Oxidized	Inactive	+
Glipizide	6	Oxidized	Inactive	+ + + +
Glyburide (glibenclamide)	6	Partially metabolized	Relatively inactive	+ + + +

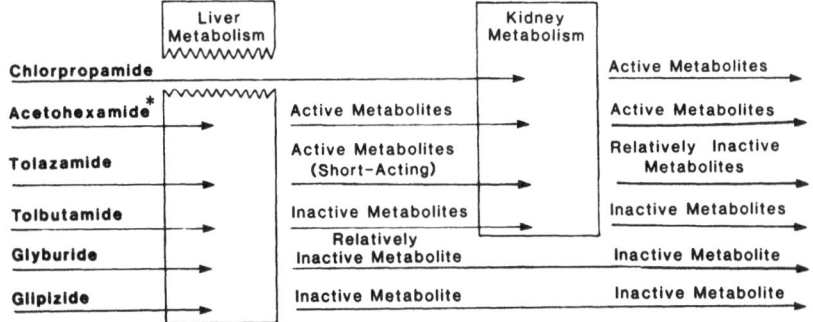

*Metabolites of Acetohexamide Found in Urine of Human Subjects

Figure 10-4. Sites of biotransformation of sulfonylureas.

glucose. In normal subjects, but not diabetics, these agents may enhance the peripheral utilization of glucose. The sulfonylureas are ineffective in the management of severe diabetes or juvenile diabetes, since the number of viable β cells in this form of diabetes is sparse. Thus the sulfonylureas are capable of increasing meal-evoked insulin secretion in most NIDDM patients. While it was once postulated that the primary mechanism of action of the sulfonylurea was enhancement of meal-stimulated insulin secretion, the insulinotropic effect of these oral hypoglycemic drugs is perhaps less important than the extrapancreatic effects.

Table 10-10 lists some of the more widely used sulfonylurea-type oral hypoglycemic agents. Dose regimens and the duration of hypoglycemic actions vary among the sulfonylurea drugs. The doses employed

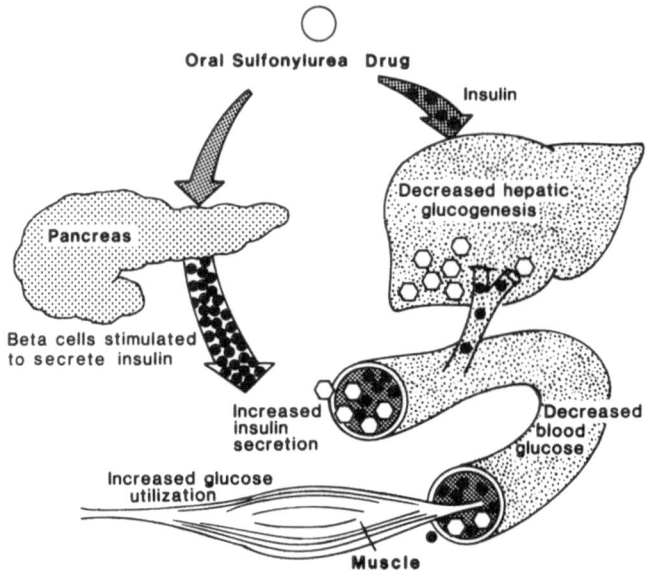

Figure 10-5. Proposed mechanism of action of sulfonylurea agents.

will depend on the severity of the diabetes as well as other factors, such as diet and exercise (or lack thereof).

Acetohexamide is usually administered orally in an initial dose of 250 mg/day, with the dosage adjusted until desired blood glucose levels are attained. Total daily doses should not exceed 1.5 g. Acetohexamide is teratogenic in animals and is therefore not recommended for use

Table 10-10. Oral Hypoglycemic Drugs Used in Diabetes Mellitus

Generic name	Trade name	Average daily dose[a] (mg)	Average duration of action (hr)
Acetohexamide	Dymelor	125–1000 (single or divided dose)	12–24
Chlorpropamide	Diabinese	100–510 (single dose)	~60
Tolazamide	Tolinase	100–1000 (single dose)	12–24
Tolbutamide	Orinase	500–3000 (divided dose)	6–24
Glyburide	DiaBeta, Micronase	2.5–20	24
Glipizide	Glucotrol	2.5–45	24

[a] Representative doses only; individualized therapies must be suited to patient's requirements.

during pregnancy. Acetohexamide is excreted in breastmilk and can produce hypoglycemia in the nursing infant.

Chlorpropamide displays not only hypoglycemic actions but an antidiuretic action as well. As an antidiabetic agent, chlorpropamide is administered orally in initial doses of 100–250 mg/ day, with the dosage being increased by increments of 50–125 mg/week. Total daily doses should rarely exceed 750 mg. Like acetohexamide, chlorpropamide is teratogenic in animals and can be excreted in breast milk.

Tolazamide is administered orally in doses of 100–250 mg/day initially, with the dosage titrated to accommodate the patients needs. The total daily dose seldom should have to exceed 1 g. Like other sulfonylureas, ethanol ingestion should be avoided when taking tolazamide.

Tolbutamide is administered orally in dosages of 500 mg, one or two times per day initially, with subsequent doses adjusted until the diabetic is therapeutically controlled or the total daily dose reaches 3 g. Like the other sulfonylurea agents, tobutamide is not effective in insulin-dependent (i.e., juvenile-onset) diabetes mellitus (IDDM).

Glyburide and glipizide, the so-called second generation of oral sulfonylurea oral hypoglycemic agents, are well absorbed following oral administration. Both drugs are extensively metabolized in the liver. In type II diabetes, glyburide and glipizide seem to be at least as effective as chlorpropamide and tolazamide.

The sulfonylureas exhibit a number of side effects (see Table 10-11). Fortunately, cross-reactions and sensitivities are rare among compounds in this class, and therefore a different sulfonylurea may be tried in order to achieve better therapeutic results while minimizing a particular side

Table 10-11. Common Side-Effects of Sulfonylureas

Severe or prolonged hypoglycemia (overdose)
  Muscular weakness
  Diarrhea, nausea, and vomiting
  Ataxia
  Dizziness, headache
  Mental confusion
  Heartburn
  Stomach pain or discomfort
Skin reactions (rashes) (rare)
Photosensitivities (rare)
Erythema
Blood dyscrasias (e.g., leukopenia thrombocytopenia)
Hepatic dysfunction (cholestatic jaundice)
Water retention (chlorpropamide)
Increased risk of cardiovascular disorders (?)

effect. The oral antidiabetics interact with many other classes of drugs (see Chapter 11). Aside from the more commonly seen side effects of the sulfonylureas, there has been a continued interest and controversy surrounding the findings of the University Group Diabetes Program (UGDP), which indicated a higher mortality in diabetic patients receiving oral hypoglycemic drugs compared with those receiving insulin. Future studies may resolve these controversies surrounding the use of the oral hypoglycemic drugs in the management of maturity-onset diabetes. Glyburide and glipizide do not appear to offer major therapeutic advantages over first-generation oral sulfonylurea hypoglycemic agents.

10.2.2. Biguanides

A second chemical class of oral hypoglycemic agents is the biguanides. The United States Food and Drug Administration (FDA) has banned the sale of phenethylbiguanide (phenformin, DBI). Phenformin and metiformin are still available in other countries.

Phenformin has a shorter duration of action than that of the sulfonylurea agents, but timed disintegration tablets can prolong its hypoglycemic actions. The mechanism of action of the biguanides has not been clearly established, but it does not involve stimulation of β-cell secretion of insulin. The biguanides may bring about an inhibition of hepatic gluconeogenesis, block respiratory enzymes, interfere with the absorption of carbohydrates, and/or possibly accelerate the peripheral utilization of glucose.

Before its withdrawal from the U.S. market, phenformin was used in the management of maturity-onset diabetes. Phenformin causes nausea and vomiting. More importantly, phenformin usage has been associated with severe and sometimes fatal disturbances in lactate metabolism. The use of phenformin has been associated with an increased risk of cardiovascular disease.

10.3. GLUCAGON

Glucagon was originally termed a hyperglycemic factor and was at one time considered a contaminant of insulin preparations. Glucagon is a polypeptide hormone with a molecular weight of 3450 (see Figure 10-6). It is secreted by the α cells of the islets of Langerhans. Glucagon is a very potent hepatic glycogenolytic agent that produces a marked hypoglycemia and hypoaminacidemia. Although pharmacological doses of glucagon can transiently elevate blood sugar levels, it is of questionable

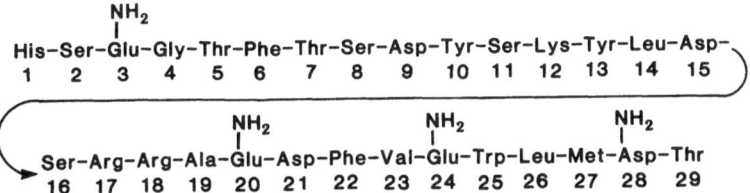

Figure 10-6. Amino acid sequence of pork glucagon.

use in the management of hypoglycemic states. Glucagon promotes lipolysis and stimulates the adenyl cyclase–cAMP system in a number of different tissues.

Several physiological and pharmacological factors can affect blood glucose levels. Glucagon can also stimulate β cells of the islets of Langerhans, hence aid in the modulation of blood glucose levels. Recent interest in glucagon has centered on its role in the genesis of diabetes mellitus. Glucagon may have a significant role in the maintenance of euglycemia in normal individuals; a deleterious role in some of the metabolic aberrations seen in the patient with diabetes mellitus. It has been proposed that in juvenile diabetics some α cells lose their glucose-sensing capacity, and therefore insulin therapy cannot completely stabilize the metablic balance between the two hormones. Theoretically, a glucagon-suppressing agent that does not enhance glucose utilization might be of therapeutic benefit.

Although there seems little indication for the pharmacological use of glucagon in causing hypoglycemia, it has been used for some of its nonmetabolic properties. Glucagon causes some degree of coronary vasodilation and can reduce renal vascular resistance. Since glucagon can exert a positive inotropic action on the myocardium, it has been tried with limited success in the treatment of congestive heart failure. Neither the metabolic nor the nonmetabolic pharmacological properties of glucagon are of any significant therapeutic value at this time.

One USP unit of glucagon is equivalent to 1 IU of glucagon and also about 1 mg of glucagon. The usual antihypoglycemic dose in adults (IM, i.v., or SC) is approximately 0.5–1 mg of glucagon, repeated in 20 min if necessary. The usual pediatric doses (IM, i.v., or SC) is equivalent to 0.025 USP units (0.025 mg) of glucagon/kg of body weight, repeated in 20 min if necessary. Glucagon is contraindicated in the management of birth asphyxia or hypoglycemia, in premature infants, or in infants who exhibit intrauterine growth retardation (IUGR). Glucagon is commercially available in 1 and 10 USP units (1 and 10 mg, respectively).

10.4. SOMATOSTATIN

As a result of the search for a hypothalamic releasing factor for growth hormone, a contaminating substance was discovered that actually caused an inhibition of somatotropin release. This compound was named growth hormone-release inhibiting hormone (GH-RIH), somatotropin-release-inhibiting factor (SRIF), or somatostatin (see also Chapter 2). Somatostatin has now been isolated and synthesized; it is a tetradecapeptide (see Figure 10-7).

Somatostatin exerts a number of biological actions on different tissues. This polypeptide inhibits growth hormone responses to all known physiological and pharmacological stimuli. Somatostatin prevents the growth hormone release ordinarily observed following arginine, L-DOPA and insulin administration. Somatostatin inhibits the secretion of both insulin and glucagon. Somatostatin can reduce fasting hyperglycemia in insulin-deficient juvenile diabetes. Elevated levels of growth hormone seen in patients with acromegaly can also be reduced by somatostatin. It has also been shown to alter aggregation of platelets and to block leukocytosis in response to endotoxin. On the basis of a number of the inhibitory actions of somatostatin on the kidney and on skeletal muscles, it has been suggested that this hormone would more appropriately be termed panhibin.

Natural and synthetic somatostatin exhibit similar biological actions. The biological half-life of either natural or synthetic somatostatin is very brief (about 5 min), as these polypeptides are quickly inactivated in the plasma. A host of somatostatin analogues, e.g., Des-(Ala^1-Gly^2)-somatostatin, Des-(Ala^1-Gly^2-Asn^5)-somatostatin, D-Trp^8-somatostatin, have been synthesized in an effort to extend their biolgoical half-life and have therefore made them more pharmacologically useful. Although some of these analogues, e.g., D-Trp^8-somatostatin, are more potent inhibitors of growth hormone, none possesses significantly longer durations of action then the parent polypeptide.

The therapeutic implications for somatostatin appear to be in the management of acromegaly, pancreatic islet cell tumors, and diabetes mellitus. In diabetes, somatostatin can acutely improve fasting and post-

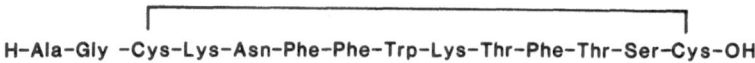

H–Ala–Gly –Cys–Lys–Asn–Phe–Phe–Trp–Lys–Thr–Phe–Thr–Ser–Cys–OH

Figure 10-7.   Primary chemical structure of somatostatin.

prandial hypoglycemia in insulin-requiring diabetics by suppressing glucagon secretion. Because growth hormone has been implicated in the genesis of diabetic retinopathy, the suppression of growth hormone secretion may reduce ocular changes. It is possible that somatostatin may ameliorate the severity of diabetic ketoacidosis. Clearly, the clinical implications for somatostatin have not been fully realized, but an understanding of the role played by this polypeptide in the management of diabetes mellitus represents a significant challenge to the physician.

10.5. NONHORMONAL HYPERGLYCEMIC AGENTS

The hypoglycemoses, i.e., disorders characterized by hypoglycemic states, have a wide variety of etiologies. Although several exogenous agents (e.g., salicylates, alcohol) can produce subnormal blood glucose levels, several other causes can produce spontaneous hypoglycemia and are attributable to aberrant endogenous metabolic processes. Pancreatic disorders (e.g., islet cell adenoma), hepatic disease (e.g., cirrhosis), hypopituitarism, and a host of other genetic and nongenetic pathological states can be characterized by hypoglycemia (see also Table 10-5).

Diazoxide (Proglycem) is an agent that can produce hyperglycemia that has been used in the therapeutic management of certain types of insulin-secretory tumors. Its actions appear to be due to its ability to decrease insulin section and to diminish the peripheral utilization of glucose. Diazoxide also possesses antihypertensive properties and may exert α-adrenergic-type effect on pancreatic β cells. The usual daily dose of diazoxide ranges from 3 to 8 mg/kg, administered in divided doses. Lower doses are used in small children and neonates. This nondiuretic thiazide does posses side effects, including GI irritation, thrombocytopenia, neutropenia, and excessive hair growth. Diazoxide is reportedly teratogenic in animals.

RECOMMENDED READINGS

Brink, S. J., Stewart, C., Insulin pump treatment in insulin-dependent diabetes mellitus, *JAMA* **255**:617, 1986.

Brownlee, M., and Cerami, A., The biochemistry of the complications of diabetes mellitus, *Annu. Rev. Biochem.* **50**:385, 1981.

Boyden, T., and Bressler, R., Oral hypoglycemic agents, *Adv. Int. Med.* **24**:53, 1979.

Cheng, K., and Lorner, J., Intracellular mediators of insulin action, *Ann. Rev. Physiol.* **47**:405–425, 1985.

Czech, M. P., Nature and regulation of the insulin receptor, structure and function, *Ann. Rev. Physiol.* **47**:357–383, 1985.

Flier, J. S., Insulin receptors and insulin resistance, *Annu. Rev. Med.* **34**:145, 1983.

Heding, L. G., Human insulin. Facts and perspectives, *Acta Med. Scand. (Suppl.)* **671**:107, 1983.

Home, P. D., and Alberti, M. G. M. M., Human insulin, *Clin. Endocrinol. Metab.* **11**:453, 1982.

Horwitz, D. L., Insulin pump therapy, rationale and principles of use, *Postgrad. Med.* **76**:80, 1984.

Jackson, J. E., and Bressler, R., Clinical pharmacology of sulphonylurea hypoglycemic agents, *Drugs* **22**:211, 1981.

Jacobs, S., and Cuatrecasas, P., Insulin receptors, *Annu. Rev. Pharmacol. Toxicol.* **23**:461, 1983.

Kahn, C. R., Molecular mechanism of insulin action, *Ann. Rev. Med.* **36**:429–451, 1985.

Larkin, R. G., Pharmacological principles of treatment in diabetes, *Med. J. Aust.* **142**:117, 1985.

Lebovitz, H. E., and Reaven, G. M., New perspectives in noninsulin-dependent diabetes mellitus and the role of glipizide in its treatment, *Am. J. Med.* **75**:1, 1983.

McCann, S. M., Physiology and pharmacology of LHRH and somatostatin, *Annu. Rev. Pharmacol. Toxicol.* **22**:491, 1982.

Predergast, B. D., Glyburide and glipizide, second-generation oral sulfonylurea hypoglycemic agents, *Clin. Pharm.* **3**:473, 1984.

Roth, J., Insulin receptors in diabetes, *Hosp. Pract.* (May), p. 98, 1980.

Seltzer, H. S., Efficacy and safety of oral hypoglycemic agents, *Annu. Rev. Med.* **31**:261, 1980.

Skillman, T. G., Oral hypoglycemic agents for treatment of NIDDM, *Geriatrics* **39**:77–83, 1984.

Unger, R. H., and Orci, L., Glucagon and the A cell. Physiology and pathophysiology, *N. Engl. J. Med.* **304**:1518, 1981.

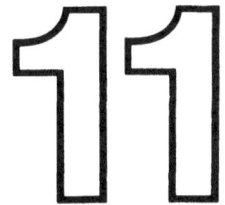

EFFECTS OF DRUGS ON THE ENDOCRINE SYSTEM

11.1. INTRODUCTION

Several synthetic steroids and hormonally active substances are able to affect the endocrine system. In such cases, the substance may possess inherent hormonal activity and therefore act rather specifically on a particular target organ of the endocrine system. Some of the so-called 19-norsteroids can effectively inhibit ovulation (e.g., norethynodrel) or can enhance protein-anabolic activity (e.g., norethandrolone). While these steroids are, in fact, drugs, they nevertheless possess inherent hormonal activity. On the other hand, drugs without inherent hormonal activity are able to affect particular target organs of the endocrine system. Some of these drugs are used for the explicit purpose of affecting an endocrine process, while still others affect a hormonal action, usually as a result of some side effect or toxic reaction. Several antithyroidal agents have no inherent hormonal activity, yet exert pharmacological effects on the endocrine system. Conversely, several CNS-depressant drugs without inherent hormonal activity are capable of affecting hormonal balance as a result of some side effect, or their ability to interfere with hypothalamic–pituitary relationships.

There are many drugs that, as a result of some secondary action, may cause alterations in endocrine activities. Such drugs are not used purposely to alter or modify hormonal states. A wide variety of pharmacological agents that affect the CNS can secondarily alter the endocrine responses of several end organs. Some of these CNS-acting drugs have been used in the study of ovulation for quite some time by reproductive physiologists. Both morphine and the barbiturates can affect pituitary–hypothalamic mechanisms involved in the process of ovulation. It is not necessary for a particular pharmacological agent to be endowed with CNS activity in order for it to affect endocrine responses. Many drugs used in the management of cancer, as well as other protein-cytotoxic antibiotics, will interfere with the process of spermatogenesis. Cancer chemotherapeutic agents are not selective enough to direct their inhibitory actions only on the rapidly dividing cells of a neoplasm. Indeed, rapidly dividing cells of the gonads are also inhibited by certain antineoplastic drugs. Different alkylating agents are known to suppress the process of spermatogenesis. Gonadal mitosis in the female may likewise be inhibited by protein-inhibitory antibiotics and antitumor agents. While its extreme toxicity ordinarily precludes its therapeutic usefulness, alloxan is somewhat specific in destroying pancreatic β cells. Also, synthalin A may damage the α cells of the pancreas. Several chemicals, some closely related to the pesticide DDT, can inhibit steroidogenesis in the adrenal cortex.

Not all drugs that affect the endocrine system do so by exerting secondary actions on the hypothalamic–pituitary axis or by destroying particular cellular components in a target tissue. Some drugs without inherent hormonal activity can alter endocrine responses by interacting with the protein-binding sites normally responsible for transporting endogenous hormones. Salicylates and phenytoin can affect the binding of thyroid hormone in the blood. Oral contraceptives and other synthetic steroids can also influence the amount of circulating thyroid hormone. Likewise, synthetic glucocorticoids can modify the degree of binding of endogenous steroidal hormones.

11.2. BASIC MECHANISMS OF DRUG–HORMONE INTERACTIONS

During the past decade, there has been a growing recognition of the problem of drug interactions. It is also important to note that many of these drugs can also effect the endocrine system. Many of the same basic mechanisms involving drug–drug interactions can be extended to drug–hormone interactions. These interactions can potentially alter the effectiveness of the pharmacological agent or can modify the normal state (see Table 11-1). The basic mechanisms involved in drug–hormone interactions include (1) interference with absorption, (2) displacement from binding sites, (3) augmentation of metabolism, and (4) facilitation or inhibition of excretion.

A number of agents can interfere with the absorption of drugs. Some

Table 11-1. Representative Drug–Hormone Interactions

Hormone	Drug	Effects of interaction
Oral contraceptives (progestin–estrogen)	Barbiturates	Accelerate metabolism of the steroid
	Phenylbutazone	Accelerate metabolism of the steroid
	Clofibrate	Reduction of cholesterol-lowering action
Androgens	Barbiturates	Accelerate metabolism of the steroid
	Phenylbutazone	Accelerate metabolism of the steroid
	Chlorcyclizine	Accelerate metabolism of the steroid
	Anticoagulants	Potentiated by norethandrolone
Anti-inflammatory steroid	Barbiturates	Accelerate metabolism of the steroid; increased activity of sedative
	Phenytoin	Reduce endogenous secretion of corticoids
	Antihistamines	Accelerate metabolism of the steroid
	Cholinergics	Accelerate metabolism of the steroid
Antidiuretic hormone (e.g., ADH, vasopressin)	Chlorpropamide	Enhanced activity of ADH
	Phenformin	Enhanced activity of ADH
	Acetaminophen	Enhanced activity of ADH
	Cyclophosphamide	Enhanced activity of ADH
Antidiuretic hormone (e.g., ADH, vasopressin)	Tolbutamide	Enhanced activity of ADH
	Opiates	Enhanced activity of ADH
	Barbiturates	Enhanced activity of ADH
	Clofibrate	Enhanced activity of ADH
	Carbamazepine	Enhanced activity of ADH
	Tricyclic antidepressants	Enhanced activity of ADH
	Vinca Alkaloids	Enhanced activity of ADH
	Lithium	Enhanced activity of ADH
Thyroxine	Phenobarbital	Reduced rate of metabolism
	Clofibrate	Reduced rate of metabolism
	Sulfonylureas	Enhanced effect
Insulin	Sulfonylureas	Enhanced hypoglycemia
	Biguanides	Enhanced hypoglycemia
	Adrenergic blockers	Enhanced hypoglycemia
	MAO inhibitors	Enhanced hypoglycemia

(Continued)

Table 11-1.   (*Continued*)

Hormone	Drug	Effects of interaction
Oxytocin	Sympathomimetics	Prolonged hypertension
Desoxycorticosterone	Barbiturates	Accelerate metabolism of the steroid
	Phenylbutazone	Accelerate metabolism of the steroid

of these drugs possess inherent hormonal properties. The gastrointestinal GI absorption of synthetic steroids (e.g., oral contraceptives) can be impeded by mineral oil as well as by fatty foodstuffs. Furthermore, antibiotics such as the tetracyclines can interfere with the absorption of calcium and hence potentially affect parathormone secretion. Factors interfering with the absorption of iron can likewise affect the levels of transferrin.

Several drugs are reversibly bound to plasma proteins during their transport and biodistribution. Two different classes of drugs can also compete for the same or similar binding sites on plasma proteins and, depending on their inherent avidity for such binding sites, can exaggerate (or inhibit) the action(s) of the other class. Drugs such as phenylbutazone and indomethacin can frequently displace the sulfonylurea oral hypoglycemic agents from plasma protein-binding sites leading to an exaggerated lowering in blood glucose levels. Phenylbutazone is strongly bound to plasma protein and has the ability to displace tolbutamide from plasma protein-binding sites. Similarly, phenylbutazone can displace corticosteroids from nonspecific binding sites on plasma proteins.

Mention should also be made of the displacement of one hormone from a specific binding site in particular target organs. A number of synthetic steroids can mimic the action of naturally occurring steroids and can compete with or otherwise displace endogenous hormones from target organ receptor sites. Drugs can either stimulate or inhibit certain hepatic microsomal enzyme systems, thereby altering the metabolism of endogenous hormones. It is well known that the barbiturates can stimulate a number of hepatic mixed-function oxidases (MFO) and that many of these same enzyme systems are involved in the metabolism of both endogenous and exogenous steroids. Likewise, phenytoin can enhance hepatic microsomal steroid hydroxylase enzymes.

Drugs that modify the excretion or urinary elimination of either endogenous substances or other drugs can also affect the endocrine system. For example, the potassium-lowering side effects of certain oral hypoglycemic agents can be exaggerated by diuretics. The biliary excretion of several drugs including many steroids constitutes still another potential site for drug–hormone interaction. Finally, the excretion of drugs and/or hormones into milk (see later section) is governed by many of the same physicochemical principles as those involving renal elimination.

In summary, pharmacological interactions between hormones and nonendocrine active drugs are poorly understood. The barbiturates can stimulate hepatic microsomal enzymes and thereby alter the biological activity of steroids such as the androgens or estrogens. In a somewhat similar fashion, pesticides of both the organochloride and organophosphate classes can alter hepatic steroid hydroxylase enzymes systems. Although hormones can be transported by specialized blood proteins, they can also bind rather nonspecifically to plasma albumins. A variety of drugs and hormones can apparently bind nonselectively to sites on blood proteins. If one agent has a greater affinity than another for these protein-binding sites, it is readily understandable how these interactions can produce altered pharmacological effects. The antibacterial sulfonamides, for example, can displace the oral hypoglycemic sulfonylurea agents from protein-binding sites and can thereby cause exaggerated hypoglycemia. In such a case, more unbound sulfonylurea is available to exert its blood glucose-lowering action. These same oral antidiabetic agents can enhance the effects of thyroxine, presumably by displacing the hormone from its binding sites on blood proteins. Still another mechanism of hormone interaction may occur at the target organ itself and not in the liver or blood. Androgen–estrogen antagonism is a well-documented example of hormonal interactions, yet the precise mechanism involved has not been established. Oral contraceptives containing estrogenic constituents might also be expected to interfere with the protein-anabolic actions of synthetic steroids like norethandrolone. It should be evident that there are many diverse examples of drug–hormone interactions, and in many instances the basic mechanisms of such interactions remain to be elucidated.

11.3. EFFECTS OF DRUGS ON ADENOHYPOPHYSEAL FUNCTION

The hypothalamic–adenohypophyseal system contains a number of functional units and integrates cortical, vegetative, and hormonal regulation. Many agents, both with hormonal or nonhormonal properties, can affect the secretion and/or release of pituitary trophic hormones. Because many of the neurotransmitters within the CNS involve acetylcholine (ACh) or catecholamines, it is not surprising that cholinergic and adrenergic drugs can profoundly affect those centers in juxtaposition to the adenohypophysis. Anticholinergic agents and those drugs that can interfere directly or indirectly with the sympathetic nervous system might be expected to modify the secretion of adenohypophyseal hormones.

Autonomic agents that deplete catecholamines (e.g., reserpine) or that mimic their actions (e.g., amphetamine) may affect the secretion of ACTH. Moderate doses of exogenous epinephrine itself, however, do not substantially alter ACTH secretion. Monoamineoxidase (MAO) inhibitors (e.g., α-ethyltryptamine, etryptamine) decrease the catabolism of catecholamines and can reduce ACTH secretion. This decrease in ACTH secretion is probably related to the pressor response elicited by the MAO inhibitors. It is also possible that this decrease in ACTH is mediated *via* the carotid and aortic baroreceptors.

Chlorpromazine and certain closely related compounds possess α-adrenergic-blocking activities. The endocrine-induced changes produced by this phenothiazine have already been discussed in some detail in the section dealing with tranquilizers. The ergot alkaloids also demonstrate α-adrenergic-blocking activity. The uterine-stimulating properties of these agents are well known. Ergocornine seems particularly endowed with endocrine-altering activities. This substance is capable of suppressing implantation. It may terminate pseudopregnancy in experimental animals. Ergocornine inhibits lactation, presumably by increasing hypothalamic levels of prolactin-inhibitory factor (PIF) (see Chapter 2).

Imidazole is capable of antagonizing certain actions of the catecholamines. It also produces changes in ACTH activity and alters levels of calcium and phosphorus. Imidazole appears to mimic the actions of thyrocalcitonin. Many of the endocrine changes produced by imidazole are related to its ability to stimulate phosphodiesterase activity and thereby enhance the breakdown of cAMP.

Agents that affect the parasympathetic division of the autonomic nervous system are likewise responsible for causing changes in various hormonal activities. Studies on isolated seminal vesicles from a variety of experimental animals have shown that this organ exhibits an increase in tone and muscular contraction upon exposure to parasympathomimetic agents. The sex accessory organs also react to sympathomimetic agents. Such cholinergic agents as carbamylcholine and pilocarpine enhance the secretory activity of sex accessory gland products. Morphine and closely related opiates are capable of altering adenohypophyseal secretion. The extent of the changes in pituitary hormone secretory activity is related to both the dose and duration of administration of these narcotics. Morphine is capable of inhibiting ovulation under certain experimental conditions. In the male it seems to interfere with luteinizing hormone (ICSH) activity. It seldom affects the process of spermatogenesis. Heroin or diacetylmorphine addicts sometimes demonstrate reduced fertility and impotence, but other factors may be involved in this loss of reproductive function.

Several nonsteroidal drugs can affect ACTH secretion, but morphine is quite consistent in causing inhibition of the release of this trophic hormone. Such an inhibition ordinarily results in diminished plasma levels, as well as urinary levels, of adrenocortical steroids. Morphine interferes at the level of the pituitary–hypothalamic axis and does not appear to directly suppress the adrenal cortex.

Chlorpromazine, and other phenothiazines exert a direct action on the hypothalamus. Chlorpromazine may affect the response of several trophic hormones. It will produce a reduction in the urinary levels of both follicle-stimulating hormone (FSH) and luteinizing hormone (LH). It also lowers the levels of estrogens and progestins found in the urine. This tranquilizer has been shown to suppress ovulation in a number of different mammalian species. It is known to interfere with estrous cycles and to lead to infertility. While it seems to inhibit ovarian function generally, it may actually induce lactation. In these respects, chlorpromazine's actions are much like those of reserpine, which also interferes with ovulation and enhances lactation. Thus these two different types of tranquilizers are capable of causing inhibition of pituitary gonadotropins and of affecting the release of prolactin. Chlorpromazine also inhibits the secretion of both STH and ACTH. The action of these drugs on the neurohypophysis is not entirely clear. While chlorpromazine seems to inhibit the release of oxytocin, its effects on antidiuretic hormone (ADH) remain unresolved. Perphenazine can profoundly enhance the process of lactation.

Reserpine is known for its tranquilizing action and as an effective antihypertensive drug. It is used to lower blood pressure, since it can generally be administered in smaller doses than can drugs used to achieve tranquility. With small doses, the complicating side effects of reserpine are reduced. Reserpine exerts a variety of complex changes in the endocrine system. Like those of chlorpromazine, the doses of reserpine required to affect these changes in the endocrine system are usually quite high. The duration of administration or the total dosage is also important to alterations in hormonal activity. Also, the endocrine changes produced by reserpine are more commonly manifest in females than in males. The underlying cause for this sex difference in the actions of reserpine is not clearly understood.

Certain analogues of reserpine are more effective in causing changes in endocrine activity than reserpine itself. Tetrahydropyranyl methyl-reserpine appears to be particularly effective in suppressing the reproductive function, whereas syrosingopine does not have much effect on these endocrine processes.

The actions of reserpine on ACTH secretion appear to vary according to the dose and duration of administration. Reserpine causes depletion of brain catecholamines without increasing the release of active catecholamines. It is associated with enhanced secretion of ACTH. Depending somewhat on the nature of the experimental conditions, reserpine may stimulate steroidogenesis and lead to adrenal hypertrophy.

Reserpine has long been known to evoke the secretion of luteotropic (prolactin) hormone. If prolactin is secreted when the mammary glands have been primed by sex steroids, lactation may ensue.

Reserpine is not the only agent that can affect blood levels of prolactin (see Table 11-2). It should be evident that a wide spectrum of hormones and drugs can effect the blood levels of prolactin. Some agents can increase levels of prolactin, while others can lead to a reduction in this tropic hormone.

Table 11-2. Effect of Various Agents on Prolactin Levels[a]

Increased blood levels	Decreased blood levels
Reserpine	Acetylcholine
Methyl-DOPA	Apomorphine
α-Methyl-p-tyrosine	Dopamine
Chlorpromazine	L-DOPA
Atropine	Iproniazid
Perphenazine (and other phenothiazines)	β-Hydroxy-GABA
Haloperidol	Somatostatin
Tricyclic antidepressants	Bromocriptine
Sulpiride	
Diethyl ether	
Nicotine	
Vasopressin	
Estrogens	
Thyroxine (and triiodothyrine)	
Histamine	
Prostaglandin E (PGE)	
β-Endorphin	
Met-enkephalin	
TRH	
Opiates	

[a] Response may vary quantitively, depending on the dose and the particular species.

Depending on the species, and to some extent the particular analogue, the ergot alkaloids can affect the secretion and/or release of a number of different trophic hormones of the adenohypophysis (see Table 11-3). Ergot drugs, regardless of their route of administration, inhibit prolactin secretion in all vertebrate species examined, including man. The inhibitory action of the ergot alkaloids on prolactin secretion does not require the presence of an intact hypothalamic–pituitary connection. The mechanism whereby ergot alkaloids affect adenohypophyseal hormone secretion seems to be due to the stimulation of dopamine receptor sites in the pituitary gland or in the central nervous system.

Several drugs or hormones can also affect the circulating levels of growth hormone (see Table 11-4). It is noteworthy that different classes of hormones can lead to increased levels of growth hormone and that no common mechanism of action is readily apparent.

Barbiturates, like a number of tranquilizers and atropine, are capable of affecting the secretion of adenohypophyseal hormones. In particular, these sedatives and tranquilizers appear to suppress the secretion of FSH and/or LH in a variety of species. The barbiturates have been shown to effect alterations in the hormonal state in both males and females of several experimental animals. The effects of barbiturates on reproductive activity in man are less evident. Phenobarbital has been demonstrated to block ovulation if administered during the critical period just before the ovulatory event takes place. The ovulatory-inhibiting action of this barbituate might be due to its ability to interfere with the conversion of pregnenolone to progesterone (and subsequent metabolites), thus disrupting the optimal steroid environment necessary for the regulation of ovulation. The barbituates may also alter hypothalamic–pituitary thresholds involved in the ovulatory mechanism.

Barbituates also produce changes in reproductive function in the male. Phenobarbital inhibits the growth-promoting actions of androgens on the seminal vesicles of immature animals. It may also reduce nucleic acid levels in other sex accessory organs. In experimental animals, an increase in the percentage of nonviable spermatozoa has been reported. It remains to be established whether the barbiturates exert these deleterious actions directly on androgenic target organs or through enhanced metabolism of male sex hormones by hepatic microsomal enzyme systems.

Since the isolation of the enkephalins, there has been considerable interest in the effects of the opiates and opioid peptides. It is now known that the opiates exert a host of effects on pituitary hormone secretion. In experimental animals, the opiates stimulate growth hormone, prolactin, and ACTH. They appear to stimulate the secretion of thyroid-

Table 11-3. Effects of Ergot Alkaloids on the Secretion of Various
Adenophypophyseal Hormones[a]

Species	FSH/LH	TSH	GH	ACTH	PRL
Subprimates	↔		↔	↑	↓
Humans	↔	↔	↑	↔	↓

[a] Absolute responses may vary, depending on the specific experimental circumstances.

stimulating hormone (TSH), FSH, and LH. In man, the role of endogenous opiates seems to involve the secretion of ACTH and FSH/LH (see also Chapter 2).

Because numerous drugs and related factors can affect the secretion and/or release of adenohypophyseal hormones, it is important to be aware of such factors or conditions when attempting to clinically assess pituitary function. With the advent of radioimmunoassays (RIA), it is now possible to assess the blood levels of most trophic hormones. Drug-induced alterations of pituitary function tests, if not realized by the

Table 11-4. Effects of Various Agents on
Growth Hormone Levels

Increased blood levels	Decreased blood levels
Norepinephrine	Somatostatin
Epinephrine	
Serotonin	
TRH	
Vasopressin	
Substance P	
Endorphins	
Enkephalins	
Arginine[a]	
Prostaglandins	
Insulin	
(hypoglycemia)[a]	
α-Desoxyglucose	
Apomorphine	
L-DOPA[a]	
Clonidine[a]	

[a] Use a provocative test for the diagnosis of growth hormone
disorders.

Table 11-5. Effects of Various Drugs on Pituitary Function Tests

Drug	GH Basal	GH Stim.	FSH/LH Basal	FSH/LH Stim.	PRL Basal	PRL Stim.	TSH Basal	TSH Stim.	ACTH Basal	ACTH Stim.
Progestins	↓	↓	↓						↓	↓
Estrogens	↑	↑	↓		↑	↑		↑		↓
Glucocorticoids	↓		↓	↓			↓	↓		↓
Phenothiazines	↓	↓			↑					
L-DOPA		↑			↓					
Phenytoin									↓	↓
Propanolol		↑								
Morphine	↓				↑					
Ethanol		↓								↓

clinician, can lead to misinterpretations and therapeutic misadventures. Indeed, the results of pituitary function can be altered by many endogenous and exogenous factors (see Table 11-5). It is particularly important for the physician to obtain a complete medication history from the patient before undertaking any assessment of anterior pituitary function.

11.4. EFFECTS OF DRUGS ON NEUROHYPOPHYSEAL FUNCTION

Many drugs are known to alter posterior pituitary function either by affecting the release of vasopressin (ADH) or by modifying its peripheral actions (see also Chapter 3). The interactions of vasopressin involve not only its release (or inhibition of release) but those drugs that affect its peripheral effects as well (see Table 11-6). It is noteworthy that ethanol can affect the secretion of either of the two neurohypophyseal hormones.

Ethanol influences endocrine activity by interfering with neurohypophyseal secretion of ADH and possibly with the release of ACTH. Alcohol produces a rather striking effect on diuresis by inhibiting the release of ADH. Experiments demonstrating an increase in adrenocortical secretions, presumably by increasing ACTH release, are not particularly convincing. The hyperglycemia produced by ethanol ingestion appears to be related to the ability of ethanol to release epinephrine and/or norepinephrine.

Large doses of atropine cause antidiuresis. Such an action is prob-

Table 11-6. Effects of Various Drugs on the Release and/or Action of Neurohypophyseal Hormones

Enhanced release	Inhibition of release	Blockage of peripheral action
Vasopressin		
Acetylcholine	Ethanol	Lithium
Nicotine		β-Adrenergic agonists
α-Adrenergic agonists		Tetracyclines
β-Adrenergic agonists		
Vincristine		
Clofibrate		
Oxytocin		
Prostaglandin E_2	Ethanol	Propranolol
Prostaglandin $F_{1\alpha}$	Methallibure	Vasopressin analogues
		Oxytocin analogues

ably related to the effects that this drug exerts on the release of ADH. Diethyl ether and several ether derivatives are capable of affecting the endocrine system. It is difficult to state whether such endocrine alterations are due solely to the anesthetic itself or to the stress reaction associated with the use of such agents. Ether is known to stimulate several endocrine glands. It is able to increase the plasma levels of thyroxine, hydrocortisone, and norepinephrine. These changes in blood constituents are probably related to stress reactions. Ether is also capable of affecting the secretion of ADH. The stimulatory actions of ether on ADH secretion result in a decrease in urinary output. Another endocrine alteration caused by ether is that of hyperglycemia. Ether-induced hyperglycemia is probably due to enhanced sympathetic nervous system activity. Ether may act by stimulating the sympathetic nerves innervating the liver. The hyperglycemia produced in this way is not caused by either insulin antagonism or an inhibition of the peripheral utilization of glucose. Ether-induced changes in endocrine activity are generally transient, and hormonal balance is restored reasonably soon after the administration of ether.

Morphine and other narcotics are able to cause a release of ADH. This results in a decrease in urinary output. The primary mechanism, albeit not the only one, seems to reside in the ability of morphine to affect the supraoptic nuclei of the hypothalamus.

11.5. EFFECTS OF DRUGS ON LACTATION AND THEIR PRESENCE IN MILK

Most of the same pharmacokinetic principles involved in the renal excretion of drugs are also operant in the excretion of drugs into milk. Because milk is more acidic than plasma, basic compounds (or drugs) may be somewhat more concentrated in plasma. Therefore, the concentration of acidic compounds in milk is lower than in the plasma. Fortunately, not all drugs are able to pass into the mother's milk in pharmacologically significant amounts. The passage of a drug across the membrane between plasma and milk is influenced by its pk_a (or its degree of ionization), its solubility in lipids (or lack of) and the presence of any specific transport system. Ionized forms of the drug pass slowly into these secretions (*viz.* lactation products). Nonelectrolytes (e.g., ethanol, urea) readily enter milk and quickly reach the same concentration as in the plasma. A wide variety of chemical and pharmacological classes of drugs, when ingested by the mother, can be excreted into breast milk (see Table 11-7). Many of the effects mediated into the infant consist of CNS-acting properties.

Antibiotics, by virtue of their widespread use in both veterinary medicine and human medicine, constitute a particular problem insofar as their presence in milk. A number of antibiotics have been detected in human milk (see Table 11-8). In addition to those drugs excreted into milk (see Table 11-7) and those antibiotics that can secondarily exert pharmacological actions on the infant, still other agents warrant special

Table 11-7. Drugs Excreted in Breast Milk

Drug ingested by mother	Pharmacological effect on infant
Ethanol	Sedation
Chloral hydrate	Sedation
Diazipam (Valium)	Sedation
Diacetylmorphine (heroin)	Dependence and sedation
Iodides	Goitrogenic
Laxatives	Increased bowel activity
Phenobarbital	Sedation
Propylthiouracil	Thyroid suppression
Reserpine	Nasal stuffiness
Methyprylon	Sedation

Table 11-8. Presence of Antibiotics in Milk

Drug	Pharmacological effect on infant
Ampicillin	Possible diarrhea and candidiasis; allergic reaction
Chloramphenicol	Excreted into milk as inactive metabolite
Erythromycin	Detected in trace amounts only
Isoniazid	No reported effect on infant
Kanamycin	Infant ototoxicity??
Metronidazole	No reported effect on infant
Nitrofurantoin	No reported effect on infant
Nalidixic acid	Hemolytic anemia in infant (rare)??
Penicillin	Allergic reactions
Streptomycin	Ototoxicity at high doses
Sulfonamide	Neonatal hyperbilirubinemia; hemolytic anemia
Tetracyclines	Possible tooth staining

consideration. Smoking (and presumably nicotine) reportedly reduces the volume of milk excreted in lactating mothers. It is likely that tetrahydrocannabinol (THC) appears in breast milk. Finally, a number of environmental toxins, such as DDT, PCBs, methylmercury, and certain heavy metals (e.g., cadmium), have reportedly been detected in human milk.

11.6.   EFFECTS OF DRUGS ON HORMONE TRANSPORT

Characteristic of the endocrine system is the fact that the chemical mediator is released from specific cells into the systemic circulation. Upon release into the systemic circulation, the chemical mediator or hormone may undergo a variety of metabolic fates. The biological half-life of hormones in the blood may be only a few minutes or it may be several days. Hormonal biological half-life may be influenced by a number of factors, including the individual rates of biotransformation of the hormones and the degree of excretion. Another factor that can influence the biological half-life of some hormones is their ability to complex or bind with larger molecules found in the blood. This binding to larger molecules provides not only a reservoir but also a vehicle for the hormone. Many hormones have specific transporting protein molecules attached to them as they circulate in the bloodstream. These carrier molecules permit the hormone to be transported from its site of synthesis or release to its target organ.

Despite the presence of hormone-transporting proteins, a particular hormone may exist in either a free (i.e., unbound) or bound state. In some instances, the hormone may be bound to a specific carrier protein. Some hormones will also bind nonspecifically to plasma proteins. In general, if the binding sites on a specific carrier molecule are occupied by a particular hormone, the hormone associates nonspecifically with plasma albumins. Regardless of whether a hormone binds specifically or nonspecifically to plasma proteins, the binding is reversible, so that the hormone can be released and subsequently assimilated by its target organ. Little is known about the dissociation of a hormone from its carrier protein except that the process probably occurs at the target cell, the liver, and the kidney.

Many hormones have specific carrier proteins that can transport them in body fluids (see Table 11-9). Hormones with smaller molecular weights are usually more apt to be bound to a carrier protein. Insulin is perhaps the hormone with the largest molecular weight associated with plasma proteins, but there is a controversy over whether this association is highly specific. Polypeptides of the posterior pituitary gland appear to be bound to transporting proteins. Smaller hormones, such as steroids and thyroxine, also are readily bound to specific transporting proteins found in the blood.

Various physiological and pathological factors can affect hormone–carrier interactions. Pharmacological agents, some with inherent hormonal activity, can also affect the interaction between endogenous hormones and their specific transporting proteins. The binding of thyroid hormones to plasma proteins can be altered by several different types of drugs. Many of the synthetic steroids used as anti-inflammatory drugs or those steroids used as oral contraceptives can interfere with the binding of endogenous steroids to their carrier proteins in the blood.

Very little is known about how the different anterior pituitary hormones are transported in the blood. Since these trophic hormones are

Table 11-9. Hormone-Transporting Proteins

Hormone	Transporting protein nomenclature
Cortisol	Transcortin (CBG)
Estrogen	Sex hormone-binding globulin (SHBG)
Progesterone	Progesterone-binding globulin (PBG)??
Testosterone	Testosterone-binding globulin (TeBG)
Thyroxine	Thyroxine-binding globulin, thyroxine binding prealbumin (TBG, TBPA)
Vasopressin/oxytocin	Neurophysins I, II

generally large proteins or glycoproteins, it is unlikely that any specific transporting substances are necessary in order for them to reach their respective target organs. Whether fractions or subunits of these trophic hormones bind to proteins is not really understood. ACTH is the smallest-molecular-weight trophic hormone in the adenohypophysis. Apparently, it does not bind to any specific transporting protein in the blood. The biological half-life is not attributable to increased binding to a carrier protein. Rather, such an increase in biological activity of certain of the synthetic ACTH molecules is due to increased resistance to degradation by aminopeptidases.

It is now generally accepted that the neurohypophyseal hormones are synthesized with their binding protein. Oxytocin and vasopressin (also known as ADH) are octapeptides. Oxytocin and vasopressin can be separated from their larger binding proteins. These neurohypophyseal hormones are bound to carrier proteins called neurophysin I and neurophysin II. A number of mammalian species appear to have two distinct carrier molecules for these posterior pituitary hormones. Unlike other smaller-molecular-weight hormones (e.g., steroids), these octapeptides of the neurohypophysis appear to be complexed with their binding proteins at their sites of synthesis in hypothalamic areas. On the other hand, steroids are not ordinarily complexed to their specific carrier molecules until they have reached the bloodstream. Plasma neurophysins are elevated by stimuli, which customarily cause the release of oxytocin and/or vasopressin. The physiological significance of these carrier proteins remains to be fully understood. Presumably, drugs that affect oxytocin and/or vasopressin release could enhance the plasma levels of neurophysin I and neurophysin II. Several drugs that act on the CNS can influence the blood levels of vasopressin or ADH (see Chapter 3).

The thyroid hormones circulate in the blood in association with transporting proteins. The specific role of these carrier proteins in thyroid gland physiology is not clearly appreciated, but they do have an important function in determining body distribution and circulating levels of hormone.

The thyroid gland secretes both thyroxine (T_4) and triiodothyronine (T_3). Three serum proteins transport thyroxine: albumin, thyroxine-binding prealbumin (TBPA), and T_4-binding α-globulin (TBG). TBG is found in very small concentrations in the blood, yet it has a very great affinity for T_4. Nevertheless, TBG also can transport a sizeable amount of T_3. The affinity of TBPA for T_3 is minimal.

The hormones of the thyroid are bound to these transporting proteins by noncovalent interactions. Only small amounts of either T_3 or

T_4 remain in a free or unbound state, but these small circulating levels may be important in controlling the disappearance from the blood and the biological activity of the hormones. Parathyroid hormone is not bound to discrete carrier proteins, but it is bound reversibly to α-globulins in the blood.

Several factors can effect the interaction between thyroid hormones and their binding to specific proteins. Both physiological and pathological factors can alter the transport of thyroidal hormones. Pharmacological agents also produce changes in thyroid hormone transport (see Tables 11-10 and 11-11). It may be that many steroids can alter the interaction of T_4 with its transporting proteins.

Certain thyroid-function tests, such as protein-bound iodine (PBI) and T_3 uptake, are affected by different drugs and steroid hormones. Such drug effects on these thyroid-function test results are frequently responsible for erroneous estimates of PBI and/or T_3 uptake.

Several steroid hormones exist in both a free (i.e., unbound) and a protein-bound state. It is probably the free or unbound form of the hormone that is biologically active. Albumins can bind steroid hormones. Albumins are present in rather high concentrations in the blood. These proteins exhibit a high capacity for steroids (i.e., they will bind substantial amounts), but they possess a rather low affinity for most steroids. Globulins are found in much lower concentrations in the blood, but they ordinarily possess an unusually high affinity for steroids; that is, the globulins have a low capacity, but a high affinity, for smaller-molecular-weight hormones such as the steroids.

Steroid hormones in the circulating blood are partly associated with serum proteins; this association is by noncovalent bonding. Such bond-

Table 11-10. Effects of Drugs or Synthetic Hormones on Thyroid-Transporting Proteins

Agent (hormone/drug)	TBG	TBPA
Drugs affecting thyroxine binding		
Phenytoin (DPH)	+	—
Salicylates	—	+
Steroids affecting thyroxine-binding capacity		
Anabolic steroids	↓	↑
Corticosteroids	↓	↑
Estrogens/oral contraceptives	↑	—
Testosterone	↓	↑

Table 11-11. Drugs That Affect Thyroid Function Tests

Drug	Effect on test
Aminosalicylic acid (PAS)	Decreased ^{131}I uptake
Protein anabolic steroids	Decreased TBG; decreased T_4; increased T_3 uptake
Anticoagulants (coumarins)	Increased T_3 uptake
Nonsteroid anti-inflammatory agents (e.g., phenylbutazone)	Increased T_3 uptake; decreased ^{131}I uptake
Anti-inflammatory steroids (also ACTH)	Decreased TBG, decreased ^{131}I uptake
Phenytoin (Dilantin)	Decreased T_4; increased T_3 uptake
Estrogens, progesterone, oral contraceptives	Increased TBG; increased T_4 decreased T_3 uptake
Sulfonamides	Decreased ^{131}I uptake
Salicylates	Decreased total T_4
Phenothiazines	Decreased TBG; decreased ^{131}I uptake

ing is dissociable, so that the steroid–protein complexes are subject to a binding equilibrium. This equilibrium is determined by the concentration and by the affinities of the components. At least four types of serum proteins interact spontaneously with steroid hormones. These serum proteins are (1) albumins, or human serum albumin (HSA); (2) α-acid glycoproteins, or α-acid globulin orosomucoid (AAG), (3) corticosteroid-binding globulin (CBG), or transcortin; and (4) β-globulins, or sex hormone-binding globulin (SHBG).

The physicochemical properties and the serum concentrations of the different steroid-binding proteins will vary considerably. The transporting proteins also differ in their affinities for different steroid hormones. For example, HSA is found in much higher concentrations than CBG, yet HSA has considerably less affinity for the corticosteroids. It should be noted that the affinity of a carrier protein for a hormone is not absolutely specific. In other words, while CBG has the highest affinity for cortisol or corticosterone, it also binds to other steroids, such as progesterone.

Steroid–protein complexes not only provide a physiological vehicle for transporting hormones, but such an interaction provides a reservoir for circulating steroids as well. The hormone–protein complex also may delay the metabolic breakdown of various steroids by the liver. A steroid that is complexed to a carrier hormone cannot be biotransformed or converted to more polar metabolites. Polar metabolites can be more readily excreted by the kidneys. Therefore, the hormone–protein complex results in a prolongation of the biological half-life of the steroid. While the free form of the hormone is most likely the biologically active form, it also is more vulnerable to metabolic alterations by the liver or the kidney. Precisely how a hormone dissociates itself from its specific carrier is unknown.

Many endocrine factors can affect not only the concentration of transporting protein but also the affinity of a hormone for its specific carrier. For example, pregnancy causes an increase in the levels of circulating CBG as well as an increase in the levels of testosterone-binding globulin (TeBG). Interestingly, TeBG levels are higher in normal females than in normal males.

Synthetic steroids used for different therapeutic indications also can affect transporting proteins. Estrogen therapy produces an elevation in the circulating levels of TeBG. The management of cancer of the prostate gland by diethylstilbestrol (DES) frequently leads to increased levels of TeBG. Many synthetic 19-norsteroids can likewise elevate TeBG levels. Progestational agents or oral contraceptive drugs can cause a rise in the circulating levels of CBG.

Corticosteroid-binding globulin, formerly referred to as transcortin, was perhaps the first of the special hormone-carrying proteins to be discovered. Many of the physicochemical characteristics of CBG have been established for several mammalian species including man. In humans, CBG has a molecular weight of about 50,000 and is composed of a carbohydrate-containing moiety. CBG has a high affinity for most major adrenocortical hormones, but progesterone and estrogen also can interact with this transporting protein. CBG does not show the same degree of affinity with sex steroids as it does with cortisol or corticosterone. While albumins may contain several active binding sites for a given steroid, CBG appears to possess only a single site for the interaction of a hormone. This single site, however, has a particularly high affinity for corticosteroids.

CBG is affected by several endocrine factors. Levels of CBG are usually higher in mature females than in mature males. Removal of the testes results in an increase in the levels of CBG. Normal males treated with estrogen exhibit levels of CBG comparable to those seen in females. Pregnancy causes an increase in CBG; a sharp decline is observed soon after parturition. Extirpation of the pituitary gland in female experimental animals causes a significant decrease in levels of CBG. Only anterior pituitary extracts or TSH tend to restore circulating levels of CBG to normal in the hypophysectomized animal. Thyroidectomy results in a loss in CBG activity, indicating that T_4 somehow assists in maintaining the level of this transporting protein.

Several pharmacological agents have been found to alter the activity of CBG. Estrogens and progesterone (including oral contraceptives) therapy can affect CBG activity. Likewise, androgen therapy can alter CBG levels. The treatment of hypothyroidism or hyperthyroidism also can be expected to interfere with CBG activity. Many of the synthetic antiinflammatory steroids have an affinity for CBG. However, their affinity for CBG is not as great as that demonstrated for the naturally occurring adrenocortical hormones. In general, synthetic adrenocortical-like steroids that are highly halogenated (e.g., fluorinated) do not significantly compete with natural corticoids for CBG. Rather, halogenated antiinflammatory steroids tend to remain free or unbound in sera. The 17 α-alkylated anabolic steroids may produce significant increase in CBG levels.

Testosterone possesses a specific plasma-binding protein (TeBG), although estrogens may also have an affinity for this protein. Progesterone also may interact with a specific serum globulin. In the case of estrogens, it is reasonably clear that despite a blood-transporting protein, the action of female sex hormones on their target organs, e.g., uterus and vagina, can occur in the absence of this transporting substance.

Albumin has a very high capacity for binding testosterone and estrogens. Such albumins, however, have a low affinity for these sex hormones. The plasma also contains low concentrations of globulins that interact with androgens or estrogens. These globulins have a low capacity for either androgens or estrogens but a high affinity for the sex steroids.

While a specific transporting protein may have a high affinity for testosterone, evidence indicates that estradiol can displace this androgen from its binding sites on the carrier molecule. It has been suggested that both androgens and estrogens are bound to the same protein in human plasma. Testosterone and estradiol bind to a single homogeneous protein over a wide range of experimental conditions. The estimated molecular weight of SHBG is nearly 100,000, or approximately twice the weight of CBG. It has been estimated that each SHBG possesses a single binding site for either testosterone or estradiol. The globulin that appears to specifically transport progesterone may possess as many as three distinct binding sites for the steroid. Progesterone also has an affinity for CBG.

Testosterone-binding globulin is increased during pregnancy and by estrogens. Similarly, the degree of binding of testosterone or dihydrotestosterone is increased in hyperthyroidism. Oral contraceptives can likewise enhance SHBG levels.

11.7. EFFECTS OF DRUGS ON STEROIDOGENESIS

Drugs that alter the secretory activity of the adrenal cortex have been classified according to their sites of action (see Figure 11-1). Such drugs as morphine, reserpine, the phenothiazines, and autonomic agents affect the central regulatory processes involved in ACTH release. These centrally acting agents somehow alter the release of ACTH and secondarily affect adrenocortical secretions. The degree of alteration of ACTH secretion depends on the experimental circumstances and the duration of drug administration.

A number of drugs can exert a direct inhibitory action on adrenal steroidogenesis (Figure 11-2; see also Figure 1-5 in Chapter 1). The an-

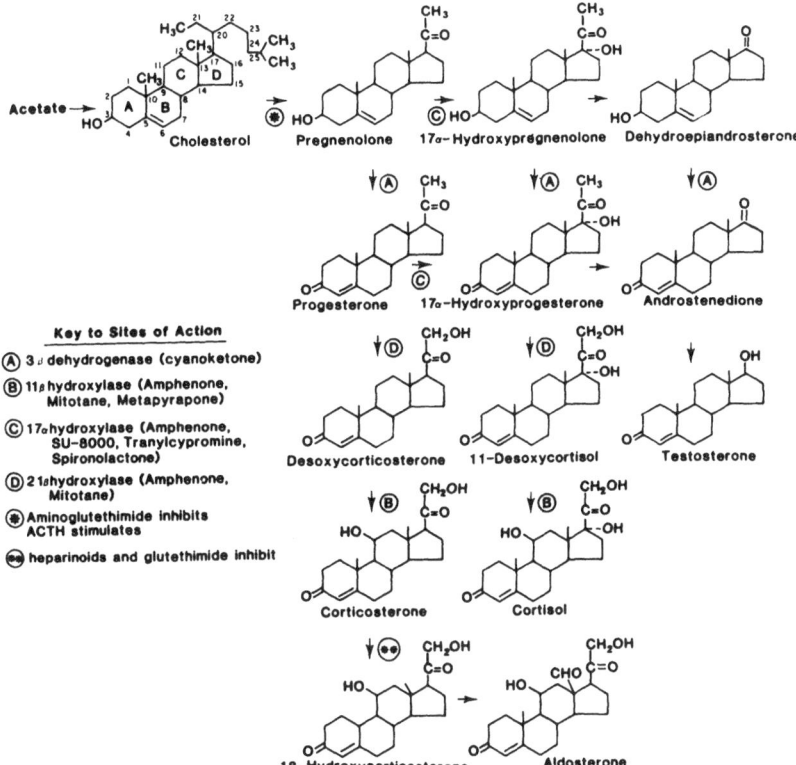

Figure 11-1. Principal pathways for the biosynthesis of adrenocorticoids and adrenal androgens—sites of action of adrenal inhibitors.

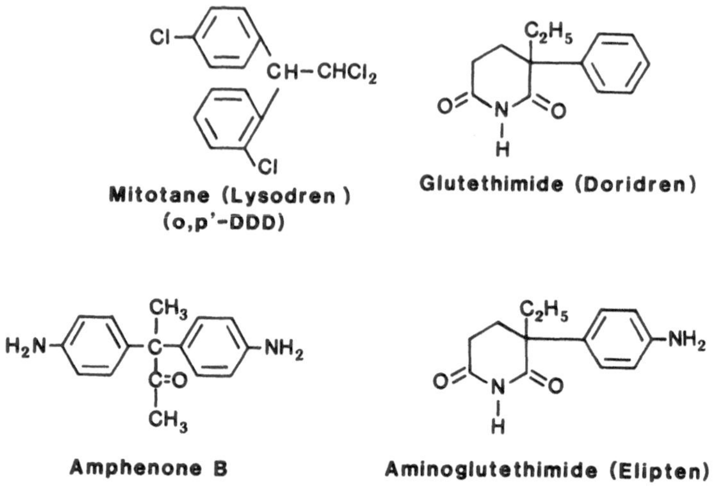

Figure 11-2. Chemical structures of agents known to affect steroidogenesis.

ticonvulsant gluthemide can inhibit the conversion of corticosterone to 18-hydroxycorticosterone and can increase the rate of excretion of 6β-hydroxycortisol. Perhaps the first substance demonstrated to be particularly cytotoxic to adrenal tissue was o,p′-DDD (Mitotane). This agent, as well as some of its isomers, appears to inhibit most pathways of adrenal steroidogenesis, but is slightly more toxic to glucocorticoid synthetic pathways. While o,p′-DDD proved too toxic for use in the treatment of adrenal carcinoma, it was found to be useful as an insecticide. It is unfortunate that DDD and its derivatives are so toxic, because they do appear to exhibit a certain degree of specificity for the adrenal gland. Such specificity would be desirable for the treatment of adrenal neoplasms.

Aminoglutethimide inhibits the conversion of cholesterol to 20α-hydroxycholesterol. These actions of aminoglutethimide cause an inhibition in the synthesis of both cortisol and aldosterone. This experimental drug has been used to decrease the hypersecretion of cortisol emanating from certain tumors.

The adrenal-inhibitory actions of methapyrapone were reported several years ago. This agent is of no value in long-term treatment of adrenal hyperfunction, but it is a very useful diagnostic agent. The classic response to the metapyrapone test (i.e., a decrease in the secretion of cortisol and corticosterone and an increase in the secretion of 11-desoxycorticosterone) indicates that this agent is a preferential inhibitor of

11β-hydroxylase enzyme systems. In other words, metapyrapone is an 11β-hydroxylase inhibitor and prevents the conversion of 11-desoxy-cortisol (Compound S) to cortisol. Compound S is unable to inhibit the pituitary release of ACTH. As cortisol levels fall (due to metapyrapone blockade of 11β-hydroxylase), ACTH is released and cortisol precursors appear in increased amounts. The metapyrapone test is thus a diagnostic tool used to determine the pituitary reserve of ACTH. Several drugs (e.g., phenytoin, chlorpromazine, meprobamate), as well as the condition of pregnancy (or estrogen administration), reduce both urinary 11-desoxycorticosterone and 11-desoxycortisol, hence alter the response of the metapyrapone test.

Large doses of salicylates not only activate the adrenal medulla but also stimulate the secretion of adrenocortical hormones. The effect is mediated by the hypothalamic–pituitary axis, since levels of ACTH are increased. The anti-inflammatory actions of salicylates are not, however, due tot heir ability to stimulate endogenous adrenocortical steroids.

A host of experimental compounds (e.g., SU-800, SU-9055, and SU-10603) are capable of inhibiting the secretion of cortisol. These compounds are considered to be inhibitors of 17α-hydroxylase enzymes. In addition to inhibiting the secretion of cortisol, these agents will impair the synthesis of testosterone. SU-9055 may have the additional property of interfering with aldosterone secretion.

MAO inhibitors may affect adrenal activity by centrally mediated actions and possibly by some direct adrenal gland-interfering action(s). Not all MAO inhibitors are able to alter adrenal–pituitary relationships. Furthermore, some MAO inhibitors seem to possess only a central inhibitory component, while still others exert only a direct adrenal gland-inhibitory action. Ethyltryptamine and nialamide appear to exert an indirect action on the adrenal gland. Their action appears to be centrally mediated. On the other hand, tranylcypromine apparently acts directly on the adrenal gland and may block the 17 α-hydroxylation step in steroidogenesis.

Heparin and closely related compounds can inhibit the secretion of aldosterone. It has been suggested that they act by blocking some biochemical step in the conversion of corticosterone to 18-hydroxycorticosterone. It is possible that heparinoids may exert their inhibitory action by denying the adrenal gland of its calcium requirement. Furthermore, heparinoids can affect the secretion of angiotensin. An inhibition of angiotensin secretion is manifested by the inhibition of steroidogenesis. Angiotensin itself exerts a direct action on the adrenal cortex, leading to an increased secretion of aldosterone. It has little effect on the secretion of glucocorticoids.

Spironolactone is a mineralocorticoid antagonist known to bind to cytosol receptors for mineralocorticoids. It possesses progestational activity and is antiandrogenic because of its ability to bind to dihydrotestosterone receptors. Spironolactone decreases 17-hydroxylase activity through its action on cytochrome p-450.

A number of experimental and clinically useful agents can interfere with cholesterol synthesis. Clofibrate and cholestyramine are able to suppress steroidogenesis by altering cholesterol metabolism. Triparanol (MER-29) also is capable of affecting steroidogenesis. None of these agents produces any profound changes in endocrine states despite an ability to alter cholesterol synthesis.

It has been reported that the protein-inhibitory antibiotics, cycloheximide and puromycin, block steroidogenesis of a regulatory protein with a rapid turnover time, which mediates the activity of enzymes acting at rate-limiting steps in steroidogenesis.

Phenytoin not only stimulates hepatic microsomal P-450 enzyme systems but reportedly increases the hepatic turnover of cortisol. Phenytoin enhances the activity of 6β-hydroxysteroid.

Rifampicin, a macrocyclic antibiotic widely used in the therapy of tuberculosis, increases the catabolism of cortisol. Cortisol production rates are increased in patients being treated with rifampicin. Rifampicin also promotes the activity of hepatic estrogen-2-hydroxylase, causing an increased rate of oxidation of ethinyl estradiol.

Anticholinesterase inhibitors, particularly certain of the organophosphate compounds, produce changes in hepatic microsomal enzymes involved in steroid metabolism. Insecticides of the organophosphate class have been reported to produce alterations in sexual activity in males. The impotence caused by these agents seems to be due to their ability to affect the neural regulatory mechanisms of reproductive organs. On the other hand, the organochloride pesticides seem to alter reproductive activity by interfering with hormonal rather than neural processes.

Cyanoketone is used primarily as a research tool. It is too toxic for use in humans. This steroid-type drug is a potent inhibitor of 3β-hydroxysteroid dehydrogenase. This enzyme catalyzes the conversion of pregnenolone to progesterone. Cyanoketone is particularly potent. Its action is believed to be a function of its ability to form a long-lasting complex with the enzyme it inhibits. Not only will it effectively block glucocorticoid secretion, but it will also suppress androgen and estrogen secretion. Thus, this agent will block both adrenal and gonadal steroidogenesis. It is an effective inhibitor of ovulation.

Amphenone, a diphenylmethane derivative related to o,p'-DDD, produces a generalized reduction in the secretion of corticosteroids. It appears to reduce steroidogenesis by blocking the 11-, 17-, and 21-hydroxylation of pregnenolone. It may also interfere with the dehydrogenation of 3-hydroxyl groups on the steroid molecule. Like many adrenocortical inhibitory agents, its degree of toxicity precludes clinical use.

It should be evident that a number of chemicals and/or drugs having very different pharmacological mechanisms of action can affect steroidogenesis. Some of these agents have rather specific sites of actions along the metabolic pathways involving steroid synthesis.

11.8. EFFECTS OF DRUGS ON GONADAL FUNCTION

Studies using experimental animals clearly demonstrate the detrimental effects of alkylating agents, antimetabolites, and a variety of cytotoxic substances on the seminiferous epithelium. The degree of spermatogenic arrest and its subsequent reversibility depends to a large extent on the particular agent employed and on the dose and duration of its use. The damage to the gonads varies from complete and permanent sterility through subfertility to a return of fertility with production of phenotypically normal offspring.

Perhaps the most frequently encountered side effects of drugs on the hypothalamic–pituitary–testicular axis are loss of libido, as well as impotence, impaired spermatogenesis/infertility, and gynecomastia. In rare instances, drug-induced priapism can occur. Those drugs that interfere principally at the hypothalamic–adenohypophyseal axis are considered in Chapter 2, while those agents that interfere with the process of ovulation are discussed along with the oral contraceptives in Chapter 8.

It is well recognized that inhibitors of mitosis, e.g., colchicine and vinblastine, can cause oligospermia or azoospermia. Alkylating agents, e.g., chlorambucil and cyclophosphamide, can also cause oligospermia or azoospermia. In general, drugs used in the treatment of cancer are usually quite toxic to the host. Since rapidly dividing cells of a neoplasm are the therapeutic target, it is not surprising that side effects extend to the process of spermatogenesis. Other reproductive functions may also be affected by these agents.

Busulfan may cause impotence, sterility, and amenorrhea. When used for extended periods, several cancer chemotherapeutic agents may lead to amenorrhea. Impairment of spermatogenesis occurs in several different species, including man. The deleterious actions on the germinal epithelium produced by alkylating agents resemble the damaging action produced by X rays. Busulfan, like X rays, affects the earlier stages of spermatogenesis. Triethylenemelamine and aliphatic nitrogen mustard alter the later stages in the process of spermatogenesis.

The pyrimidine analogue, 5-fluorouracil, (5-FU), interferes with reproductive function. This antimetabolite can interfere with the growth-promoting actions exerted by testosterone on sex accessory organs. Another cancer chemotherapeutic agent, cyclophosphamide, can produce destructive changes in germinal epithelium and thereby lead to sterility. Arrest of spermatogenesis by the various types of antineoplastic agents (e.g., alkylating agents, antimetabolites) is reversible upon discontinuation of the drug. In this respect, colchicine-induced spermatogenic arrest is also reversible.

Certain diamine derivatives, originally investigated for their amebicidal activity, produce spermatogenic arrest in both man and animals. The deleterious actions produced by the diamines appear to be similar to those produced by the nitrofurans.

The systemic use of derivatives of nitrofurane and thiophene leads to varying degrees of altered spermatogenesis. In the rat, spermatogenesis is arrested by furadroxyl mainly at the stage of the primary spermatocyte. Nitrofurane derivatives and some antibiotics and chemotherapeutic agents (e.g., gentamycin, oxytetracycline, trimethoprim) may exert similar mechanisms of toxic actions on the process of spermatogenesis.

Estrogens are particularly effective in causing oligospermia or azoospermia. Some nonsteroidal agents can inhibit spermatogenesis by suppressing FSH/LH, thereby interfering with the biosynthesis of testosterone. For example, methallibar, a derivative of bisthiourea, can cause inhibition of spermatogenesis, atrophy of accessory sex organs and a loss of libido. The linear or cyclic phenylmethylpolysiloxanes, which inhibit FSH/LH, can cause spermatogenic arrest and atrophy of accessory sex organs.

Certain antihypertensive agents (e.g., reserpine), diazepam, chlopromazine, and barbiturates can interfere with the secretion of gonadotropins. Reserpine can cause alterations in gonadal activity in male rodents. High doses of reserpine produce a retardation of spermatogenesis and a reduction in sex accessory gland metabolism. These regressive changes are seen in both adult and immature animals. The infertility produced by reserpine is generally attributed to its ability to inhibit pituitary gonadotropins.

Several potent protein-inhibitory antibiotics (*viz.* puromycin, antinomycin D, cyclohexamide) can affect either the testes or the ovary. They can interfere with the actions of sex steroids on their respective target organs. These agents can also inhibit ovulation in experimental animals.

Alkane sulfonic esters, e.g., methylene dimethane sulfonate (MDS), a close analogue of busulfan, produces spermatogenic arrest and seems to act primarily during the early stages of the process. Conversely, ethyldimethylsulphonate (EDS) exerts its inhibitory effects during later stages of spermatogenesis. Accordingly, with the exception of spermatogonia and epididymal spermatozoa, all stages of spermatogenesis are impaired by EDS. Thus, the antifertility action of EDS is clearly different from that of MDS, busulfan, and dimethylbusulfan.

While chemical and/or drug-induced sterility can be brought about by inhibiting spermatogenesis, other agents can affect neural mechanisms, leading to impotence or decreased libido. A wide variety of chemical classes of drugs can lead to impairment of male sexual function (see Table 11-12). It is quite apparent that many of the agents cited exert their pharmacological actions by nonhormonal mechanisms or neural mechanisms. For example, alcohol-induced impotence often occurs in the absence of a marked reduction in libido. The chronic use of narcotics leads to a marked diminuation of male sexual activity; it is possible that both hormonal and nonhormonal mechanisms are involved in the action(s) of these agents. Antihypertensive drugs can cause impotence or failure of ejaculation.

Adrenergic blocking drugs are capable of inducing impotence and failure to ejaculate. Failure to ejaculate is undoubtedly due to inhibition of sympathetic nervous system activity. Serotonin antagonists such as methylsergide and pizotifen have occasionally been reported to induce impotence. Anticholinergic agents may interfere with penile erection. Impotence caused by the antimuscarinic effects of drugs is likely to occur with a diminution in libido.

Several agents can cause a reduction in circulating levels of testosterone, including ketoconazole, an antifungal drug, morphine (and heroin), and marihauna.

11.9. EFFECTS OF DRUGS ON PANCREATIC FUNCTION

The most important chemical class of drugs that affect pancreatic function are the sulfonylureas (see Chapter 10). The sulfonylureas are a class of clinically important oral hypoglycemic agents used in the management of diabetes mellitus. The oral hypoglycemic agents interact with numerous other classes of drugs (see Table 11-13).

Aside from the sulfonylurea agents, a number of other agents, some

Table 11-12. Drugs Affecting Male Sexual Function as a Result of Exerting a Particular Pharmacological Effect

Drug(s)	Pharmacological effect(s)
Reserpine, clonidine, methyldopa, phenytoin, carbamazepine, ethanol, phenothiazines, butyrophenones, barbiturates, morphine, β-adrenergic antagonists	Production of CNS depression, sedation
Metoclopramide, reserpine, morphine, cimetidine, phenothiazines	Elevated plasma prolactin (gynecomastia)
Atropine, metantheline, benztropine, tricyclic antidepressants, disopyramide, butyrophenones, ganglion-blocking agents	Impotence
Guanethidine, bethanidine, debrisoquine, lithium	Failure to ejaculate
Spironolactone	Gynecomastia and impotence

Table 11-13. Interaction of Various Drugs with Oral Hypoglycemic Agents and Insulin

Enhanced Effect (i.e., greater hypoglycemic action)	
Ethanol	Phenylbutazone
Anabolic steroids	Phenyramidol
Chloramphenicol	K^+ salts
Bishydroxycoumarin	Propranolol
Guanethidine	Probenecid
Oxytetracycline	Salicylates
MAO inhibitors	Sulfonamides
	Sulfinpyrazone
Antagonist Effect	
Acetazolamide	Marihuana
D-Thyroxine	Oral Contraceptives
Corticosteroids	Diuretics (e.g., chlorthalidone, ethacrynic,
Phenothiazines	acid, furosemide, thiazides,
Epinephrine	triamterene)
Phenytoin	

quite toxic, can affect pancreatic function. Some of the agents that affect the pancreas are very cytotoxic and can destroy specific cells within this organ.

Some agents that can rather selectively destroy pancreatic β cells have been used to study experimental diabetes mellitus in laboratory animals. Such compounds that destroy pancreatic β cells produce some of the signs and symptoms of diabetes mellitus, particularly hyperglycemia and glycosuria. Such agents include alloxan, uric acid, dialuric acid, dehydroascorbic acid, quinolones, and streptozotocin. Interestingly, alloxan and α-D-glucose are chemically similar, and they may interact with a common receptor on the β cells. Like alloxan, streptozotocin, the N-nitroso derivative of glucosamine synthesized by the microorganism *Streptomyces achromogenes*, is cytotoxic to pancreatic β cells. The early β-cell damage is accompanied by the release of insulin. Unfortunately, the renal toxicity of either alloxan or streptozotocin is too great for these agents to be of any clinical use in the chemical treatment of insulin-secreting tumors. In experimental animals, some agents are also known to rather selectively destroy pancreatic α cells. The injection of cobalt chloride has been shown to cause degranulation and vacuolization of the α cells in rabbits, dogs, and guinea pigs. Synthalin A can also cause destruction of pancreatic α cells (see Figure 11-3).

Some compounds (e.g., diazoxide) can cause hyperglycemia by apparently decreasing insulin secretion as well as diminishing the peripheral utilization of glucose. Diazoxide (Proglycem) seems to possess some

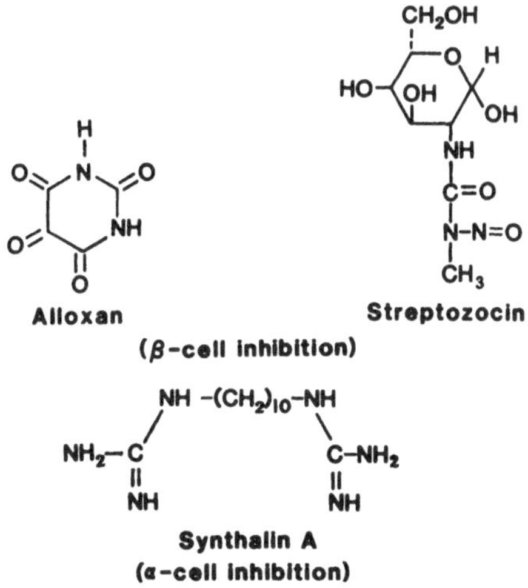

Figure 11-3. Agents known to affect pancreatic function.

α-adrenergiclike actions—a property that leads to the enhancement of its actions by propranolol (see also Chapter 10).

11.10. EFFECTS OF DRUGS ON THYROID FUNCTION

Those drugs that are clinically useful in the management of thyroid disorders have already been discussed (see Chapter 4), but a number of other agents can influence thyroid function (see Table 11-11). It may be seen that no particular chemical moiety is required insofar as affecting certain thyroid gland activities. In addition to those agents cited as affecting TBG, T_4 and ^{131}I, drugs such as cholestyramine can interfere with the absorption of T_4. Salicylate can also cause a decrease in plasma-bound iodine levels and actually decrease the uptake of iodine by the anionic pump of the thyroid gland. A number of drugs, such as aminosalicylate, thiazolsulfene (antileprosy agent), and certain sulfonamide antibacterials can produce goiters and may lead to myxedematous states.

11.11. EFFECTS OF DRUGS ON LABORATORY ANALYSES

Laboratory analyses of a number of blood or plasma constituents play an important part in the correct diagnosis of a specific disease process. Certainly blood chemistries are an important consideration in the diagnoses of a number of pathological states.

Several agents or drugs affect these routine biochemical determinations (see Tables 11-14 and 11-15). A number of nonpituitary hormones such as the estrogens, androgens, adrenocorticoids, and T_4 can interfere with biochemical analyses and lead to erroneous interpretations of laboratory results. Synthetic steroids, such as the oral contraceptives and the so-called protein-anabolic steroids, are also able to affect blood levels in several routine biochemical analyses.

Pharmacological amounts of ACTH can interfere with certain standardized clinical laboratory tests. The alterations produced by exogenous amounts of this trophic hormone are generally mediated through the adrenal cortex. Excessive exogenous amounts of other trophic hormones, such as growth hormone, could readily affect the laboratory values of blood glucose. Similarly, vasopressin-induced release of ACTH could lead to hyperglycemia and erroneously high laboratory results. Needless to say, both insulin and glucagon would affect blood sugar determinations.

Of the variety of pharmacological agents capable of influencing the

Table 11-14. Effect of Various Hormones or Endocrine-Acting Agents on Laboratory Blood Chemistry Determinations

Blood determination	Effect on determination	
	Increased value	Decreased value
Bilirubin	Acetohexamide Tolbutamide Androgenic/anabolic steroids	None reported
Bromsulphalein clearance	Acetohexamide Chlorpropamide Tolbutamide Oral contraceptives Androgenic/anabolic steroids	None reported
Calcium	Androgenic/anabolic steroids Calciferol Dihydrotachysterol Oral contraceptives Parathyroid hormone	Corticosteroids
Cephalin–cholesterol flocculation	Chlorpropamide Tolbutamide	None reported
Chloride	None reported	ACTH/Corticosteroids
Total cholesterol	ACTH/Corticosteroids Androgenic/anabolic steroids	ACTH Estrogens Thyroid hormones
Glucose	ACTH/Corticosteroids Oral contraceptives Thyroid hormones Morphine	Chlorpropamide Tolbutamide Phenformin Metformin Insulin
Acid phosphatase	Androgens (in females)	None reported
Alkaline phosphatase	Acetohexamide Chlorpropamide Tolazamide Tolbutamide Oral contraceptives Androgenic/anabolic steroids	None reported

many blood chemical analyses, the oral hypoglycemic drugs seem to be particularly susceptible to such interactions. The sulfonylurea class of oral hypoglycemic agents appear to exert a more widespread effect on these determinations than do the biguanides. Despite the fact that the oral hypoglycemic drugs could alter a considerable number of blood biochemical constituents, there is little likelihood that such interactions would escape notice, since the user of the drug would already have been diagnosed as a diabetic. Several factors can also modify the secretion of insulin and thereby affect the actions of oral hypoglycemic agents (see Chapter 10).

Prolonged use of synthetic steroids is apt to lead to changes in several blood chemistry determinations. In many instances, such changes are related to the ability of these synthetic steroids to alter hepatic function. The oral contraceptives, both progestins and 19-norsteroids, frequently contain 17α-alkyl side groups on the steroid molecule. This particular side group is responsible for rendering these steroids orally effective and is believed responsible for causing changes in hepatic function tests. Similarly, protein-anabolic steroids with this same side-chain addition can induce hepatic changes as reflected by alterations in certain blood chemistry analyses.

Just as steroid-induced changes can affect blood chemistry, so too can different drugs influence the measurement of steroids. A host of drugs can interfere or otherwise modify the levels of blood and/or urinary corticosteroids and ketosteroids (see Table 11-16).

Table 11-15. Effect of Various Hormones or Endocrine-Acting Agents on Laboratory Blood Chemistry Determinations

Blood determination	Effect on determination	
	Increased value	Decreased value
Phosphorus	Calciferol	Insulin
		Parathyroid extract
Potassium	Phenformin	ACTH/corticosteroids
Total protein	ACTH/corticosteroids	Glucocorticoids[a]
	Androgenic/anabolic steroids	Thyroid hormones[a]
	Growth hormone	
	Insulin	
	Thyroid hormones	
SGOT	Androgenic/anabolic steroids	None reported
	Oral contraceptives	
Sodium	Androgenic/anabolic steroids	None reported
	Corticosteroids	
Thymol turbidity	ACTH	None reported
	Corticosteroids	
	Growth hormone	
	Tolbutamide	
	Insulin	
BUN	Acetohexamide	None reported
Uric acid	Acetohexamide	Corticosteroids[a]
	Corticosteroids	

[a] Variable effect, depending on the dose and duration of hormone therapy.

Table 11-16.   Pharmacological Agents Known to Interfere
with the Measurement of Corticosteroids and
Ketosteroids

Nonbarbiturate sedatives and/or tranquilizers
  Chlorpromazine
  Chlordiazepoxide
  Ethinamate
  Reserpine
  Paraldehyde
  Chloral hydrate
  Hydroxyzine
  Meprobamate
  Phenaglycodol
Antibiotics and antibacterial agents
  Triacetyloleandomycin
  Sulfamerazine
  Nalidixic acid
Monamine oxidase inhibitors
  Etryptamine
Oral hypoglycemic agents
  Acetohexamide
Miscellaneous drugs and agents
  Quinine
  Quinidine
  Phenytoin
  Colchicine
  Diagnostic dyes (e.g., BSP, PSP)
  Spironolactone
  Heparin preparations containing benzoyl alcohol preservative[a]

[a] May elevate plasma 11-hydroxycorticosteroid values.

RECOMMENDED READINGS

Arena, J. M., Drugs and chemicals excreted in breast milk, *Pediatr. Ann.* **9**:15, 1980.
Barber, H. R. K., The effect of cancer and its therapy upon fertility, *Int. J. Fertil.* **26**:250, 1981.
Brater, D. C., Drug–drug and drug–disease interactions with nonsteroidal anti-inflammatory drugs, *Am. J. Med.* **80**:62, 1986.
Cohen, K. L., Metabolic, endocrine and drug-induced interference with pituitary function tests: A review, *Metabolism* **26**:1165, 1977.
Elias, A. N., Gwinup, G., Effects of some clinically encountered drugs on steroid synthesis and degradation, *Metabolism* **29**:582, 1980.
Fody, E. P., and Walker, E. M., Effects of drugs on male and female reproductive systems, *Ann. Clin. Lab. Sci.* **15**:451–458, 1985.
Horowitz, J. D., and Goble, A. J., Drugs and impaired male sexual function, *Drugs* **18**:206, 1979.

Ribelin, W. E., The effects of drugs and chemicals upon the structure of the adrenal gland, *Fund. Appli. Toxicol.* **4**:105, 1984.

Roeser, R. A. P., Stocks, A. E., and Smith, A. J., Testicular damage due to cytotoxic drugs and recovery after cessation of therapy, *Aust. N. Z. J. Med.* **8**:250, 1978.

Sandow, J., Toxicological evaluation of drugs affecting the hypothalamic–pituitary system, *Pharmacol. Ther.* **5**:297, 1979.

Steinberger, E., The etiology and pathophysiology of testicular dysfunction in man, *Fertil. Steril.* **29**:481, 1978.

Stockley, I. H., Mechanisms of drug interaction, *Am. J. Hosp. Pharmacol.* **27**:977, 1970.

Thachib, J. V., Jewett, M. A. S., and Rider, W. D., The effects of cancer and cancer therapy on male fertility, *J. Urol.* **126**:141, 1981.

Thomas. J. Reproductive hazards and environmental chemicals: A review, *Toxic Subst. J.* **2**:318, 1981.

Thomas, J. A., Korach, K. S., and McLachlan, J. A., (ed), *Endocrine Toxicology*, Target Organ Toxicology Series, Raven Press, New York, 1985.

Thomas, J. A., Shahid-Salles, K. S., and Donovan, M. P., Effects of narcotics on the reproductive system. Regulatory mechanisms affecting gonadal hormone action, in: *Advances in Sex Hormone Research* (J. A. Thomas, and R. L. Singhal, eds.) Vol. 3, University Park Press, Baltimore, p. 69, 1977.

INDEX